Mometrix
TEST PREPARATION

AF834732

Fundamentals of Nursing Secrets Study Guide

Part 2 of 2

Dear Future Exam Success Story

First of all, **THANK YOU** for purchasing Mometrix study materials!

Second, congratulations! You are one of the few determined test-takers who are committed to doing whatever it takes to excel on your exam. **You have come to the right place.** We developed these study materials with one goal in mind: to deliver you the information you need in a format that's concise and easy to use.

In addition to optimizing your guide for the content of the test, we've outlined our recommended steps for breaking down the preparation process into small, attainable goals so you can make sure you stay on track.

We've also analyzed the entire test-taking process, identifying the most common pitfalls and showing how you can overcome them and be ready for any curveball the test throws you.

Standardized testing is one of the biggest obstacles on your road to success, which only increases the importance of doing well in the high-pressure, high-stakes environment of test day. Your results on this test could have a significant impact on your future, and this guide provides the information and practical advice to help you achieve your full potential on test day.

Your success is our success

We would love to hear from you! If you would like to share the story of your exam success or if you have any questions or comments in regard to our products, please contact us at **800-673-8175** or **support@mometrix.com**.

Thanks again for your business and we wish you continued success!

Sincerely,
The Mometrix Test Preparation Team

Printed in the United States of America

TABLE OF CONTENTS

Physiological Integrity: Basic Care and Comfort

Hygiene

ADLs, Dressing, and Grooming

Activities of daily living (ADLs) are tasks that are required to keep a person healthy and functional. Often, a person's level of health is determined by their ability to perform ADLs. The tasks are divided into two subgroups:

- **Basic ADLs** are tasks people must be able to perform in order to care for themselves. These include bathing, dressing, feeding, toileting, and walking.
- **Instrumental ADLs** are tasks people must be able to perform in order to live independently within the community. These include shopping, cooking, housework, medication management, and money management.

Dressing and grooming are important basic activities of daily living, and a patient that is unable to perform these independently requires assistance. Prior to conducting any elements of dressing or grooming, the patient should be greeted. Next, hands must be washed and the procedure explained to the patient. Gloves should be worn if any risk of exposure to bodily fluid exists.

Dressing a Stroke Patient

When the patient has suffered a **stroke**, it can result in weakness on one side of the patient's body, and the patient often requires assistance with daily activities as a result. It is important to teach the patient how to safely dress and undress to promote independence and decrease the risk of falling. Before beginning to assist the patient in undressing, make sure the clean set of clothes is within easy reach. When putting on clothing, the patient should be taught to dress the weakened side of the body first, using their strong side to do so. For example, a patient with weakness on the right side should insert the right arm into the sleeve first. When removing clothes, the patient should be taught to undress the strong side first.

Shaving a Patient

If a patient needs their face to be shaved, first apply a pair of gloves and then follow the below procedure.

1. Use a wet washcloth to moisten the hair on the patient's face and neck.
2. Check the razor to make sure it does not have any loose blades or jagged edges.
3. Drape the patient with a towel and apply shaving cream to the area that needs to be shaved.
4. Use one hand to pull the skin taut, while moving the razor with firm strokes in the direction that the hair is growing.
5. Rinse the razor in a basin of water as often as necessary.
6. Use a moistened washcloth to rinse off all remaining shaving cream.

Of note, if a patient requires shaving before a surgical procedure, this should be done by a specialist.

Although hygiene care in most facilities is performed by the nurse aide, this care may be handled by either the nurse or the nurse aide depending on the level of assistance needed by the patient.

Morning and Evening Care

Morning care is typically done prior to any scheduled medical procedures. It involves a complete bath, shaving, dressing, hair care, oral care, and nail care, and may require changing of the bed linens. Evening care is done at bedtime and involves an abbreviated form of skin care, including washing the patient's face and hands. Oral care should also be performed. A back rub may be given for 5–10 minutes to ensure the patient is relaxed and ready for sleep. Additional tasks may be performed, depending upon the patient's level of health and activity.

Hair Care

Hair care is a procedure that helps to improve patient comfort and morale. It stimulates blood circulation within the scalp. Hair washing also removes excess oils and bacteria. Frequency of hair care depends upon the amount of oil that has accumulated in the patient's hair, as well as the level of dryness of the scalp.

Vigilance is required while performing hair care. Head lice, an excessive amount of dandruff, or sores on the scalp should be **reported immediately**. Such findings may require special precautions to be taken while performing hair care in the future.

Procedure for Performing Hair Care

The procedure for performing hair care is as follows:

1. Raise the head of the bed to a comfortable level and place a towel beneath the patient's head.
2. Part the patient's hair into manageable sections, and run the comb or brush slowly through it. If the hair is tangled, hold the strand of hair above the tangle while combing it to prevent pulling the patient's hair.
3. While combing, carefully inspect the scalp for any lesions, lice, or signs of dryness.
4. Try to shape the hair into the patient's preferred style; even parting the hair on the correct side can provide a greater level of comfort for the patient.
5. After hair care is complete, remove the towel and reposition the patient for comfort.

Nail Care

Nail care is important for a number of reasons. The primary purpose of nail care is to remove bacteria and dirt from the patient's nail beds, preventing the spread of microorganisms. Appropriate nail care also ensures the patient's nails are not sharp or jagged, which increases the risk of infection from breakage of the skin. While performing nail care, there is also the opportunity to inspect the patient's nail beds for any signs of inflammation or fungal growth. Any signs of infection or discoloration should immediately be reported and documented.

For some patients in some facilities, nail care must be performed by a specialist. Before beginning nail care, verify whether you are permitted to perform nail care on the patient. These classes of patients require special care:

- **Patients who are receiving anticoagulation therapy**: This type of medication puts the patient at an increased risk for bleeding.
- **Patients with diabetes or peripheral vascular disease that decreases circulation to the feet**: Diabetes and low circulation affect the ability of the tissue to repair itself. As a result, even the smallest cut on the skin places the patient at risk for severe ulcers on the feet.

Procedure for Proper Nail Care

The procedure for proper nail care is as follows:

1. Soak the patient's hands and feet in warm water to soften them and prevent the nails from cracking.
2. Carefully remove any dirt from beneath the patient's nails.
3. Trim each nail by cutting straight across with a pair of nail clippers, then round the edges using an emery board. Be careful not to cut the nails too short as this may cause irritation to the nail bed.
4. If desired, apply lotion to the patient's nails.
5. After nail care has been completed, reposition the patient for comfort and wash hands.

Oral Care

Abnormal Findings

Performing oral care presents an ideal opportunity to examine the patient's oral mucosa for **abnormalities**. The patient's mouth should be examined for any sores, redness, or bleeding on the patient's lips or gums. Cracking may occur on the patient's lips as a result of dryness. The health care team should also be observant for any odor that may occur as a result of infection. Thrush is a fungal infection that can develop as a result of poor oral care or after taking certain medications. If thrush is present, the patient may appear with white patches covering the tongue or gums. The patient may also complain of a thick, furry feeling in the mouth.

Unconscious Patients

When performing oral care on the **unconscious patient**, first drape a towel over the patient's chest. Adjust the level of the bed to a comfortable height and raise the head of the bed greater than 30 degrees. Turn the patient's head toward oneself and hold the mouth open with a tongue depressor in one hand. Clean the patient's teeth, gums, and tongue. After cleaning has been completed, suction the secretions out of the patient's mouth. Position the patient for comfort, remove the gloves, and wash one's hands.

Conscious Patients

Some **conscious patients** may not be able to perform oral care on themselves as a result of palsy or weakness in the upper extremities. When assisting a conscious patient with oral care, the following procedure should be followed:

1. After donning gloves, drape a towel over the patient.
2. Raise the level of the bed to a comfortable height, and position the head of the bed greater than 30 degrees.
3. Using a toothbrush, thoroughly clean the patient's teeth, gums, and tongue.
4. While performing oral care, carefully inspect the patient's mouth for any lesions or signs of infection.
5. If the patient is able to take small amounts of water without aspirating, allow them to rinse their mouth and spit the water into an emesis basin.
6. Position the patient for comfort and wash hands.

Denture Care

Denture care is a common requirement for elderly patients. The procedure is as follows:

1. Obtain the patient's dentures, which are often kept in a specific cup if they are not already in the patient's mouth.
2. Place a towel or washcloth in the sink to prevent breakage if the dentures are accidentally dropped.
3. Using a toothbrush, clean the surface of the patient's dentures.
4. Place the dentures in a denture cup filled with cool water.
5. Provide oral care to the patient using sponge swabs and mouthwash; carefully observe for any lesions or signs of infection.
6. After the procedure has been completed, ask the patient if they would like to wear their dentures. If not, place the dentures in the denture cup and place it on the patient's bedside table.
7. Position the patient for comfort and wash hands.

Bathing

Purpose

Over time, irritants can build on the patient's skin, which can cause a rash or skin breakdown. These irritants can also cause itching, which may provoke the patient to scratch the skin, creating a source of infection. **Bathing** cleanses the patient's skin of these irritants. Bathing can also promote patient relaxation and increase circulation. Bathing presents an opportunity to perform a thorough assessment of the patient's skin. Any signs of breakdown or lesions should be immediately reported. Furthermore, the patient's skin should be closely monitored for dryness, as this can cause cracking of the patient's skin, an additional portal of entry for infection.

Bed Bath, Tub Bath, and Partial Bath

A **tub bath** is preferred when the patient is strong enough to get into and out of the bathtub. It involves completely washing the patient, including performing perineal care. A tub bath can be given daily. However, if the patient's skin is showing signs of dryness, the frequency may be reduced to two or three times a week.

A **bed bath** is given to a patient when they are unable to ambulate. A complete bed bath involves cleansing the patient's skin and changing the patient's linens.

If the patient is incontinent of urine or stool, a **partial bath** may be given. This involves cleansing only those parts of the body that have been soiled and changing only those linens that are dirty.

Necessary Supplies for a Bed Bath

A bed bath can be a time-consuming procedure, depending upon the patient's level of activity. One way to facilitate a bed bath is to make sure that all of the **necessary supplies** are present prior to starting the bath. A basin of water, soap, and lotion will be required in addition to several washcloths and at least two towels. The water should be warmed to 105–115 °F. Those assisting with the bath must also have a pair of gloves to wear. Linens should be changed while the bed bath is being performed. In order to change the bed, a fitted sheet, a bed pad, a flat sheet, a blanket, and pillowcases will be required.

Procedure for Performing a Bed Bath

The procedure for performing a **bed bath** is as follows:

1. Fill a basin with water at a temperature of 105–115 °F.
2. Remove as much medical equipment from the patient as possible.
3. Keep the patient covered to maintain dignity.
4. Allow the patient to bathe as much of himself or herself as possible.
5. Begin by washing the patient's face, moving downward to the arms, the chest, abdomen, legs, back, and perineal area.
6. Use a different washcloth for each area of the body.
7. If necessary, change the patient's bed linens while washing the back.
8. Apply lotion if desired.
9. After the bath has been completed, reposition the patient for comfort and wash hands.

Procedure for Performing Tub Bath

The procedure for performing a **tub bath** is as follows:

1. Prior to performing a tub bath, the bathtub should be cleaned.
2. Place towels in the tub and on the floor outside the tub to prevent slipping.
3. Ambulate the patient to the tub, observing all precautions.
4. Once the patient is in the tub, fill it to the desired level. Make sure the water temperature is no greater than 115 °F.
5. Provide privacy while the patient washes, but maintain close supervision to make sure the patient does not slip.
6. Wash the patient's back and any area they are unable to reach.
7. Drain the water and dry the patient.
8. Assist the patient into a standing position and carefully help them out of the tub.
9. Assist the patient in putting on clothes.
10. Position the patient for comfort, clean the tub, and wash hands.

Procedure for Providing Perineal Care During the Bath

Perineal care is an important part of bathing because it allows the patient's skin and perineal area to be assessed. If done properly, it also decreases the risk for urinary tract infections. Perineal care should be done during a complete bath and should also be performed after the patient is incontinent. Hands should be washed and a pair of gloves donned. Instruct the patient to open their legs. Cleanse the skin of the perineal area, using front to back movements. Never wash from back to front as this can introduce germs from the anus to the urethral area. After the skin has been cleansed, completely dry the area. Do not reuse the linens that were used to wash the perineal area. Obtain a clean towel and washcloth to complete the bath.

Procedures to Prevent Skin Irritation

Skin irritation can result in sores and infection. There are a number of measures that can be taken to **prevent skin irritation** from occurring.

- One way to avoid skin rash or irritation is to completely **cleanse the skin of any urine or feces** if the patient has soiled himself. Because urine and stool are acidic in nature, skin breakdown can occur quickly if they are left close to the patient's skin.
- If the patient is incontinent, applying **water resistant lotion** will protect the skin by creating a barrier that will prevent rashes or breakdown.
- **Frequent repositioning** should also be performed to prevent skin breakdown. A bedridden patient should be turned every two hours to prevent breakdown over bony prominences.

Nutrition and Oral Hydration

Nutrients

Nutrients are elements in nature that are necessary for humans to consume in order to live. Our bodies absorb the nutrients from the foods we eat. Nutrients are divided into the following groups:

- **Carbohydrates** are composed primarily of sugar and serve as the main source of energy.
- **Protein** is made primarily of amino acids and aids in tissue repair.
- **Fats** are composed of fatty acids and are essential for cell membrane integrity and thermal regulation.
- **Minerals** and **vitamins** are needed to aid metabolism and a number of other body processes.
- **Water** acts as a solvent and is also required for a number of body processes.

Water

Water is a vitally important nutrient. It aids in metabolism, temperature regulation, and elimination of body waste. Water is constantly lost through normal sweating, elimination, and exhalation. Certain states, such as illness and increased activity, can cause increased water loss. It is recommended that the patient take in at least 1500–2000 mL or 8–10 glasses of water every day to maintain hydration and replace lost body fluids. If the patient does not receive an adequate volume of fluids, dehydration may occur. If left uncorrected, dehydration can be a fatal condition.

Feeding Patients

Assessing the Meal and the Need for Feeding Assistance

Before taking the tray into the patient's room, it is imperative to confirm that the patient is **receiving the correct tray**. Check the patient's armband and compare it to the name and room number on the tray. Check to make sure the patient's tray contains foods that are appropriate for the patient's ordered diet.

The **amount of feeding assistance** that should be provided depends upon the individual patient. Some patients will not require assistance to feed themselves. If the patient is able to feed themselves, they should be allowed to do so as a means of encouraging independence. Some assistance may be required, such as cutting larger portions and opening beverages. Some patients, such as those who suffer from blindness, may only need verbal cues to eat. Some patients are unable to feed themselves as a result of weakness or paralysis of the upper body. These patients will require their food to be cut and each bite fed to them. Care should be taken to not rush the feeding and to ensure the patient has chewed and swallowed each bite of food before offering the next.

Process for Feeding a Patient

The process for feeding a patient is as follows:

1. Wash hands and raise the head of the patient's bed.
2. Explain to the patient what foods are being served on the tray and allow the patient to select what foods will be fed first.
3. When providing a bite to the patient, ensure the spoon is only half full. Use only the tip of the spoon to feed the patient.
4. Feed the patient slowly, ensuring the patient has swallowed all of the food in their mouth before offering the next bite.

5. Make sure the patient has had enough food to eat before taking the tray away.
6. If the patient appears to be having difficulty swallowing, stop feeding the patient immediately and report this issue. The patient may require a swallow study and be placed on NPO status until this study is conducted.

Clock Method of Feeding Patients

The clock method is a way of describing the placement of food on a plate to a visually impaired patient who is able to feed oneself. The patient should be instructed to picture the plate as a clock face, with positions of food located at corresponding numbers. For example, the meat can be at the 12 o'clock position, the vegetables at the 3 o'clock position, bread at the 6 o'clock position, and the fruit at the 9 o'clock position. This pattern should be repeated at every meal so that the patient is familiar with the locations of each type of food.

Tasks Performed After Assisting the Patient with Eating

After the patient has finished eating, remove the meal tray and calculate the amount of food the patient took in. If the patient is on a calorie count diet, calculate the percentage of food eaten and tolerance to the food. If the patient's intake and output is being monitored, calculate the amount of fluid the patient took in. Document these findings in the patient's chart as required. Position the patient for comfort and place the call light within reach. Make sure any necessary items, such as the tray table and personal items, are within reach. Hand hygiene should then be performed.

Fluid Intake

Dehydration

Dehydration is a life-threatening condition that occurs when the body does not have enough water to perform normal body functions. Patients who are dehydrated may present with sunken eyes and dry mucous membranes. Dehydrated patients will often complain of generalized weakness and constant thirst. Their skin may lose its elasticity as a result of dehydration. In cases of severe dehydration, additional symptoms may include a weak rapid pulse and low blood pressure. The urine will become darker and more concentrated when patients are dehydrated; a result of the kidneys conserving as much water as possible.

Causes of Dehydration

Dehydration can be caused by too little intake or too much output. Limited intake may result if the patient is unable to take in fluid as a result of chronic nausea or difficulty swallowing. The patient may be unable to obtain an adequate amount of fluid if they are confused or kept NPO. Dehydration may also result if the patient is excreting too much fluid. The most common cause of over-excretion of fluid is frequent diarrhea or vomiting. Excessive sweating from fever or exercise may also result in excessive fluid loss if that fluid is not being actively replaced. Blood loss after surgery, hemorrhage, or fluid loss after a burn may also cause dehydration, in addition to some medical conditions such diabetes insipidus.

Encouraging Fluids

If a patient is dehydrated, they must increase the volume of fluids that they consume in order to restore fluid balance. To encourage more fluid intake, explain to the patient why it is important to consume more fluids and make sure a water pitcher and glass is within reach. Fluids should be encouraged each time the patient's room is entered unless that patient is on fluid restriction orders. Other fluids may also be made available, such as fruit juice or decaffeinated tea or coffee. Try to avoid sugary sodas or caffeinated beverages as these may not quench the patient's thirst. If the patient has family present, ask them to also encourage the patient to drink more. If patients are unable to take in sufficient fluid volume, IV fluids may be initiated.

Therapeutic Diets

NPO, Clear Liquid, and Mechanical Soft

NPO (nothing by mouth) is a diet that is ordered for patients who are not allowed to eat. It is typically ordered in anticipation of medical testing or a surgical procedure. Patient status will also be made NPO if it is unsafe for the individual to eat, such as a patient who is intubated, sedated, or unable to swallow properly.

A **clear liquid** diet is the first diet prescribed after a patient is taken off NPO status. It is typically ordered to allow the patient to eat without experiencing nausea.

A **mechanical soft diet** is prescribed for patients who have difficulty chewing, such as patients who do not have their dentures. It is also intended to help patients to transition from NPO to a regular diet.

Condition-Specific Diets

The diet that is prescribed for a patient depends upon the individual's health history and current diagnosis:

- A **regular diet** has no dietary restrictions; patients can eat whatever they like.
- A **calorie count diet** is typically ordered for diabetic patients; it limits the amount of sugar the patient takes in and counts the number of calories and carbohydrates the patient consumes.
- **A low-sodium diet** is prescribed to limit the amount of salt ingested by patients with a history of renal impairment or hypertension.
- A **cardiac diet** is ordered for patients with a history of cardiac problems; while on this diet, they are served low-fat, low-calorie, and low-sodium foods.

Aspiration

Indications

Aspiration occurs when small amounts of food or water move down the trachea and into the patient's lungs instead of traveling through the esophagus to the stomach as they should. This is extremely dangerous and can result in aspirational pneumonia. Certain patients are at a significant risk for aspirating food. This includes sedated patients, patients with altered mental status, patients with a current or past stroke with weakness of the face/mouth/tongue, patients experiencing delirium, as well as others. Forceful coughing or a wet-sounding voice after swallowing a bite of food may be an indication of aspiration. If a patient needs to chew food for long periods of time or requires multiple attempts to swallow food, they may be aspirating. Other indications include unusual head movements while trying to swallow, difficulty breathing, drooling while eating, or pocketing food in the cheeks. All of these signs should be reported and documented.

Aspiration Precautions

Aspiration precautions are steps that are to prevent aspiration in patients having difficulty swallowing or having other risk factors for aspiration. Prior to being fed, the patient should be positioned with the head of the bed at a 90° angle. The patient's food and drinks must be checked to make sure they are thickened to the prescribed consistency. The patient should be fed slowly, with small amounts of food being offered on a spoon. The patient should be allowed an adequate amount of time to chew and swallow. After the meal has been completed, the patient should remain upright for at least half an hour to prevent reflux. After the half hour has passed, the patient can be repositioned for comfort.

Meeting Patient's Personal Dietary Needs

Upon admission to the hospital or long-term care facility, any cultural or religious requests that the patient may have regarding **personal dietary needs** should be confirmed. The facility dietary service should be notified as soon as possible to ensure the patient is provided with appropriate foods. Prior to taking the tray in to the room, the tray must be checked to make sure the food on the tray meets the patient's dietary restrictions. If it does not, the dietary service should be notified regarding the problem, and a replacement meal should be obtained as soon as possible.

Mobility and Immobility

Deep Vein Thrombosis (DVT)

A deep vein thrombosis (DVT), is a blood clot that develops in the larger veins in an extremity. DVTs most commonly form in the legs, though the risk of developing a DVT in the arms does increase if the patient has an intravenous line. DVTs are most commonly caused by immobilization, though other factors such as obesity, infection, tobacco use, and advanced age can increase the patient's risk for developing a clot. The most common signs of a DVT include swelling and redness of the affected extremity. The patient may also complain of pain in the affected extremity. DVTs present a heavy risk for embolism, when part of the clot breaks apart and travels in the bloodstream to the heart, lungs, or brain. This can result in pulmonary embolism, heart attack, or stroke. If a patient presents with any signs of a DVT, that extremity should be elevated and rubbing/massaging of the extremity should be avoided (as this can create an embolism). This should be escalated immediately.

Sequential Compression Device (SCD)

A sequential compression device (SCD) is a pair of cuffs that are placed on the patient's legs to prevent the formation of blood clots. While the SCDs are on, the device applies pressure to different parts of the legs over time. The increased pressure encourages blood flow within the legs, preventing blood clots. Care should be taken while the SCDs are in place to ensure the tubing does not become kinked as this prevents the SCDs from working. The circulation in the patient's feet should also be monitored. Frequent skin care should be performed as the skin underneath the cuffs can become damp and hot. SCDs should not be used on extremities that have an existing DVT, as it could encourage the formation of an embolism.

Anti-Embolism Stockings and Elastic Bandages

Anti-Embolism Stockings

Anti-embolism stockings or T.E.D. (thrombo-embolic deterrent) hose are tight elastic stockings that are applied to the patient's legs. They are typically prescribed for patients who have undergone surgery or have decreased activity. When a patient is unable to move, blood pools in the legs, which increases the risk of developing blood clots and edema. Anti-embolism stockings work by placing pressure on the legs, which encourages blood flow. With improved circulation in the lower extremities, the patient's risk for developing a blood clot or edema is decreased. Care should be taken to frequently monitor circulation in the patient's legs while the anti-embolism stockings are in place.

Applying Anti-Embolism Stockings

The process for applying anti-embolism stockings is as follows:

1. Prior to applying anti-embolism stockings, verify that the anti-embolism stockings are the proper size for the patient based upon height and weight; they should be tight without cutting off circulation.
2. Place the patient in a supine position.
3. Gather the fabric of the anti-embolism stocking and slide it onto the patient's foot.
4. Roll the stocking upward until the upper edge is placed above the patient's knee.
5. Check to make sure there are no wrinkles in the stocking and that the stocking is placed properly so that the toes and heels are in the appropriate spots.
6. Once the stocking is in place, position the patient for comfort, remove the gloves, and wash hands.

Applying Elastic Bandages

The process for applying elastic bandages is as follows:

1. Prior to applying an elastic bandage, check the order to confirm where the bandage is to be placed.
2. Wash the hands and apply a pair of gloves.
3. Hold the end of the bandage in place with one hand and wrap it around the extremity twice to secure it.
4. Continue to wrap the bandage around the area that needs to be covered, working from bottom to top.
5. While wrapping, overlap the bandages to keep them from sliding down and to ensure the area is covered.
6. Once the elastic bandage is in place, secure it with tape, clips, or Velcro.
7. Remove the gloves and wash hands.

Monitoring Patients Wearing Elastic Bandages or Anti-Embolism Stockings

While patients are wearing anti-embolism stockings or elastic bandages, it is important to **monitor** them closely to ensure they receive an appropriate amount of circulation to their extremities. Frequently assess the patient's toes (or fingers, if the elastic bandage is on the arm) to check for signs of decreased circulation. Any complaints of numbness, tingling, or decreased sensation in the extremity should be escalated and investigated immediately. Make sure to remove the patient's anti-embolism stockings every 8 hours to allow for circulation. Elastic bandages should be removed per the doctor's order.

Pressure Injuries

Stages

Pressure-related injuries result from pressure with or without shear and/or friction over bony prominences. The National Pressure Injury Advisory Panel developed a staging system to ensure that definitions for pressure injuries were standardized:

- **Suspected deep tissue injury**: Skin discolored, intact or blood blister
- **Stage I**: Intact skin with non-blanching reddened area
- **Stage II**: Abrasion or blistered area without slough but with partial-thickness skin loss
- **Stage III**: Deep tissue injury with exposed subcutaneous tissue; tunneling or undermining may be evident with or without slough or epibole (rolling inward of wound edge)
- **Stage IV**: Deep tissue injury, full thickness, with necrosis into muscle, bone, tendons, and/or joints
- **Unstageable**: Eschar and/or slough prevents staging prior to debridement

Prevention

There are a number of methods available to **prevent** the formation of pressure injuries:

- The primary method of prevention is **frequent repositioning**. The patient should be turned and repositioned at least every two hours to prevent skin breakdown. Pillows may be used to provide additional support.
- The patient's **feet should be elevated** to prevent breakdown on the ankles, and the head of the bed should be kept at less than a 30° angle to reduce pressure on the buttocks.
- The patient's **skin should be assessed** frequently.
- The patient's **nutritional status** should be closely monitored as well since patients who have poor nutrition are at an increased risk of developing a pressure sore.

Air Mattresses and Egg Crate Mattresses

Pressure injuries typically develop when the patient is unable to move as a result of illness or injury. As the patient lies in bed, their weight causes breakdown over bony prominences, such as over the shoulder blades and coccyx. When inflated, an **air mattress** decreases the amount of pressure placed upon the bony prominences. An **egg crate mattress** is a foam cushion that has alternating raised areas and grooves that decrease the area of pressure on bony prominences. Though these items do not replace turning the patient, they can aid in preventing pressure sores in high-risk patients.

Treatment

Pressure injuries are difficult to heal as a result of the patient's compromised health status. If a patient develops a pressure injury, it is important to ensure it does not get worse by frequently turning and repositioning the patient. The patient should be placed on a support surface, such as an air mattress. This helps to decrease the amount of pressure on bony prominences. The skin over the affected area should be kept clean and dry. Dressings can be applied to the pressure sore, though the type of dressing depends on the severity of the pressure injury. It is also important to ensure the patient maintains good nutrition to ensure healing.

Caring for a Patient with Contractures

Patients that are immobile have a high risk for **contractures**, the permanent shortening of muscles/tendons that results in frozen joints and deformities. There are a number of treatment options for a patient with contractures. When a patient first develops a contracture, the physician and the physical therapist should be notified. Attempts should be made to mobilize the joint using range-of-motion techniques. Heat therapy may be used prior to initiating activity to ease pain and increase flexibility. In some cases, the affected joint may be placed in a splint, which will continuously stretch the joint. Care of the splint should be performed as ordered by the doctor. If the contracture does not respond to other treatments, the patient may be taken to surgery to manipulate the tendon.

Preventing Edema

Edema can develop in the patient's extremities as a result of fluid overload or inactivity, so the patient should be encouraged to move regularly to prevent swelling. If the patient is unable to walk, range-of-motion exercises should be frequently performed. While in bed or in the chair, the patient's legs should be elevated on pillows to prevent swelling in the lower extremities. Massaging the patient's extremities using lotion can also prevent edema. If the patient has a history of heart or kidney failure, their fluid and sodium intake should be closely monitored, as too much can result in increased edema.

Effects of Immobility on Self-Image and Activity Tolerance

Patients may be immobile for a number of reasons, including edema, weakness, trauma, pain, severe infection, and neuromuscular disease. **Immobility** prevents the patient from interacting normally with the environment and others, so the patient may become focused on body and health concerns, becoming demanding or, in some cases, passive. The patient may begin to feel powerless because of the necessity of relying on others to meet needs and may develop a negative body image and lowered self-esteem. The patient may become depressed, angry, and withdrawn, especially if immobility is prolonged.

Additionally, immobility interferes with the patient's ability to carry out activities of daily living without assistance. Muscles weaken from disuse, bones lose calcium and are more prone to fractures, and the patient may experience a sudden fall in blood pressure when sitting or standing (orthostatic hypotension). The patient may tire easily and is at increased risk of falls.

ADLs

Activities of daily living (ADLs) are a group of activities that are used to evaluate a patient's return to normal function; these are activities that the patient had performed on a daily basis before hospitalization, and will be expected to perform once he or she has completed rehabilitation. The **rate** at which the patient accomplishes these activities, in addition to the **level of independence** maintained by the patient when performing the activities, can help caregivers determine the amount of rehabilitation required, and can also be used to monitor the progress of the patient during the rehabilitation process. ADLs are grouped into 3 different areas: **personal or physical**, **instrumental**, and **occupational**.

Grouping ADLs

The first group of ADLs, the **physical or personal group**, contains those daily activities that relate to the patient's ability to take care of him or herself. Included in this group are activities related to health management, nutritional needs, elimination of bladder and bowel contents, exercise, self-esteem, coping/stress management, cognitive abilities, communication, sexual health and ability, and relationship roles. The second group of ADLs, the **instrumental group**, contains activities such as shopping, answering the phone, and other activities that involve leaving home. The third group, **occupational activities**, includes activities that are required of being a parent, husband, or wife, as well as those required on the job.

Rehabilitation

Rehabilitation is an area of health care that is dedicated to helping patients improve and/or restore functions and abilities after a disease or injury. Although rehabilitation is usually thought of in relation to **physical therapy** (which is one of the many areas of rehabilitation), it also encompasses **drug and alcohol rehabilitation**, as well as **occupational therapy** for physically and mentally ill patients. The general goals of all types of rehabilitation include an improvement in overall function; the promotion of independence, satisfaction, and well-being; and the preservation of the individual's self-esteem in the face of illness or debilitating disease or injury.

Assessing Potential for Rehabilitation

There are various factors that are considered when assessing a patient to determine whether he or she will benefit from **rehabilitation**. A patient with the inability to perform any of the ADLs will automatically be considered for rehabilitation. At this point, however, other factors must be considered. First and foremost is whether or not the patient has a **desire to improve his or her functions** through rehabilitation; if the patient is not interested in improvement, the rehabilitation potential is poor. If the patient wants to improve function and increase independence, the potential for rehabilitation is greater. Another factor is whether or not the patient has **support at home**; even if the patient improves greatly during his or her rehabilitation stay, he or she will still most likely need some support at home. If the patient has no support at home, rehabilitation may eventually fail.

Diseases and Illnesses That Commonly Require Rehabilitation

There are some diseases, illnesses, and injuries that almost always require rehabilitation at some point during their course; in these cases, rehabilitation may be initiated before the patient even leaves the hospital to be transferred to a rehabilitation facility. It is important to know which diseases usually require rehabilitation, because the sooner evaluation and rehabilitation are initiated, the better the patient's chance of recovery. The following are diseases, illnesses, and injuries that **commonly require rehabilitation**: AIDS, amyotrophic lateral sclerosis (ALS), limb amputation, traumatic or ischemic brain injury, spinal cord injury, burns, Guillain-Barré syndrome, hip or knee replacement, multiple sclerosis (MS), and most types of cancer.

Rehabilitation Settings

There are various kinds of rehabilitation settings, depending on the needs of the patient. Once the need for rehabilitation has been determined and the patient has been evaluated regarding specific rehabilitation needs, he or she can be placed in an appropriate rehabilitation setting. A **long-term acute care hospital** is a rehabilitation facility that is best for patients who are physically and psychologically stable but are receiving medical treatment such as dialysis or ventilation and thus require medical support. A **subacute care unit** is appropriate for patients who require more limited treatment, such as cancer patients. A **comprehensive inpatient rehabilitation facility** is just what the name suggests; it addresses the needs of a broad range of different patients, from burn victims to amputees. The comprehensive rehabilitation center has a "team" of medical specialists that includes a rehabilitation medicine physician, nurses trained in rehabilitation, occupational therapists, physical therapists, social workers, and speech-language pathologists. **Outpatient rehab** is designed for the high-functioning patient who can return home after rehab sessions.

Interventions to Consider When Beginning Rehabilitation Process

When a patient is to be considered for rehabilitation, he or she must undergo a rather extensive **evaluation** in order to increase the likelihood that he or she will succeed during rehabilitation. This process of evaluation, which includes various interventions, should take place in the early stages of illness, when the patient is still in the hospital. The goal is to forestall any **secondary complications** that may inhibit the rehabilitation process. These **interventions** include health management, in which the patient and family are educated about his or her disease(s); nutritional status assessment and support; initiation of bowel and bladder management in order to prevent infection; exercises; assessment of cognitive function; and education involving self-esteem, relationship roles, sexual activity, and coping mechanisms.

Occupational Therapy

Occupational therapy is defined as the use of creative activities in the treatment of individuals with disabilities, whether physical or mental. The purpose of occupational therapy is to provide those individuals with the skills that are necessary to live life as fully and independently as possible; after completion of occupational therapy, the individual should be able to perform at his or her **maximum potential**. The occupational therapist will typically provide the patient with **interventions** tailored to his or her disability. The OT will also visit the patient's home and/or place of employment in order to assess potential problems and provide **adaptive solutions**. As part of occupational therapy, the patient will receive regular **assessments** of his or her skills, as well as specific training. The occupational therapist is also responsible for educating the patient's family, caretakers, friends, and coworkers.

The philosophy of occupational therapy is based on the idea that **occupation** (meaning, loosely, either an activity or activities in which an individual engages) is a **basic human need**, one that is important to an individual's health and overall well-being in that it is in and of itself therapeutic in nature. The basic assumptions of occupational therapy are based on the idea of occupational therapy as stated by its creator, **William Rush Dunton**. Dunton states that occupational therapy is a human need because an individual's occupation has an effect on his or her health and general well-being. It creates **structure** in the individual's life and allows for him or her to manage and organize time. Another assumption is that individuals have different sets of values and, therefore, will value different occupations; for each person, however, the occupation that he or she chooses is meaningful to him or her.

Areas in Which Occupational Therapy May Be Instituted and Practiced

Although occupational therapy is an important part of the overall rehabilitation process for hospitalized individuals, it is also beneficial in other areas because occupational therapy deals not only with physical disabilities but with **emotional and cognitive disabilities** as well. Occupational therapy as related to **physical disabilities** may be practiced in outpatient clinics, pediatric hospitals or units, acute care rehabilitation facilities, and long-term, or comprehensive, inpatient rehabilitation centers. Occupational therapy as related to **mental disabilities** may be practiced in mental health clinics, acute and long-term psychiatric hospitals, prisons, and gateway or halfway houses. Occupational therapists may also work at schools, childcare facilities, workplaces, or shelters, or they may even work with individuals in their own homes.

Assistive Devices

Crutches should be properly fitted before client attempts ambulation. Correct height is one hand-width below axillae. The handgrips should be adjusted so the client supports the body weight comfortably with elbows slightly flexed rather than locked in place. The client should be cautioned not to bear weight under the axillae as this can cause nerve damage but to hold the crutches tight against the side of the chest wall. The type of gait used depends on the type of injury.

A **cane** should be held in the opposite hand of the side of injury. When holding the cane in neutral position, the elbow should be bent at about a 15-degree angle and if holding the cane straight down to the side of the body, the top of the cane should be in line with the crease of the wrist.

The same is true of a **walker**, the elbow should be bent at 15 degrees when standing up straight and grasping the handles, and the handle grasps should be in line with to the crease of the wrists. The client should be able to move the walker forward without leaning over.

Pain Management

Temperature-Controlled Therapies

Methods of Heating and Cooling

There are a number of different ways to **heat** (thermotherapy) or **cool** (cryotherapy) for **healing**:

- **Conduction**: Conveyance of heat, cold, or electricity through direct contact with the skin, such as with hot baths, ice packs, and electrical stimulation.
- **Convection**: Indirect transmission of heat in a liquid or gas by circulation of heated particles, such as with whirlpools and paraffin soaks.
- **Conversion**: Heating that results from converting a form of energy into heat, such as with diathermy and ultrasound.
- **Evaporation**: Cooling caused by liquids that evaporate into gases on the skin with a resultant cooling effect, such as with perspiration or vapo-coolant sprays.
- **Radiation**: Heating that results from transfer of heat through light waves or rays, such as with infrared or ultraviolet light.

Superficial Heat

Superficial heat with externally applied heat sources penetrates only the superficial layers of the skin (1–2 cm after about 30 minutes), but it is believed to relax deeper muscles by reflex, decrease pain, and increase metabolisms (2–3 times for every 10 °C increase in skin temperature). Therapeutic temperature range is 40–45 °C. **Superficial heat modalities** include:

- **Moist heat packs** placed on the skin and secured by several layers of towels to provide insulation, applied for 15–30 minutes.
- **Paraffin baths** (52–54 °C) with the hand, foot, or elbow dipped 7 times, cooling between dippings, and then wrapping with plastic and towels for 20 minutes.
- **Fluidotherapy** uses hot-air warmed (38.8–47.8 °C) cellulose particles into which a hand or foot is submerged for 20–30 minutes.

Passive and active range of motion exercises are done after superficial heat treatment. Contraindications include cardiac disease, peripheral vascular disease, malignant tumor, bleeding, and acute inflammation.

Deep heat differs from superficial heat in that the heat is generated internally using ultrasound, short wave, and microwave diathermy rather than applied to the surface of the skin. Deep heating has penetrance to 3–5 cm.

Shortwave Diathermy

Shortwave diathermy uses radio waves (27.12 megahertz) to **increase the temperature in subcutaneous tissue** and is used along with passive and active range of motion exercises to **improve range** in painful conditions such as inflammation of the muscles, tendons, and bursae. The radio waves (eddy currents) are transmitted through a capacitor or inductor in a continuous or pulse waveform. Temperatures increase about 15 °C in fatty tissue and 4–6 °C in muscular tissue. Shortwave diathermy should not be used over any organs containing fluid, including the eyes, heart, head, or over pacemakers as the diathermy may disrupt the settings. Because this treatment may increase cardiac demand, it should be avoided in those with preexisting cardiac conditions and should not be used over malignancies. Additionally, it is contraindicated in areas of inflammation because heating the tissue increases inflammation. It cannot be used over prostheses as the metal may heat and damage tissue. Shortwave diathermy should avoid the epiphyses in children, as it may stimulate abnormal growth.

Microwave Diathermy

Microwave diathermy is used similarly to shortwave diathermy but has a lower rate of heat increase and penetrance so it is used for muscles and joints near the surface rather than deep muscles, such as the hip. Heat is created by **electromagnetic radiation** (9.15–14.50 MHz) and raises temperature in fatty tissues by about 10–12 °C and in muscular tissue by 3–4 °C. **Treatment** is usually given for 15–30 minutes per session and is followed by range of motion exercises (passive and active) to increase flexibility. Contraindications are similar to those of shortwave diathermy in that this treatment should not be used where increase in temperature may be detrimental, such as over organs containing fluid, areas of inflammation, and epiphyses of children. Additionally, it should not be used over prostheses or pacemakers and should be avoided in those with cardiac disease.

Cryotherapy

Cryotherapy uses therapeutic cold treatment to cool the surface of the skin and underlying subcutaneous tissues in order to decrease blood flow, pain, and metabolism. Initially response to cold therapy causes **vasoconstriction** to occur within the first 15 minutes but if the tissues are cooled to -10 °C, then the body responds with **vasodilation**. Cryotherapy affects sensory response so the person will at first feel cold, which progresses to burning, aching, and finally to numbness and tingling. Treatment is usually given for 15–30 minutes. **Treatment modalities** include:

- **Ice packs** such as refrigerated gel packs (-5 °C) or plastic bags filled with water and ice chips are applied directly to the skin for 10–15 minutes for superficial cooling and 15–20 minutes for greater penetrance.
- A **towel dipped in ice and water slurry** is wrapped around limb to provide cold therapy, but this is best used only for emergency situations when ice packs are unavailable, as the towel must be changed frequently as the skin warms the towel rapidly.
- **Ice massage** is applied directly to the affected area for 5–10 minutes, usually rubbing the ice in circular motions on the skin surface. An ice massager is easily made by filled a paper cup with water and freezing it with a tongue depressor or Popsicle stick (to use as a handle) inserted into the center as the water starts to freeze. Then, the paper can be torn away from the bottom and sides when the ice is solid. Ice massage is often followed by friction massage.
- **Ice baths** (13–18 °C) are used for limbs, such as the lower leg, foot, or hand. The body part is immersed for 20 minutes.

Cryotherapy is usually followed by **active and passive exercises**. Contraindications include impaired circulation or sensation, cardiac disease, Raynaud's disease, and nerve trauma.

Whirlpool Baths

Whirlpool baths are used to increase **circulation** and promote **healing**. They are tubs with a turbine that mixes air with water, which is pressurized and flows into the tub water to create turbulence. Tubs are usually large enough to accommodate the full body although smaller limb-sized whirlpool tubs are available. Water temperature is 95–104 °F (adjusted for the individual) and should be deep enough to completely submerge the affected part. The body part should be cleaned with soap and water before immersion or a shower taken. If the full body is treated, then the patient should wear a swimming suit. During the whirlpool treatment, the muscles relax from the heat and **range of motion exercises** can be done while in the water. Typically, treatments last about 20 minutes, but the patient should be monitored, especially for the first 5 minutes, as some people become lightheaded and can lose consciousness.

Contrast Baths

Contrast baths (alternating hot and cold) are used in the sub-acute phase of healing (after edema begins to subside) for **strains and sprains**. It is believed that contrast baths increase the circulation and help to further decrease edema by a pumping action as the **vasoconstriction and vasodilation** alternate. Two containers are filled with water, one with hot and the other with cold. The hot water should be maintained at about 100–110 °F and the cold at 55–65 °F. The cycle begins and ends with immersion in cold water. Cold water immersions usually last about 1 minute and hot water immersions 4 minutes. Typically, the affected limb is immersed in the cold water for 1 minute, removed, and immediately immersed in hot water for 4 minutes. This cycle is repeated about 3–4 times.

Therapeutic Ultrasound

Ultrasound treats soft-tissue injuries (such as myositis, bursitis, and tendinitis) with sound waves (frequency 0.8–3.0 MHz). Ultrasound utilizes a **piezoelectric crystal** that vibrates, producing sound waveforms, which are transmitted from the transducer through a gel substance into the tissue. The sound waves bounce off of the bone in an irregular pattern that causes an increase in temperature in the connective tissue, such as collagen fibers. Temperatures of the tissue may increase up to 43.5 °C, increasing metabolism in the area, neural conduction, as well as blood flow. Ultrasound is used to **decrease both contractures and scarring**. During treatment, the transducer passes in a circular motion about the skin surface, staying in contact with the gel medium. If a distal limb is submerged in water, the treatment is given with the head of the transducer 0.5–1.0 in from the skin surface. Treatment is followed by range of motion exercises, passive and active. Contraindications are similar to other heat-producing modalities and include peripheral vascular disease, but ultrasound may be used over metal prostheses.

TENS

Transcutaneous electrical nerve stimulation (TENS) uses electrical stimulation to stimulate **peripheral sensory nerve fibers** to reduce acute or recurrent pain. TENS machines may be 2-lead or 4-lead and have adjustments for both frequency (1–20 Hz) and pulse width (50–300 µs, 10–50 mA). Stimulation can be intermittent or continuous. TENS units are small and battery-powered with wires and adhesive electrodes attached so that they can be worn while the person goes about usual activities. The positioning of the electrodes and the settings depend upon the site and type of injury, following guidelines provided by the manufacturer. The TENS machine can be used for a number of hours, but if used for days at a time, it will be less effective. TENS treatment is contraindicated with demand pacemakers and should not be used on the head or neck or over irritated skin.

Complementary and Alternative Therapies

Complementary Therapy

Complementary therapies are often used, either alone or in conjunction with conventional medical treatment. These methods should be included if this is what the patient/family chooses, empowering the family to take control of their plan of care. Complementary therapies vary widely and most can easily be incorporated. The **National Center for Complementary and Alternative Medicine** recognizes the following:

- **Whole medical systems**: Chinese medicine (acupressure, acupuncture), naturopathic and homeopathic medicines, and Ayurveda
- **Mind-body medicine**: Prayer, artistic creation, music and dance therapy, biofeedback, focused relaxation, and visualization
- **Biological medicine**: Aromatherapy, herbs, plants, trees, vitamins and minerals, and dietary supplements
- **Manipulation**: Massage and spinal manipulation
- **Energy medicines**: Magnets, electric current, pulsed fields, Reiki, qi gong, and laying-on of the hands

Precautions

The use of alternative and complementary therapies should be thoroughly discussed by patients and their physician. Patients should be encouraged to use therapies that are shown to have a beneficial, complementary effect on conventional medical treatment. These therapies include the use of massage, superficial stimulation, relaxation, distraction, hypnosis, and guided imagery.

- Encourage patients to practice the techniques until they are proficient in their use to give them a chance to prove their value.
- Teach the patient how the therapies work to encourage the patient to believe in them to contribute to the placebo effect.
- Caution the patient against abandoning current medical treatment.
- Inform the patient of the high cost of alternate therapies that can divert needed funds and result in little or no benefit.
- Provide the patient with resources in the form of books, pamphlets, and informative websites that prove the results of scientific research so that they can evaluate alternative therapies for themselves.

Whole Medical Systems

Whole medical systems are different philosophies and methods of explaining and treating health and illness. Some systems include:

- **Homeopathic medicine**: This European system uses small amounts of diluted herbs and supplements to help the body to recover from disease by stimulating an immune response.
- **Naturopathic medicine**: This is a European system that uses various natural means (herbs, massage, acupuncture) to support the natural healing forces of the body.
- **Chinese medicine**: Centers on restoring the proper flow of life forces within the body to cure disease by using herbs, acupressure and acupuncture, and meditation.
- **Ayurveda**: This is an Indian system that tries to bring the spirit into harmony with the mind and body to treat disease via yoga, herbs, and massage.

Essential Oils

Essential oils (concentrated oils from plants) are either inhaled (aromatherapy) or diluted and applied to the skin. Essential oils are believed to reduce stress, aid sleep, improve dermatitis, and aid digestion. Commonly used essential oils include eucalyptus, lavender, lemon, peppermint, rosemary, rose, and tea tree. Oils may cause skin irritation when applied to the skin.

Cupping

Cupping is an ancient practice still used in Southeast Asia and the Middle East to reduce pain, promote healing, and improve circulation. With dry cupping, cups are heated by placing something flammable (such as paper or herbs) inside the cup and setting it on fire to heat the cup, which is then immediately placed on the back along the meridians (generally on both sides of the spine) to form a vacuum that draws blood to the skin and causes circular bruises believed to heal that part of the body. Wet cupping includes leaving the heated cup in place for three minutes, removing it, making small cuts in the skin, and then applying suction cups again to withdraw blood. Cupping should be avoided in children under 4 and limited to short periods in older children.

Acupuncture

Alternative systems of medical practice include acupuncture, homeopathy, and naturopathy. **Acupuncture**, an ancient Oriental practice, uses stainless steel or copper needles inserted into superficial skin layers at points where energy or life force called *qi* is believed to occur. The needles are supposed to restore balance and the flow of *qi*. The NIH has recognized the effectiveness of acupuncture for certain side effects of other cancer treatments, such as nausea, vomiting, and pain. However, there is no documented scientific evidence to support the principles expounded. Acupuncturists are certified through either formal coursework or apprenticeships, and there is also board certification in this area for physicians. The needles used are classified as class II, which means they have manufacturing and labeling requirements.

Herbal Remedies and Regulations

In the United States, most **herbal preparations** are classified as dietary supplements. That means that they are not subject to the same rigorous manufacturing, safety, efficacy, and control practices as pharmaceutical drugs. Herbal supplements are only governed by the Dietary Supplement and Health Education Act (DSHEA). As long as no specific disease treatment or curative claims are made, the supplement can be marketed without limitation and safety concerns must be pursued by the FDA after the fact. Nevertheless, some herbal remedies have been undergoing clinical trials in the U.S. to substantiate their health-enhancing or traditional/historical or international use claims. However, the focal point of these studies is still only on the effectiveness of the specific supplement. In Europe, there has been some movement toward greater regulation and licensing of herbal products, but not to the extent of formal drug regulations.

Toxicities Associated with Herbal Remedies

Use of herbal preparations has been associated with a variety of **toxicities**, primarily in categories such as cardiovascular problems, hypersensitivity reactions, disorientation, gastrointestinal problems, and liver malfunction. Because quality control measures are relatively lax for these remedies, contamination from infectious agents and toxic metals can potentially cause other side effects. Many of these herbal medicines **interact with conventional drugs**, thus altering their pharmacodynamics. For example, St. John's wort, which is primarily used for depressive disorders or as a sedative, interacts with a wide range of traditional pharmacologic agents and suppresses their levels in the bloodstream. Kava kava, made from dried roots of a type of pepper bush, is used as a sedative, but it also has been associated with hepatic failure and via interactions with several other drugs can actually induce a comatose state. Ginseng is an Asian remedy touted for its curative properties in a number of diseases. However, it can react with steroidal drugs and induce shaking and manic episodes. These are just a few examples of potential dangers.

Non-Pharmaceutical Pain Relief

Non-pharmaceutical methods to relieve pain that can be used exclusively or combined with medications include massage, heat, cold, electrical stimulation, distraction, relaxation, imagery, visualization, and music. Other **alternatives or adjuncts to pain medication** include hypnosis, magnets, acupuncture, acupressure, and therapeutic touch. Herbs, aromatherapy, reflexology, homeopathic medicine, and prayer may also be accepted by the patient. Any method that the patient feels may help that isn't harmful should be used to help get relief.

Mind-Body Medicine for Pain and Disease

Mind-body medicine (prayer, artistic creation, music and dance, biofeedback, relaxation, and visualization) can help distract people from pain or other symptoms if they are able to concentrate on the method. This can result in the transfer of less painful stimuli to the brain by stimulating the **descending control system**. These methods work if the patient can use them to create alternate sensations in the brain, but will not work if the patient is unable to concentrate due to intense pain.

Relaxation that occurs as a result of using these methods helps to reduce muscular tension that can make pain worse and reduces fatigue caused by chronic pain. Relaxation has been proven to be the most helpful after surgery. Postoperative patients report a greater feeling of control over their pain and tend to request fewer opioids to control pain. Biofeedback can help patients to recognize the feelings of both tension and relaxation and provide a way to indicate their success in managing muscle tension.

Use of Visualization

There are a number of methods used for **visualization** to reduce anxiety and promote healing. Some include audiotapes with guided imagery, such as self-hypnosis tapes, but the patient can be taught basic **techniques** that include:

- Sit or lie comfortably in a **quiet place** away from distractions.
- Concentrate on **breathing** while taking long slow breaths.
- **Close the eyes** to shut out distractions and create an image in the mind of the place or situation desired.
- Concentrate on that **image**, engaging as many senses as possible and imaging details.
- If the mind wanders, breathe deeply and **bring consciousness back** to the image or concentrate on breathing for a few moments and then return to the imagery.
- End with positive imagery.

Sometimes, patients are resistive at first or have a hard time maintaining focus, so **guiding** them through visualization for the first few times can be helpful.

Stimulation of the Skin to Reduce Pain

Skin, muscles, fascia, tendons, and the cornea contain **nociceptors** that are nerve endings that respond to painful stimuli. Massage, transcutaneous electrical nerve stimulation (TENS), heat and cold provide stimulation to other nerves that transfer only sensation, not pain. These signals block some of the transfer of the nociceptor impulses:

- **Massage** not only sends alternate sensation to the brain, but also results in relaxation that decreases the muscular tension that contributes to pain.
- **TENS** works well on incisional and neuromuscular pain by providing a gentle electrical stimulation that overrides the painful impulses from the area and may stimulate endorphins.
- **Heat therapy** increases blood flow and oxygen to promote healing and stimulates neural receptors, decreasing pain. Heat also helps loosen tense muscles that may be contributing to pain.
- **Cold therapy** decreases circulation and reduces production of chemicals related to inflammation, thereby reducing pain.

Bowel and Urinary Elimination

Bladder Training

Bladder training usually requires the person to keep a toileting diary for at least three days so patterns can be assessed. There are a number of different approaches:

- **Scheduled toileting** is toileting on a regular schedule, usually every 2-4 hours during the daytime.
- **Habit training** involves an attempt to match the scheduled toileting to a person's individual voiding habits, based on the toileting diary. This is useful for people who have a natural and fairly consistent voiding pattern. Toileting is done every 2-4 hours.
- **Prompted voiding** is often used in nursing homes and attempts to teach people to assess their own incontinence status and prompts them to ask for toileting.
- **Bladder retraining** is a behavioral modification program that teaches people to inhibit the urge to urinate and to urinate according to an established schedule, restoring normal bladder function as much as possible. Bladder training can improve incontinence in 80% of cases.

Prompted Voiding

Prompted voiding is a communication protocol for people with mild to moderate **cognitive impairment**. It uses positive reinforcement for recognizing being wet or dry, staying dry, urinating, and drinking liquids.

- Ask patient **every two hours** (8 a.m. to 4-8 p.m.) whether they are wet or dry.
- Verify if they are correct and give **feedback**, "You are right, Mrs. Brown, you are dry."
- **Prompt** patient, whether wet or dry, to use the toilet or urinal. If yes, assist them, record results, and give positive reinforcement by praising and visiting for a short time. If no, repeat the request again once or twice. If they are wet, and decline toileting, change and tell them you will return in two hours and ask them to try to wait to urinate until then.
- Offer **liquids** and record amount.
- **Record** results of each attempt to urinate or wet check.

Bladder Retraining

Bladder retraining teaches people to control the urge to urinate. It usually takes about three months to rehabilitate a bladder muscle weakened from frequent urination, causing a decreased urinary capacity. A short urination interval is gradually lengthened to every 2-4 hours during the daytime as the person suppresses bladder urges and stays dry.

- The patient keeps a **urination diary** for a week.
- An individual program is established with **scheduled voiding times and goals**. For example, if a patient is urinating every hour, the goal might be every 80 minutes with increased output.
- The patient is taught **techniques** to withhold urination, such as sitting on a hard seat or on a tightly rolled towel to put pressure on pelvic floor muscles, doing five squeezes of pelvic floor muscles, deep breathing, and counting backward from 50.
- When the patient consistently meets the goal, a **new goal** is established.

THE KNACK TO CONTROL URINARY INCONTINENCE

The **knack** is the use of precisely timed muscle contractions to prevent **stress incontinence**. It is "the knack" of squeezing up before bearing down. The knack is a preventive use of **Kegel exercises**. Women are taught to contract the pelvic floor muscles right before and during events that usually cause stress incontinence. For example, if a woman feels a cough or sneeze coming, she immediately contracts the pelvic floor muscles and holds until the stress event is over. This contraction augments support of the proximal urethra, reducing the amount of displacement that usually takes place with compromised muscle support, thereby preventing incontinence. It is particularly useful if used before and during stress events, such as coughing, sneezing, lifting, standing, swinging a golf club, or laughing. Studies have shown that women who are taught this technique for mild to moderate urinary incontinence and use it consistently are able to decrease incontinence by 73-98%.

BOWEL TRAINING

Bowel training for defecation includes keeping a bowel diary to chart progress:

- **Scheduled defecation** is usually daily, but for some people 3-4 times weekly, depending on individual bowel habits. Defecation should be at the same time, so work hours and activities must be considered. Defecation is scheduled for 20-30 minutes after a meal when there is increased motility.
- **Stimulation** is necessary. Drinking a cup of hot liquid may work, but initially many require rectal stimulation, inserting a gloved, lubricated finger into the anus and running it around the rim of the sphincters. Some people require rectal suppositories, such as glycerine. Stimulus suppositories, such as Dulcolax (bisacodyl), or even Fleet enemas are sometimes used, but the goal is to reduce use of medical or chemical stimulants.
- **Position** should be sitting upright with knees elevated slightly if possible and leaning forward during defecation.
- **Straining** includes attempting to tighten abdominal muscles and relax sphincters while defecating.
- **Exercise** increases the motility of the bowel by stimulating muscle contractions. **Walking** is one of the best exercises for this purpose, and the person should try to walk 1 or 2 miles a day. If the person is unable to walk, then other activities, such as chair exercises that involve the arms and legs and bending can be very effective. Those who are bed bound need to turn from side to side frequently and change position.
- **Kegel exercises** increase strength of the pelvic floor muscles. Kegel exercises for urinary incontinence and fecal incontinence are essentially the same, but the person tries to pull in the muscles around the anus, as though trying to prevent the release of stool or flatus. The person should feel the muscles tightening while holding for 2 seconds and then relaxing for 2 seconds, gradually building the holding time to 10 seconds or more. Exercises should be done 4 times a day.

Management Strategies for Constipation and Fecal Impaction

Management strategies for constipation and impaction include:

- **Enemas** and **manual removal of impaction** may be necessary initially.
- Add **fiber** with bran, fresh/dried fruits, and whole grains, to 20-35 grams per day.
- Increase **fluids** to 64 ounces each day.
- **Exercise** program should include walking if possible, and exercises on a daily basis.
- Change in **medications** causing constipation can relieve constipation. Additionally, the use of stool softeners, such as Colace (docusate), or bulk formers, such as Metamucil (psyllium), may decrease fluid absorption and move stool through the colon more quickly. Overuse of laxatives can cause constipation.
- Careful **monitoring** of diet, fluids, and medical treatment, especially for irritable bowel syndrome.
- **Pregnancy-related constipation** may be controlled through dietary and fluid modifications and regular exercise.
- **Delayed toileting** should be avoided and bowel training regimen done to promote evacuation at the same time each day. During travel, stool softeners, increased fluid, and exercise may alleviate constipation.

Purpose of Fiber in the Diet

Most constipation is caused by insufficient **fiber** in the diet, especially if people eat a lot of processed foods. An adequate amount of fiber is 20-30 grams daily. There are both soluble and insoluble forms of fiber, and both add bulk to the stool and are not absorbed into the body. Some foods have both types:

- **Soluble fiber** dissolves in liquids to form a gel-like substance, which is why liquids are so important in conjunction with fiber in the diet. Soluble fiber slows the movement of stool through the gastrointestinal system. Food sources include bananas, potatoes, dried beans, nuts, apples, oranges, and oatmeal.
- **Insoluble fiber** changes little with the digestive process and increases the speed of stool through the colon, so too much can result in diarrhea. Food sources of insoluble fiber include wheat bran, whole grains, seeds, skins of fruits, vegetables, and nuts.

Geriatric Considerations

Age Categories of the Elderly

The elderly population can be divided into three groups. The age group ranging from 65-74 years are considered the **young-old**, from 75-84 are considered the **middle-old**, and 85 and older are considered **old-old**. There are many physical and psychological changes that occur as someone moves through these age groups. As this population increases in size, so does the number of those with physical and mental illnesses.

Factors That Influence Presentation of Illness in Older Adults

There are three major factors that influence **how an illness will present in an older patient.** These factors, either alone or in combination with one another, have the potential to make an ordinarily standard clinical presentation confusing for the clinician.

- The first of these factors is **underreporting of illness or the symptoms associated** with illness. There are a number of reasons that illnesses are not reported: the patient may fear hospitalization, institutionalization, or loss of control, or the patient may be convinced that there really is no problem.
- Another factor is the **pattern of distribution of illness** amongst the elderly population. This affects presentation because there are a number of diseases and impairments that are prevalent among older adults, including congestive heart failure, arthritis, osteoporosis, and pneumonia; therefore, identifying and differentiating the primary diagnosis may be difficult.
- The last factor is an **altered response to illness**. This can make diagnosis and treatment very difficult because symptoms may be exaggerated by other problems, or they may be nonexistent.

Age-Related Considerations When Evaluating Adult Patients

Because each individual patient is exposed to different environmental, psychological, and physical stressors that can affect the aging process, it is important to consider that some patients may experience adverse health impacts, while other patients of the same age may not be affected. As individuals age, the amount of wear on the body, as well as the likelihood of pathological changes, increases at different rates for every individual. Factors affecting the aging process include proper nutrition (or the lack thereof), level of physical activity, smoking, alcohol consumption, environmental or occupational exposures, and socioeconomic standing. Also, remember that as an individual ages, a disease or impairments with one organ or organ system will have a marked effect on other systems, because the body is not able to compensate as it once was. Symptoms may not be noticeable until other functions begin to decline. Most often, health issues manifest in the elderly as confusion, so close attention must be given to this symptom and investigated when present.

Basic Patient Safety Assessments When Evaluating a Patient

There are four basic assessments that the nurse should make when **assessing a patient's safety** and identifying possible safety concerns:

- The first of these is the **mobility assessment**; different safety risks apply to patients who are mobile as opposed to those who are not. An immobile patient, for example, has a tendency to form pressure injuries, or bedsores.

- The next assessment is the evaluation of the patient's **level of awareness**; is the patient able to communicate to the nursing staff when something is wrong? If not, certain measures should be undertaken to ensure that the nursing staff is aware of a change in the patient's condition.
- An extension of this assessment is determining whether the patient is in **critical condition**; these patients must be monitored more closely for changes.
- An assessment of the patient's **mental status** is also important because the patient may not be able to make safe decisions on his or her own.

Functional Evaluation of Elderly Patient

A functional evaluation of the elderly patient examines the patient's ability to carry out activities of daily living (ADL) that are critical in gauging the patient's ability to care for oneself without the need of assistance. Use the **Index of Independence in Activities of Daily Living Scale** to check foundational tasks such as taking a shower, getting dressed, eating, and going to the bathroom. Aged patients will be more likely to overstate what they are able to do and understate their limitations, while the patient's family will likely understate what the patient is able to handle. Assess mental ability with the following exams:

- Short Portable Mental Status Questionnaire (SPMSQ)
- Mini-Mental State Exam (MMSE)

The **Tinetti Balance and Gait Evaluation** exams are also important elements of the functional evaluation of an elderly patient. These tests, along with the simple **Up-and-Go test,** are used to assess the balance and gait issues that elderly patients have. The patient has to complete certain actions, such as sitting down and standing up from a chair, turning around, bending over, etc. The entire assessment takes approximately 15–20 minutes. The **Lawton and Brody: Instrumental Activities of Daily Learning** test is used to check whether the patient can do more complex activities important to daily living, second to the ADL's required for basic function. Examples of IADLs include the ability to go shopping, wash clothes, cook, etc. The **Index of Independence of Activities of Daily Living** is utilized to find what the patient is able do independently on a regular basis.

Depression and Suicide in the Elderly

Depression commonly goes unidentified in an aging patient. Cognitive changes are often wrongly identified as dementia, confusion, or natural aging changes, rather than depression. It is important to be cognizant of the prevalence of this issue among the elderly, and treat appropriately.

Suicide rates for elderly patients are higher than any other age group. The compounding stress and emotional burden of losing loved ones, mobility, and independence often contribute to suicidal ideations. Other factors include seemingly unbearable psychological anguish, dissatisfaction, and unmet requirements. Suicide is more commonly seen in elderly males (seven times higher rate), Caucasians, unmarried individuals (divorced, separated, single), individuals who are poor and/or out of work, individuals with psychiatric or cognitive impairments, the very sick, individuals with substance additions, individuals that are grieving (particularly in the first year of loss or retirement), those without friends or community relationships, or those who have tried suicide before. Suicidal thoughts and attempts may be overt or covert.

As with patients of other age ranges, if an elderly patient hints at suicidal ideations or thoughts, this must be addressed directly by the nurse.

INDICATIONS AND ASSESSMENTS FOR DELIRIUM

Delirium (acute confusion) presents in a variety of indications. The patient may experience mental issues, including inattention or short attention span, difficulty remembering, trouble with perception, bafflement, and lack of decision-making. There may be changing moods, faulty ability to manage whims, stress, slight to moderate depression, visual or auditory hallucinations, confabulation, changing intellectual ability that worsens at night (sun-downing) and is more frequently seen in patients that have had prior dementia, psychomotor agitation including inability to sleep, tachycardia, enlarged pupils, and perspiration. The patient may appear restless, overcautious, not cautious enough, or appear lost/stunned. There may be tachycardia, high blood pressure, fever, rapid breathing, and there might be focal neurological indications.

Physical assessments include a complete history, physical examination, check of mind and neurological issues to determine what is causing the problem, foundation of lab work such as CBC, electrocardiogram, chest radiograph, urinalysis, urine toxicology, and other assessments that are deemed necessary, such as EED, CT, or blood work for drugs.

Physiologic Integrity: Pharmacological and Parenteral Therapies

Pharmacokinetics and Routes of Administration

Principles of Pharmacokinetics

Pharmacokinetics relates to the route of administration, the absorption, the dosage, the frequency of administration, the distribution, and the serum levels achieved over time.

- The **drug's rate of clearance (elimination)** and **doses needed** to ensure therapeutic benefit are considered. Most drugs are cleared through the kidneys, with water-soluble compounds excreted more readily than protein-soluble compounds.
- **Volume of distribution** (IV drug dose divided by plasma concentration) determines the rate at which the drug passes into tissue. Drug distribution depends on the degree of protein binding and ion trapping that takes place.
- **Elimination half-life** is the time needed for the concentration of a particular drug to decrease to half of its starting dose in the body. Approximately five half-lives are needed to achieve steady-state plasma concentrations if giving doses intermittently.
- **Context-sensitive half-life** is the time needed to reach 50% concentration after withdrawal of a continuously-administered drug.
- **Recovery time** is the length of time it takes for plasma levels to decrease to the point that the effect is eliminated. This is affected by plasma concentration.
- **Effect-site equilibrium** is the time between administration of a drug and clinical effect (the point at which the drug reaches the appropriate receptors) and must be considered when determining dose, time, and frequency of medications.
- The **bioavailability** of drugs may vary, depending upon the degree of metabolism that takes place before the drug reaches its site of action.

Principles of Pharmacodynamics

Pharmacodynamics relates to biological effects (therapeutic or adverse) of drug administration over time. Drug transport, absorption, means of elimination, and half-life must all be considered when determining effects. Responses may include continuous responses, such as blood pressure variations, or dichotomous responses in which an event either occurs or does not (such as death). Information from pharmacodynamics provides feedback to modify medication dosage (pharmacokinetics). Drugs provide biological effects primarily by interacting with receptor sites (specific protein molecules) in the cell membrane. Receptors include voltage-sensitive ion channels (sodium, chloride, potassium, and calcium channels), ligand-gated ion channels, and transmembrane receptors. Agonist drugs exert effects after binding with a receptor, while antagonist drugs bind with a receptor but have no effects, so they can block agonists from binding. The total number of receptors may vary, upregulating or downregulating in response to stimuli (such as drug administration). Dose-response curves show the relationship between the amount of drug given and the resultant plasma concentration and biological effects.

First Pass Metabolism and Drug Clearance

First pass metabolism is the phenomenon that occurs to ingested drugs that are absorbed through the gastrointestinal tract and enter the hepatic portal system. Drugs metabolized on the first pass travel to the liver, where they are broken down, some to the extent that only a small fraction of the active drug circulates to the rest of the body. This first pass through the liver greatly reduces the bioavailability of some drugs. Routes of administration that avoid first pass metabolism include intravenous, intramuscular, and sublingual.

Drug clearance refers to the ability to remove a drug from the body. The two main organs responsible for clearance are the liver and the kidneys. The liver eliminates drugs by metabolizing, or biotransforming, the substance or excreting the drug in the bile. The kidneys eliminate drugs by filtration or active excretion in the urine. Drugs use either renal or hepatic methods of clearance. Kidney and liver dysfunction inhibit the clearance of drugs that rely on that organ for removal. Toxicity results from poor clearance.

Enterohepatic Recirculation of Drugs and Renally Excreted Drugs

Enterohepatic recirculation refers to the process whereby a drug is effectively removed from circulation and then reabsorbed. The drug is secreted in bile, which is collected in the gall bladder and emptied into the small intestine, from which part of it is reabsorbed and part excreted in the feces. This reabsorption reduces the clearance of these drugs and increases their duration of action. Generally, drugs susceptible to enterohepatic recirculation are generally those with a molecular weight greater than 500 g/mol and those that are amphipathic (have both a lipophilic portion and a polar portion).

Renally excreted drugs are metabolized (biotransformed) by the liver to a form that can be excreted by the kidneys. Others are excreted by the kidneys unchanged. Infants with decreased renal function demonstrate decreased urine output or elevated levels of BUN and creatinine. The nurse should avoid using drugs that depend on the kidneys for clearance if the infant has renal impairment, as overdose may result.

Absorption in Relation to Routes of Medication Administration

The absorption rate of a drug depends on its transfer from its site of administration to the circulatory system. Different **routes of administration** have different absorption characteristics:

- **Oral**: Ingested medications pass from the gastrointestinal tract into the bloodstream. Most absorption occurs in the small intestine and is affected by gastric motility and emptying rate, drug solubility in gastrointestinal fluids, and food presence. Orally administered drugs are susceptible to first pass metabolism by the liver.
- **Intravenous**: Medications directly administered to the bloodstream have 100% absorption. Peak serum levels are rapidly achieved. Some drugs are not tolerated intravenously, due to vein irritation or toxicity, and others must be given as an infusion.
- **Intramuscular**: Medications injected into a muscle are absorbed fairly rapidly because muscle tissue is highly vascularized. Drugs in lipid vehicles absorb more slowly than those in aqueous vehicles.
- **Subcutaneous**: Medications injected beneath the skin absorb more slowly because the dermis is less vascularized than muscle. Hypoperfusion and edema decrease absorption further.

Effects of Pharmacokinetic Characteristics on Different Age Groups

Pediatric Age Group

Infants, in particular, have unique **absorption profiles** that can dramatically impact the use of drugs in this age group. Babies have very variable rates of absorption, which precludes the use of certain routes of administration. At birth, full-gestational infants generally have a gastric pH near neutral, but after about one day, it drops to the highly acidic range (about pH 1-3). On the other hand, premature babies cannot effectively secrete acid, have a high stomach pH, and empty their stomachs more slowly. Infants also have **immature epithelial barriers** on the skin, making the skin more permeable. Infants have a larger percentage of water weight than adults, making **water-soluble drugs** more effective. However, in turn, their low protein concentrations can depress binding and distribution. Processes involved with elimination are also not fully developed in the infant until he or she is about a year old.

Geriatric Age Group

Pharmacokinetics involves four steps: absorption, distribution, metabolism, and elimination. All of these steps are affected by the age of the patient, as the organs involved degenerate from wear and tear:

1. **Absorption** of most drugs occurs in the small intestine. Drug absorption in older adults may be delayed or decreased due to decreased blood flow to the small intestine. This could change the blood levels of drugs achieved in the geriatric patient.
2. **Distribution** of the drug is altered due to a change in body composition. Elderly patients have decreased total body water and lean muscle mass. This relative increase in total body fat may increase the duration of action of lipid-soluble drugs.
3. Most drugs are **metabolized** by either the liver or the kidneys. Decreased function of these organs leads to delayed metabolism and elimination of certain medications.
4. **Renal function** and **elimination effectiveness** diminish with age, often decreasing the kidney's ability to remove toxins and medications from the body. For this reason, drugs may remain in the body longer, therefore requiring smaller doses among the elderly.

Blood Drug Levels

Plasma drug levels are used for **therapeutic drug monitoring** because, although plasma is often not the site of action, plasma levels correlate well with therapeutic (effective) and toxic (dose-related adverse effects) responses to most drugs. The therapeutic range of a drug is that between the minimum effective concentration (level at which there is no therapeutic benefit) and the toxic concentration (level at which toxic effects occur). To achieve drug plateau (steady state), the drug half-life (time needed to decrease drug concentration by 50%) must be considered. Most drugs reach plateau with administration equal to four half-lives and completely eliminate a drug in 5 half-lives. Because drug levels fluctuate, peak (highest drug concentration) and trough (lowest drug concentration) levels may be monitored. Samples for trough levels are taken immediately prior to administration of another dose, while peak samples are taken at various times, depending on the average peak time of the specific drug, which may vary from 30 minutes to 2 hours or so after administration.

Side Effects of Medications

All drugs can have side effects, and some are toxic at certain levels or in combination with other drugs. Some side effects will be minor and may go away after a week or two. Others can be severe or life-threatening, such as anaphylaxis. Common side effects include nausea, vomiting, diarrhea, and rashes. Side effects may vary with individuals according to age, gender, and condition and may be related to non-compliance with treatment, incorrect dosage, polypharmacy, or drug interactions. Drug compendiums will list all possible side effects according to system or incidence.

Pharmacologically similar medications usually have some common side effects among the drugs in that class. Nursing actions include:

- Always question the patient about allergies or previous drug reactions before administering medication.
- Educate the patient about possible side effects of all medications.
- Watch out for drug-drug and food-drug combinations that are dangerous.

DRUG INTERACTIONS

Drug interactions occur when one drug interferes with the activity of another in either the pharmacodynamics or pharmacokinetics:

- With **pharmacodynamic interaction,** both drugs may interact at receptor sites causing a change that results in an adverse effect or that interferes with a positive effect.
- With **pharmacokinetic interaction**, the ability of the drug to be absorbed and cleared is altered, so there may be delayed effects, changes in effects, or toxicity. Interactions may include problems in a number of areas:
    - **Absorption** may be increased or (more commonly) decreased, usually related to the effects within the gastrointestinal system.
    - **Distribution** of drugs may be affected, often because of changes in protein binding.
    - **Metabolism** may be altered, often causing changes in drug concentration.
    - **Biotransformation** of the drug must take place, usually in the liver and gastrointestinal system, but drug interactions can impair this process.
    - **Clearance interactions** may interfere with the body's ability to eliminate a drug, usually resulting in increased concentration of the drug.

SPECIFIC INTERACTIONS

Some drugs will either increase or inhibit the actions of other drugs. They may interfere with receptor-site binding or the way in which the drug is metabolized or excreted. Certain drugs may cause drowsiness when taken together or with alcohol. Some foods will inhibit drug action, such as the inhibition of warfarin by vitamin-K-containing foods. Other foods may cause toxic levels of a drug to accumulate. Grapefruit juice, for example, is metabolized by the same enzyme that metabolizes about 50 drugs, including digoxin and statins, and this can prevent the liver from breaking down drugs and lead to severe reactions. The nurse should always obtain a complete medication list from the patient, including prescription and over-the-counter medications, herbals, vitamins, minerals, and dietary supplements that are taken regularly and occasionally. All medications taken should be checked for **potential interactions with drugs or foods**.

DRUG CLASSIFICATION

The following are different ways to classify drugs:

- **Therapeutic classification**: The common uses for the drug will place it in a certain therapeutic classification.
- **Pharmacological classification**: The action of the drug determines which pharmacological category a drug will be in.

All drugs have a **chemical name** and a **generic name,** which is simpler. A company making the drug can give it a **trade or brand name**. The generic form of a drug is generally cheaper but may differ in efficacy from a brand name drug due to a difference in the amount of drug that is absorbed for use in the body. The Controlled Substances Act restricts usage of certain drugs and classifies them according to schedules that include:

- **Schedule I**: Ecstasy, LSD, marijuana, peyote, mescaline, psilocybin, heroin, and others
- **Schedule II**: Amphetamine, cocaine, codeine, fentanyl, Dilaudid, Demerol, Ritalin, morphine, opium, and others
- **Schedule III**: Anabolic steroids, barbiturates, codeine, Vicodin, and pentothal
- **Schedule IV**: Xanax, Librium, Klonopin, Valium, Ativan, Versed, phenobarbital, Restoril, Ambien
- **Schedule V**: Lomotil and others

5 Rights of Medication Administration

The 5 rights of medication administration are used to prevent/reduce medication errors in the hospital setting. Often these 5 rights are integrated into the scanning requirements of electronic documentation. The **5 rights of medication administration** must also be incorporated into the prescriber's order:

- **Right Patient**: Confirm the patient's identity using two identifiers, often being their full name and date of birth. Scanning will also confirm the patient's identity with their bar code and electronic health record.
- **Right Drug**: Check the name of the drug with the prescriber's order. By scanning the medication, the drug name will also be checked against the order.
- **Right Dose**: Check the dose of the drug with the prescriber's order. Some medications require a second nurse confirm any dosage calculations utilized before administration. Ensure the dosage is appropriate and contact the prescriber if there are any concerns.
- **Right route**: Routes include oral (PO), subcutaneous, intradermal, IV, or IM, amongst others. The route must also be confirmed with the prescriber's order.
- **Right time/frequency**: The drug may be administered as a one-time dose, PRN (as needed), or recurring administration (twice daily, every 8 hours, etc.).

Clinical Situations That Have Implications for Medication Administration

It is quite important to recognize clinical situations involving patients that may have **implications for the administration of medications**. For example, many patients have co-morbid conditions that will impact decisions about their medication administration. A patient with non-insulin-dependent diabetes and coronary artery disease who is being treated for a hip fracture would require oral hypoglycemic medications, cardiovascular medications, pain medication, and anti-coagulants. Another example would be an insulin-dependent diabetic patient with concomitant hypertension and renal failure. This patient would require insulin, anti-hypertensive medications, and dosing adjustments of medications secondary to renal failure. The nurse who is responsible for the patient must ensure that the correct dosages of each prescribed medication are administered on time. Potential negative side effects and drug-drug interactions should be avoided, and the patient should be monitored for adverse reactions to newly prescribed drugs.

Routes of Drug Administration

The route of administration is the manner by which a drug is introduced into the body. The most **common routes of administration** are:

- Enteral (oral, rectal, or by feeding tube)
- Topical (on the skin, in the eyes or nose, vaginal, or inhaled)
- Parenteral (IV, subcutaneous, intramuscular, intracardiac, intraosseous, intradermal, intrathecal, intraperitoneal, transdermal, transmucosal, intravitreal, and epidural)

There are many variations on these three basic routes of administration. The FDA acknowledges 111 different routes of administration. When deciding on the route of administration, the doctor and pharmacist consider:

- How fast the patient requires the drug
- How effective it will be by a given route
- The likelihood of toxicity
- The discomfort it will cause
- How likely the patient is to comply with the route
- How likely the route is to play into the patient's addictive habits

Injections

The three most common types of injections and the preferred injection sites are as follows:

- **Subcutaneous Injection**: Deliver the drug under the skin with a ½ inch, 24- or 25-gauge needle held at a 45° angle to reach the fat. Choose the upper arm, abdomen, thigh, or lower back as the site. The maximum amount of subcutaneous medication is 0.5 mL. An example is insulin for a patient with diabetes.
- **Intramuscular Injection**: Deliver the drug into the muscle at a 90° angle to reach the deep tissue. Standard needle length is 1 to 1.5 inches depending on the weight of the individual. CDC guidelines recommend the use of a 22- to 25-gauge needle for adult intramuscular injections. Recommended sites for injection on the adult include deltoid (most recommended), vastus lateralis (thigh), ventrogluteal (hip), or dorsogluteal (buttocks). The maximum recommended amount of IM medication is 3 mL. An example is Vitamin B12 for a patient with pernicious anemia.
- **Intravenous Injection**: Deliver the drug into a vein of the arm, hand, leg, foot, scalp, or neck with an Angiocath, butterfly, or Insyte Autoguard needle. Use a size from 14 gauge to 26 gauge, depending on the fluid and the patient. The nurse sets the drip rate per minute by adjusting the clamp and monitoring the drip chamber. An example of a drug requiring intravenous injection is Zoledronate, which is given yearly to prevent bone fractures for individuals with osteoporosis.

Review Video: Calculating IV Drip Rates
Visit mometrix.com/academy and enter code: 396112

Two less frequently used forms of injection are: Intradermal (into the skin) for Mantoux TB test, and intraosseous access (IO) into the bone, which is used in emergency situations when other access sites are not available.

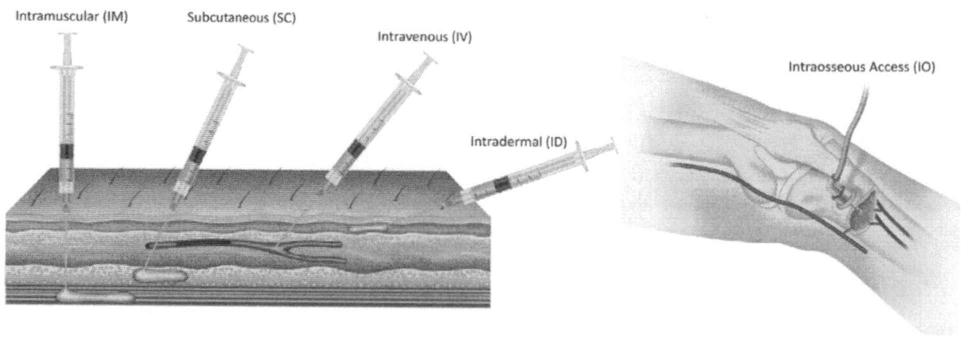

Herbal-Drug Contraindications

Patients on certain medications should not take some herbals. Some **contraindications for common herbals** include:

- **Echinacea**: Anti-anxiety meds, antifungals, heart medications, HIV medications, anabolic steroids, methotrexate, NSAIDs
- **Gingko Biloba**: Anticoagulants, NSAIDs, aspirin, acetaminophen
- **Garlic**: Anticoagulants, oral hypoglycemics, NSAIDs
- **Licorice**: Diuretics, digoxin, antihypertensives
- **St. John's Wort**: Antidepressants, anticoagulants, Tamoxifen, oral contraceptives, HIV medications, anesthetics. Action is similar to MAO inhibitor
- **Valerian**: Sedatives, anti-seizure meds, anesthetics, alcohol, opioids
- **Feverfew**: Anticoagulants, migraine meds, NSAIDs
- **Ginger**: Anticoagulants, NSAIDs
- **Ginseng**: Anticoagulants, antihypertensives, NSAIDs, opioids. Do not take when pregnant or lactating
- **Goldenseal**: Antihypertensives, diabetic medications, meds for kidney diseases. Do not take when pregnant or lactating
- **Kava-kava**: Alcohol, anti-seizure meds, antidepressants, sedatives, anesthetics, antipsychotics, NSAIDS, opioids
- **Saw Palmetto**: Hormone therapy
- **Hawthorn**: Digoxin

Abbreviations for Different Units of Measure

Abbreviation	Meaning
ss	One half, 1/2
L	Liter
mL	Milliliter
tsp	Teaspoon (5 mL)
tbsp	Tablespoon (15 mL)
Fl oz	Fluid ounce (30 mL)
gr	Grain
qs, qs ad	Dispense a sufficient quantity or add a sufficient quantity to make
aq	Water
ad	Up to

Abbreviation	Meaning
aa	Of each
gtt	Drop
G, g, gm	Gram
kg	Kilogram
mg	Milligram
mcg	Microgram
mEq	Milliequivalent
ds	Days' supply
lb	Pound
c	Cup

Roman Numerals

I	1
II	2
III	3
IV	4
V	5

VI	6
VII	7
VIII	8
IX	9
X	10

L	50
C	100
D	500
M	1000

Conversion Factors

Conversion factors are used to change from one unit of measure to another. For instance, if a drug is prescribed in milliliters and the patient wants to know their dose in teaspoons, you will have to use a conversion factor.

Conversion Factors	
1 kg	2.2 lb
1 tsp	5 mL
1 tbsp	3 tsp (15 mL)
1 fl oz	29.57 mL (often rounded to 30 mL)
1 cup	8 oz
1 L	33.8 oz
1 gr	64.8 mg

Converting Between Grams, Kilograms, Milligrams, and Micrograms

A gram (g) is the basic metric unit of mass or weight. All other metric units of mass are centered around the gram. Metric units of measure can be easily converted from one form to another by moving the decimal place. A kilogram (kg) is 10^3 or 1000 times larger than a gram. Therefore, to convert grams to kilograms, the decimal place must be moved to the left three places. Milligrams (mg) and micrograms (mcg) are smaller than a gram. A milligram is 10^{-3} or 1000 times smaller than a gram, whereas a microgram is 10^{-6} or 1,000,000 times smaller than a gram. To convert grams to milligrams, the decimal place must be moved to the right three places. To convert grams to micrograms, the decimal place must be moved to the right six places.

Unit of Measure	Kilogram	Gram	Milligram	Microgram
Conversion factor	10^3	1	10^{-3}	10^{-6}
Sample conversion	0.008	8	8000	8,000,000

Review Video: Measurement Conversions
Visit mometrix.com/academy and enter code: 316703

Adding and Subtracting Fractions

In order to **add or subtract fractions**, you must first convert the fractions to an equivalent fraction so that both fractions have the same denominator (the number on the bottom of the fraction). An easy way of doing this is to multiply the two denominators together and multiply the numerators (the top number of the fraction) by the original denominator of the opposite fraction (cross-multiplication):

$$\frac{1}{4} + \frac{1}{6} =$$

Cross-multiply the numerators by the opposite denominator, and multiply the denominators to get a common denominator:

$$\frac{6}{24} + \frac{4}{24} =$$

Once the fractions are converted to have the same common denominator, the numerators (the numbers on the top of the fraction) can simply be added:

$$\frac{6}{24} + \frac{4}{24} = \frac{10}{24}$$

Reduce the fraction by converting it to its smallest possible form. Divide each part of the final fraction by a common whole number until the numbers cannot be divided any further:

$$\frac{10}{24} \div \frac{2}{2} = \frac{5}{12}$$

Review Video: Adding and Subtracting Fractions
Visit mometrix.com/academy and enter code: 378080

Multiplying and Dividing Fractions

In order to **multiply fractions**, simply multiply the numerators (top numbers) and denominators (bottom numbers) separately. Then, reduce the final fraction to the smallest possible form by dividing the numerator and denominator by a common whole number until the numbers cannot be divided further.

Example:

$$\frac{1}{4} \times \frac{6}{8} = \frac{6}{32}$$

Reduce the fraction:

$$\frac{6}{32} \div \frac{2}{2} = \frac{3}{16}$$

In order to **divide fractions**, use the same process as multiplying fractions except flip the second fraction upside down. The mathematical term for a fraction that is flipped upside down is called the reciprocal. Then, reduce the fraction to its smallest possible form.

Example:

$$\frac{1}{4} \div \frac{6}{8} =$$

Flip the second fraction:

$$\frac{1}{4} \times \frac{8}{6} = \frac{8}{24}$$

Reduce the fraction:

$$\frac{8}{24} \div \frac{8}{8} = \frac{1}{3}$$

Review Video: Multiplying and Dividing Fractions
Visit mometrix.com/academy and enter code: 473632

Dimensional Analysis

A useful method for solving problems involving unit conversions is **dimensional analysis**. In this method conversion factors (example: $\left(\frac{1\text{ g}}{1{,}000\text{ mg}}\right)$) or their reciprocals (example: $\left(\frac{1{,}000\text{ mg}}{1\text{ g}}\right)$) may be used to obtain the required unit. Consider this drip rate example:

$$\text{Drip rate} = \frac{25\text{ mL}}{1\text{ hour}} \times \frac{10\text{ gtt}}{1\text{ mL}} \times \frac{1\text{ hour}}{60\text{ min}} = \frac{250\text{ gtt}}{60\text{ min}} = 4.2\,\frac{\text{gtt}}{\text{min}}$$

In this example, the flow rate (25 mL/hour) was given, as was the conversion factor of 10 gtt (drops) per mL. Those values plus the conversion of 1 hour = 60 minutes can be used to solve the problem.

One way to check that the problem was set up and solved correctly is to make sure the units cancel out across the problem to give the desired dimensions. This problem asked for drip rate, which is measured in drops (gtt) per unit of time (minutes in this problem). Below, the mL and hour in the numerator cancel out the mL and hour in the denominator because 1 hour ÷ 1 hour = 1 and 1 mL ÷ 1 mL = 1, so the resulting units match the units required for the answer.

$$\text{Drip rate} = \frac{25\text{ }\cancel{\text{mL}}}{1\text{ }\cancel{\text{hour}}} \times \frac{10\text{ gtt}}{1\text{ }\cancel{\text{mL}}} \times \frac{1\text{ }\cancel{\text{hour}}}{60\text{ min}} = \frac{250\text{ gtt}}{60\text{ min}} = 4.2\,\frac{\text{gtt}}{\text{min}}$$

Decimals

To **multiply decimals**, first multiply the numbers as if there were no decimals present. Then, place a decimal point at the end of the number (to the right) and move the decimal place to the left the number of spaces equal to the total number of decimal places in the original numbers.

Example: 5.68 × 1.25

The total number of decimal places = 2 + 2 = 4

At first, multiply the numbers ignoring the decimal places: 568 × 125 = 71,000

Place a decimal place at the end of this number: 71,000

Move the decimal place to the left a total number of spaces equal to the total number of decimal places in the original numbers (in this case, four spaces): 7.1

To **convert a decimal to a percent**, move the decimal two places to the *right* and add a % sign.

Example: 0.30 = 30%

To **convert a percent to a decimal**, move the decimal point two places to the *left* and remove the % sign.

Example: 65% = 0.65

Review Video: Decimals
Visit mometrix.com/academy and enter code: 837268

Review Video: How to Multiply Decimals
Visit mometrix.com/academy and enter code: 731574

Review Video: Converting Percentages to Decimals and Fractions
Visit mometrix.com/academy and enter code: 287297

Sample Ratio and Proportion Calculation Problem

You are to prepare an IV for a patient that contains potassium chloride 10 mEq in 500 mL. All you have in stock is potassium chloride 40 mEq/10 mL. How much of the stock solution should be added to the 500 mL IV bag in order to prepare the 10 mEq solution?

In order to solve this type of proportion problem, it is easiest to use cross multiplication. In cross multiplication, you summarize the information into two fractions where three values are known, and one value is unknown. Then, you cross-multiply to solve for the unknown value.

We know that the stock solution we have contains 40 mEq/10 mL, so this is our first fraction or proportion. We also know that we need to end with 10 mEq, but we don't know how much volume equates to 10 mEq. Therefore, our second fraction will be 10 mEq over an unknown volume:

$$\begin{aligned} \frac{10\text{ mEq}}{?\text{ mL}} &= \frac{40\text{ mEq}}{10\text{ mL}} \\ 10\text{ mEq} \times 10\text{ mL} &= 40\text{ mEq} \times ?\text{ mL} \\ ?\text{ mL} &= \frac{(10 \times 10)}{40}\text{ mL} \\ &= 2.5\text{ mL} \end{aligned}$$

The correct answer is 2.5 mL. This means that 2.5 mL of the 40 mEq/10 mL stock solution must be added to the 500 mL IV bag in order to prepare a 10 mEq/500 mL solution (although in reality the exact concentration would become 10 mEq/502.5 mL because nothing would be removed from the 500 mL IV bag when the 2.5 mL is added).

It's always a good idea to review your answer to ensure that it is reasonable. If the stock solution is 40 mEq/10 mL and we need 10mEq, that means that our answer will be one-fourth of 10 mL because 10 mEq is one-fourth of 40 mEq. Because 2.5 mL is one-fourth of 10 mEq, our answer is correct.

Sample IV Flow Rate/Drip Rate Problem

An IV antibiotic was prescribed for a patient to be administered at a rate of 25 mL/hour. What volume (in mL) of IV solution would be needed to last 8 hours? What is the drip rate if the IV is running through at a rate of 10 gtt/mL?

Flow rates can be expressed in mL/hour or mL/min depending upon what type of pump is being used to administer the IV:

$$\textbf{Flow rate} = \frac{\text{mL of IV solution}}{\text{hours or minutes}}$$

In this problem, the IV flow rate is given, and it is asking how many mL of solution are needed to run over an 8-hour time frame. In order to figure this out, the flow rate must be multiplied by the time period:

$$\text{Flow rate (mL/hour)} \times \text{hours} = \text{total mL administered}$$

$$25 \text{ mL/hour} \times 8 \text{ hours} = \textbf{200 mL} \text{ administered over 8 hours}$$

The drip rate is the number of drops of IV solution that are administered per minute.

$$\textbf{Drip rate} = \frac{\text{gtt of IV solution}}{\text{minute}}$$

In order to calculate the drip rate from the flow rate, the mL of solution must be converted into drops (gtt). A conversion factor will be given for this. In this problem, the rate is 10 gtt/mL. If the flow rate is given in hours, then the time must be converted into minutes to calculate the drip rate.

$$\text{Drip rate} = \frac{25 \text{ mL}}{1 \text{ hour}} \times \frac{10 \text{ gtt}}{1 \text{ mL}} \times \frac{1 \text{ hour}}{60 \text{ min}} = \frac{250 \text{ gtt}}{60 \text{ min}} = 4.2 \frac{\text{gtt}}{\text{min}}$$

Review Video: Calculating IV Drip Rates
Visit mometrix.com/academy and enter code: 396112

Sample Amount of Glucose in Solution Problem

How many grams of glucose are there in a 500 mL bag of glucose 5% solution? How many grams are contained in a 500 mL bag of glucose 0.5% solution?

A concentration is the amount of substance in a volume of solution. Concentrations can be expressed as weight to volume (g/100 mL), volume to volume (mL/100 mL) or weight to weight (g/100 g).

A percentage is the quantity of substance in 100. Because concentrations are also expressed as an amount per 100, no conversion or decimal place movement is required to convert the percentage into a concentration. To solve this problem, multiply the concentration of the solution by the volume of the bag to find the total amount of glucose contained within the bag:

$$\text{Glucose } 5\% = \frac{5\text{ g}}{100\text{ mL}} \times \frac{500\text{ mL}}{\text{bag}} = \frac{(5 \times 500)}{100} = 25\text{ g}$$

$$\text{Glucose } 0.5\% = \frac{0.5\text{ g}}{100\text{ mL}} \times \frac{500\text{ mL}}{\text{bag}} = \frac{(0.5 \times 500)}{100} = 2.5\text{ g}$$

Ensure that these answers are reasonable and make sense. If there is 5% glucose in a solution (5 g/100 mL), then a 500 mL bag will have five times as much as a 100 mL bag. Because 5 × 5 = 25, our answer of 25 g makes sense. For the 0.5% solution, move the decimal place to the left one place to find the answer in comparison to the answer for a 5% solution. Therefore, 2.5 g is a reasonable answer.

Child Dosage Calculation

In most cases, the manufacturer's instructions will provide children's (pediatric) dosing for a medication. However, there are some instances in which pediatric dosing is not provided and must be calculated. Formulas for estimating a pediatric dose will typically use age, weight, or body surface area.

Young's Rule (Age, >2 yr)

$$\text{child dose} = \frac{\text{age of child (yr)}}{\text{age of child (yr)} + 12} \times \text{adult dose}$$

Fried's Rule (Age, <2 yr)

$$\text{child dose} = \frac{\text{age of child (mo)}}{150 \text{ mo}} \times \text{adult dose}$$

Clark's Rule (Weight)

$$\text{child dose} = \frac{\text{weight of child (lb)}}{150 \text{ lb}} \times \text{adult dose}$$

Mosteller Formula (BSA)

All BSA calculations are based on the general formula below:

$$\text{child dose} = \frac{\text{child BSA}}{\text{average adult BSA}} \times \text{adult dose}$$

The Mosteller formula is specifically a way to estimate a child's BSA based on height and weight. Plugging the Mosteller formula into the general equation gives the following formula:

$$\text{child dose} = \frac{\sqrt{\text{height (in)} \times \text{weight (lb)}}}{96.8} \times \text{adult dose}$$

BSA-based calculations tend to provide the most reasonable estimates, followed by weight-based. Age-based calculations are rarely used. BSA-based calculations are sometimes used in dosage calculations for chemotherapy regimens.

Geriatric Dosage Calculation

Children are not the only patients who require dosing adjustments. Elderly (geriatric) patients also have a reduced ability to metabolize medications and may require dosage decreases. Geriatric dosage adjustments are usually listed in the manufacturer's instructions but can also be found in the *Geriatric Dosage Handbook*. Patient who are very frail or who have gastrointestinal diseases (e.g., Crohn's disease, ulcerative colitis) may also absorb and metabolize medications differently and may require dosage adjustments.

Safe Medication Administration and Error Reduction

Hazardous Materials

Hazardous materials, those that are ignitable, corrosive, reactive, or toxic, are any that are harmful to humans or the environment and may be solids, liquids, solid gases, or sludges. Hazardous wastes are generally transported by hazardous waste transporters in special hazardous waste containers to Treatment Storage and Disposal Facilities (TSDFs) where they are stored, inactivated, and/or recycled. Each facility should have a plan in place for appropriate **handling of hazardous materials**:

- Staff must be trained in safe handling of hazardous materials with training repeated at least annually.
- Appropriate personal protective equipment (PPE) should be available for staff members handling hazardous materials.
- Hazardous materials should be clearly labeled for easy identification.
- All hazardous materials must be safely and securely stored in appropriate environmental temperatures and conditions.
- Safety Data Sheets (SDS) must be readily available for all hazardous materials.
- Decontamination procedures must be reviewed and appropriate decontamination facilities (such as eyewash stations and showers) must be available.
- Records must be maintained for any accidental exposures (with or without injury) and reported to the appropriate authorities.

Biohazard Symbol

Biological/Biohazardous Waste

Biological wastes are those that contain or are contaminated with pathogens (human, plant, animal); rDNA; and blood, cell, or tissue products; and cultures. Biological wastes that are, or may, be infectious or rDNA contaminated (biohazardous waste) must be inactivated before disposal in hazardous waste containers. Typically, inactivation is carried out with autoclaving or treating with hypochlorite solution (bleach). Contaminated sharps must be maintained in special sharps containers to avoid injury to handlers, and inactivated before disposal. Non-infectious biological wastes, such as uncontaminated gloves, do not require deactivation and are disposed of in biological waste containers.

Routes Biological Hazards May Take to Enter the Body

Biological hazards may **enter the body** through the following avenues:

- Airborne (through the nasal passage into the lungs)
- Ingestion (eating/drinking)
- Subcutaneous (broken skin/open wounds)
- Percutaneous (through intact skin)
- Mucosal (through the lining of the mouth and nose)

Cleaning up Small Blood Spills

The best way to clean a small blood spill is to absorb the blood with a paper towel or gauze pad. Then disinfect the area with a disinfectant. Soap and water are not considered a disinfectant nor is alcohol. Never scrape a dry spill; this may cause an aerosol of infectious organisms. If blood is dried, use the disinfectant to moisten the dried blood.

Internal Radiation Therapy

Internal radiation therapy **(brachytherapy)** may be utilized to treat a variety of cancers, including prostate, breast, and cervical cancer. Radiation implants may be permanent or temporary. Temporary implants may have high-dose radiation (HDR) or low-dose radiation (LDR). Systemic brachytherapy may be administered per IV with radioactive isotopes; intraluminal and intracavity, per catheters or tubes; and interstitial, per seeds, needles, small implants, or wires. Symptoms relate to the area being irradiated, but the skin and GI tract are usually the most sensitive. Bone marrow suppression may occur if the source of radiation is near bone marrow, and patients may experience fatigue and weakness. Because patients emit radiation during therapy, safeguards include:

- Specific limitations and safeguards posted at room by x-ray department outlining requirements, such as time limits for contact time
- Visitors limited to non-pregnant adults who must be 6 feet from the patient and remain in room no longer than 30 minutes each day
- Staff, limited to those who are non-pregnant, wear dosimeters for contact with patient
- Patient placed in private room
- Staff limit time in room to only that necessary to carry out care (in accordance with posted guidelines)

Drugs, Adverse Effects, Interactions, and Contraindications

Anti-Hypertensive Medications

The classes of anti-hypertensive medications are as follows: Diuretics, sympatholytics, vasodilators, calcium channel blockers, and angiotensin-converting enzyme inhibitors (ACE inhibitors).

- Diuretics include hydrochlorothiazide, chlorthalidone, chlorothiazide, indapamide, metolazone, amiloride, spironolactone, triamterene, furosemide, bumetanide, ethacrynic acid, and torsemide.
- Sympatholytics are clonidine, methyldopa, guanabenz, guanadrel, guanethidine, reserpine, labetalol, prazosin, and terazosin.
- Vasodilators include diazoxide, hydralazine, minoxidil, and nitroprusside sodium.
- Calcium channel blockers include amlodipine, nimodipine, isradipine, nicardipine, nifedipine, bepridil, diltiazem, and verapamil.
- ACE inhibitors include benazepril, captopril, enalapril, fosinopril, lisinopril, moexipril, quinapril, ramipril, and losartan.

Review Video: Side Effects of ACE Inhibitors and ARBs
Visit mometrix.com/academy and enter code: 525864

Diuretics

Diuretics increase **renal perfusion and filtration**, thereby reducing preload and decreasing peripheral and pulmonary edema, hypertension, CHF, diabetes insipidus, and osteoporosis. There are different types of diuretics: loop, thiazide, and potassium sparing.

Loop Diuretics

Loop diuretics inhibit the reabsorption of sodium and chloride (primarily) in the ascending loop of Henle. They also cause increased secretion of other electrolytes, such as calcium, magnesium, and potassium, and this can result in imbalances that cause dysrhythmias. Other side effects include frequent urination, postural hypotension, and increased blood sugar and uric acid levels. They are short-acting so are less effective than other diuretics for control of hypertension.

- **Bumetanide** (Bumex) is given intravenously after surgery to reduce preload or orally to treat heart failure.
- **Ethacrynic acid** (Edecrin) is given intravenously after surgery to reduce preload.
- **Furosemide** (Lasix) is used for the control of congestive heart failure as well as renal insufficiency. It is used after surgery to decrease preload and to reduce the inflammatory response caused by cardiopulmonary bypass (post-perfusion syndrome).

Review Video: Diuretics
Visit mometrix.com/academy and enter code: 373276

Thiazide Diuretics

Thiazide diuretics inhibit the **reabsorption of sodium and chloride** primarily in the early distal tubules, forcing more sodium and water to be excreted. Thiazide diuretics increase secretion of potassium and bicarbonate, so they are often given with supplementary potassium or in combination with potassium-sparing diuretics. Thiazide diuretics are the first line of drugs for treatment of **hypertension**. They have a long duration of action (12–72 hours, depending on the drug) so they are able to maintain control of hypertension better than short-acting drugs. They may be given daily or 3–5 days per week. There are numerous thiazide diuretics, including:

- Chlorothiazide
- Chlorthalidone
- Hydrochlorothiazide

Side effects include, dizziness, lightheadedness, postural hypotension, headache, blurred vision, and itching, especially during initial treatment. Thiazide diuretics cause sensitivity to sun exposure, so people should be counseled to use sunscreen.

Potassium-Sparing Diuretics

Potassium-sparing diuretics inhibit the **reabsorption of sodium** in the late distal tubule and collecting duct. They are weaker than thiazide or loop diuretics, but do not cause a reduction in potassium level; however, if used alone, they may cause an increase in potassium, which can cause weakness, irregular pulse, and cardiac arrest. Because potassium-sparing diuretics are less effective alone, they are often given in a combined form with a thiazide diuretic (usually chlorothiazide), which mitigates the potassium imbalance. Typical side effects include dehydration, blurred vision, nausea, insomnia, and nasal congestion, especially in the first few days of treatment.

- **Spironolactone** (Aldactone) is a synthetic steroid diuretic that increases the secretion of both water and sodium and is used to treat congestive heart failure. It may be given orally or intravenously.
- **Eplerenone** is an antimineralocorticoid similar to spironolactone but with fewer side effects.

Antidysrhythmic Drugs

Antidysrhythmic drugs include a number of drugs that act on the conduction system, the ventricles and/or the atria to control dysrhythmias. There are four classes of drugs that are used as well as some that are unclassified:

- **Class I:** 3 subtypes of sodium channel blockers (quinidine, lidocaine, procainamide)
- **Class II:** β-receptor blockers (esmolol, propranolol)
- **Class III:** Slows repolarization (amiodarone, ibutilide)
- **Class IV**: Calcium channel blockers (diltiazem, verapamil)
- **Unclassified:** Miscellaneous drugs with proven efficacy in controlling arrhythmias (adenosine, electrolyte supplements)

Pharmacological Agents Used for Asthma

Numerous pharmacological agents are used for control of asthma, some that are long-acting to prevent attacks and others that are short-acting to provide relief for acute episodes. Listed with each are the standard med and dosage used for urgent care:

- **β-Adrenergic agonists** include both long-acting and short-acting preparations used for relaxation of smooth muscles and bronchodilation, reducing edema, and aiding clearance of mucus. Medications include salmeterol, sustained-release albuterol and short-acting albuterol, and levalbuterol. Albuterol 2.5–5.0 mg every 20 minutes, 3 doses by nebulizer.
- **Anticholinergics** aid in preventing bronchial constriction and potentiate the bronchodilating action of β-Adrenergic agonists. The most commonly used medication is ipratropium bromide 500 mcg every 20 minutes, 3 doses by nebulizer.
- **Corticosteroids** provide anti-inflammatory action by inhibiting immune responses and decreasing edema, mucus, and hyper-responsiveness. Because of numerous side effects, glucocorticosteroids are usually administered orally or parenterally for ≤5 days (prednisone, prednisolone, methylprednisolone) and then switched to inhaled steroids. If a person receives glucocorticoids for more than 5 days, then dosages are tapered. Methylprednisolone 60–125 mg IV is the standard dose for respiratory failure. The Global Initiative for Asthma (GINA) recommends daily inhaled corticosteroids for all individuals with severe asthma to reduce the risk of exacerbations.
- **Methylxanthines** are used to improve pulmonary function and decrease the need for mechanical ventilation. Medications include aminophylline and theophylline.
- **Magnesium sulfate** is used to relax smooth muscles and decrease inflammation. If administered intravenously, it must be given slowly to prevent hypotension and bradycardia. When inhaled, it potentiates the action of albuterol. Standard dosage: 2 g (8 mmol), 1 dose by IV over 20 minutes.
- **Heliox** (helium-oxygen) is administered to decrease airway resistance with airway obstruction, thereby decreasing respiratory effort. Heliox improves oxygenation of those on mechanical ventilation.
- **Leukotriene inhibitors** are used to inhibit inflammation and bronchospasm for long-term management. Medications include montelukast.

Additional Pulmonary Pharmacology

There is a wide range of agents used for pulmonary pharmacology, depending upon the type and degree of pulmonary disease. Agents include:

- **Opioid analgesics**: Used to provide both pain relief and sedation for those on mechanical ventilation to reduce sympathetic response. Medications may include fentanyl or morphine sulfate.
- **Neuromuscular blockers**: Used for induced paralysis of those who have not responded adequately to sedation, especially for intubation and mechanical ventilation. Medications may include pancuronium and vecuronium. However, there is controversy about the use of such blockers, as induced paralysis has been linked to increased mortality rates, sensory hearing loss (pancuronium), atelectasis, and ventilation-perfusion mismatch.
- **Human B-type natriuretic peptides**: Used to reduce pulmonary capillary wedge pressure. Medications include nesiritide.
- **Surfactants**: Reduces surface tension to prevent the collapse of alveoli. Beractant (Survanta) is derived from bovine lung tissue and calfactant from calf lung tissue. They are administered as inhalants.
- **Alkalinizers**: Used to treat metabolic acidosis and reduce pulmonary vascular resistance by achieving an alkaline pH. Medications include sodium bicarbonate and tromethamine (THAM).
- **Pulmonary vasodilator (inhaled nitric oxide)**: Used to relax the vascular muscles and produce pulmonary vasodilation. Some studies show it reduces the need for extracorporeal membrane oxygenation (ECMO).
- **Methylxanthines**: Used to stimulate muscle contractions of the chest and stimulate respirations. Medications include aminophylline, caffeine citrate, and doxapram.
- **Diuretics**: Used to reduce pulmonary edema. Medications include loop diuretics such as furosemide and metolazone.
- **Nitrates**: Used for vasodilation to reduce preload and afterload, which in turn reduces myocardial need for oxygen. Medications include nitroglycerin and nitroprusside sodium.
- **Antibiotics**: Used for treatment of respiratory infections, including pneumonia. Medications are used according to the pathogenic agent and may include macrolides such as azithromycin (Zithromax) and erythromycin.
- **Antimycobacterials**: Used for treatment of TB and other mycobacterial diseases. Medications include isoniazid, ethambutol, rifampin, streptomycin sulfate, and pyrazinamide.
- **Antivirals**: Used to inhibit replication of a virus early in a viral infection. Effectiveness decreases as time passes because the replication process has already begun. Medications include ribavirin and zanamivir.

Oral Hypoglycemic Agents

Oral hypoglycemic agents are **anti-diabetic treatments** generally used in the treatment of Type II Diabetes. There are five classic categories of oral hypoglycemic agents: sulfonylureas, biguanides, meglitinides, competitive inhibitors of alpha-glucosidases (located in the intestinal brush border), and thiazolidinediones. More recently, two additional novel classes of oral hypoglycemics, DPP-4 inhibitors and SGLT2 inhibitors, were introduced with proven effectiveness when used in conjunction with changes in diet and exercise. Some examples of sulfonylurea oral hypoglycemic agents include the first-generation agents tolbutamide, tolazamide, chlorpropamide, and acetohexamide; and second-generation agents glyburide, glimepiride, and glipizide. The biguanide oral hypoglycemic agent is metformin. Metformin has the distinct advantage of not causing weight gain or hypoglycemic reactions. The meglitinide agent is repaglinide. Examples of alpha-glucosidase inhibitors are acarbose and miglitol. Alpha-glucosidase inhibitors bind tightly to intestinal alpha-glucosidases and decrease the postprandial rise in glucose levels. The only available thiazolidinedione oral hypoglycemic agent is currently pioglitazone; troglitazone was removed from US market in 2000, and rosiglitazone was removed from US market in 2011. Examples of DPP-4 inhibitors include linagliptin, vildagliptin, sitagliptin, and saxagliptin. Examples of SGLT2 inhibitors include canagliflozin, dapagliflozin, and empagliflozin.

Insulin Used to Treat Glycemic Disorders

There are a number of different types of **insulin** with varying action times. Insulin is used to metabolize **glucose** for those whose pancreas does not produce insulin. People may need to take a combination of insulins (short- and long-acting) to maintain glucose control. Duration of action may vary according to the individual's metabolism, intake, and level of activity:

- **Humalog** (Lispro H) is a fast-acting, short-acting insulin with onset in 5–15 minutes, peaking at 45–90 minutes and lasting 3–4 hours.
- **Regular** (R) is a relatively fast-acting insulin with onset in 30 minutes, peaks in 2–5 hours, and lasts 5–8 hours.
- **NPH** (N) insulin is intermediate-acting with onset in 1–3 hours, peaking at 6–12 hours, and lasting for 16–24 hours.
- **Insulin Glargine** (Lantus) is a long-acting insulin with onset in 3–6 hours, no peak, and lasting for 24 hours.
- **Combined NPH/Regular** (70/30 or 50/50) has an onset of 30 minutes, peaks at 7–12 hours, and lasts 16–24 hours.

Immunosuppressant Drugs

Drugs	Actions	Side effects
Corticosteroids	Depress cell-mediated immune response, humoral immune response, and inflammation, reducing proliferation of T cells and B cells. Used with transplantations and to prevent GVHD disease.	Weight gain, edema, Cushing syndrome, hyperglycemia, bruising, and osteoporosis. Abruptly stopping drugs may trigger Addisonian crisis.
Ciclosporin (cyclosporine)	Inhibit activation of T cells. Used to prevent transplantation rejection and to treat autoimmune diseases and nephrotic syndrome.	Tremor, excessive facial hair, gingivitis, bone marrow suppression with increased risk of infection and cancer, especially skin cancer.
Intravenous immuno-globulin G (IVIG)	Used to combat immunosuppression by increasing antibodies to prevent infection or treat acute infection, such as Guillain-Barre. Used off-label for many different disorders and infections.	Dermatitis, headache, renal failure, and venous thrombosis. Infections can occur because IVIG is extracted from pooled plasma.

Review Video: Immunomodulators and Immunosuppressors
Visit mometrix.com/academy and enter code: 666131

Chemotherapy

Chemotherapy may be offered during palliative care to enhance patient comfort, wellbeing, and symptom control for **enhanced quality of life**. It is understood that the treatment is not expected to provide a cure and should not be given as a means to maintain a sense of false hope within the patient or family. It should be clear that the expectation of treatment is **prolonged survival** and **control of cancer-related symptoms**. Not all patients will benefit from palliative chemotherapy. The decision to provide chemotherapy is based on the clinical indicators and the patient's wishes. The benefit and cost ratios of treatment need to be considered. Tumor response to treatment, metastasis, and other disease specific factors will help define chemotherapy's usefulness for an individual patient. Patients also need to be aware that chemotherapy involves a commitment to repeated travel, hospitalizations, invasive procedures, and assessments in order to make an informed decision.

Chemotherapeutic Agents

The major chemotherapy agents are alkylating agents, antimetabolites, plant alkaloids, antitumor antibiotics, and steroid hormones.

- **Alkylating agents** work directly by attacking the DNA of cancers such as chronic leukemias, Hodgkin's disease, lymphomas, and lung, breast, prostate, and ovary cancers.
- **Nitrosoureas** inhibit repair in damaged DNA. They are able to cross the blood-brain barrier and are frequently used to treat brain tumors, lymphomas, multiple myeloma, and malignant melanoma.
- **Antimetabolites** block cell growth. This class of chemotherapeutic drugs is used to treat leukemias, choriocarcinoma, and gastrointestinal, breast, and ovary cancers.
- **Antitumor antibiotics** are a broad category of agents that bind to DNA and prevent RNA synthesis and are used with a wide variety of cancers.
- **Plant (vinca) alkaloids** are extracted from plants and block cell division. These are used to treat acute lymphoblastic leukemia, Hodgkin and non-Hodgkin lymphomas, neuroblastomas, Wilms tumor, and lung, breast, and testes cancers.
- **Steroid hormones** have an unclear action but may be useful in treating hormone-dependent cancers such as ovary and breast cancer.

Routes of Delivery

Chemotherapy treatments may be provided orally, intramuscularly, intravenously, intra-arterially, intralesionally (directly into the tumor), intraperitoneally, intrathecally, or topically. **Oral chemotherapy** is the easiest and often used in the home. **Intravenous delivery** is the most common chemotherapy route but **intramuscular delivery** may have more lasting effects. The goal of **intra-arterial chemotherapy** is to introduce the agent directly into the blood supply feeding the tumor or affected organ. Ovarian cancer with tumors greater than 2 cm in diameter may be treated with **intraperitoneal therapy**. Acute lymphocytic leukemia is primarily treated with **intrathecal administration. Intralesional treatments** are used for melanoma and Kaposi sarcoma. **Topical treatment** is most common with skin cancers.

Side Effects

Not every patient will experience every symptom, or in the same degree. **Side effects** can vary greatly; some can be easily controlled with additional medications. Many side effects are due to the effects of the chemotherapy on **cells**, such as bone marrow, hair, and gastrointestinal cells, which have a rapid mitotic rate and rapid turnover. Common side effects can include bone marrow suppression, hair loss (alopecia), mouth ulcers, sore throat and gums, heartburn, nausea, vomiting, loss of appetite, weight loss, anorexia and cachexia, anemia, nerve and muscle problems, dry or discolored skin, kidney and bladder irritation, fatigue, and increased bruising, bleeding, and infection. The patient's sexual function can also be affected, including possible infertility.

Risks

Infection is a common concern of chemotherapy because of the decreased number of **neutrophils** in the patient's system. **Neutropenia** is silent but dangerous, leaving no neutrophils to fight the threat of infections. Neutropenia can cause a septic situation, which can be life-threatening. Severe **anemia** may result in the need for blood transfusions. **Neurological damage** may include mild alterations in taste or smell, peripheral neuropathy, mental status changes, or seizures. Some anticancer drugs can cause **heart damage** if not monitored closely. Many anticancer drugs cause **kidney damage**, as well as increasing the risk of drug toxicity from decreased renal function. Anticancer drugs can also cause **cataracts** and **retina damage**.

Palliative Sedation

Palliative sedation is a treatment method focused on controlling and easing symptoms that have proven otherwise refractory or unendurable in nature. This process was originally named **terminal sedation**. It was changed to palliative sedation to emphasize the differences between symptom management and euthanasia. The purpose of palliative sedation is **symptom control**; it does not hasten or cause death. Through the monitored use of medications such as midazolam or propofol, relief can be provided through varying levels of unconsciousness. Among terminally ill patients, palliative sedation is most often used to calm persistent agitation and restlessness. The second most frequent need is for pain control, followed by confusion, shortness of breath, muscle twitching or seizures, and anguish.

Anticoagulants

Common anticoagulants used at home and in the hospital setting are discussed below, including possible complications and the antidotes for each:

- **Antithrombin activators**: Heparin (unfractionated) and derivatives, LWM (Dalteparin, Enoxaparin, tinzaparin), and Fondaparinux.
    - Possible complications: Thrombocytopenia, bleeding/hemorrhage, osteopenia, hypersensitivity.
    - Antidote: Protamine sulfate 1% solution—dosage varies according to drug and drug's dosage. (1 mg protamine neutralizes 100 units of heparin or 1 mg of enoxaparin.)
- **Direct thrombin inhibitors**: Hirudin analogs (bivalirudin, desirudin, lepirudin). Others: Apixaban, Argatroban, and dabigatran.
    - Possible complications: Bleeding/hemorrhage, GI upset, backpain, hypertension, headache.
    - No antidote is available.
- **Direct Xa inhibitor**: Rivaroxaban
    - Possible complications: Bleeding/hemorrhage.
    - No antidote is available.
- **Antithrombin (AT)**: Recombinant human AT, Plasma-derived AT
    - Possible complications: Bleeding/hemorrhage, hypersensitivity.
    - No antidote is available.
- **Warfarin**
    - Possible complications: Bleeding/hemorrhage. Drug interactions may cause thrombosis or increased risk of bleeding.

- Antidote: Vitamin K_1 usually at 2.5 mg PO or 0.5–1.0 mg IV. If ineffective, FFP or fresh whole blood may be administered.

Heparin

Pharmacology

Heparin is an **anticoagulant** derived from the intestinal mucosa of the pig and the lung of the pig. The mechanism of action of heparin is to bind to the surface of the endothelial cell membrane. The activity of heparin depends upon plasma protease inhibitor antithrombin III. Antithrombin III inhibits thrombin and other anti-clotting proteases. In addition, heparin binding causes a change in antithrombin III inhibitor form, resulting in increased antithrombin-protease complex formation activity. After antithrombin-protease complex formation, heparin is subsequently released and is available to bind to more antithrombin molecules.

Risk Factors

The major risk factor of heparin use is hemorrhage. Predisposing factors for hemorrhage include advanced age and renal failure. Prolonged use of heparin can result in osteoporosis and fractures. Other risk factors of heparin use include transient thrombocytopenia, severe thrombocytopenia, paradoxical thromboembolism, and heparin-induced aggregation of platelets. These risks can be reduced by careful selection of patients who receive heparin therapy, careful control of the dosage of heparin, and meticulous monitoring of the partial thromboplastin time, or PTT. It is important to remember that thrombocytopenia or the development of a thrombus may be due to heparin itself.

Contraindications

There are numerous contraindications to the use of heparin, including: hypersensitivity to heparin; diseases of the hematologic system (hemophilia, purpura, or thrombocytopenia); uncontrolled hypertension; intracranial bleed; infectious endocarditis; active tuberculosis; gastrointestinal ulcers; cancer of the gastrointestinal visceral organs; severe liver dysfunction; severe kidney dysfunction; and threatened miscarriage or abortion. Heparin is contraindicated in the following medical procedures: following brain surgery; following spinal cord surgery; following eye surgery; after a lumbar puncture; and after regional anesthesia blocks. The effects of heparin may be reversed by stopping heparin or by the use of a specific antagonist (protamine sulfate).

Review Video: Heparin – An Injectable Anti-Coagulant
Visit mometrix.com/academy and enter code: 127426

Warfarin

Pharmacology

Warfarin causes a deficiency in prothrombin in the plasma and is used as an **anti-thrombotic agent** and to decrease the risk of embolism in humans. This agent causes the liver to manufacture less of the proteins necessary for blood coagulation. Since it is 99% bound to albumin in the plasma, warfarin has a high bio-availability. The mechanism of action of warfarin involves prothrombin, factor VII, factor IX, factor X, and protein C. Warfarin inhibits the g-carboxylation of the glutamate residues in the aforementioned factors. The mechanism of action of warfarin also involves vitamin K. Warfarin has a slow onset of action, usually 24 hours, and a typical duration of 2–5 days. Using increased dosages of warfarin as loading dosages will serve to speed up the onset of anti-coagulation. Patients on warfarin must discontinue this medication five days before planned surgery due to its longer duration.

DRUG-DRUG INTERACTIONS

Warfarin has many drug-drug interactions, the most serious of which increases the risk of bleeding. Sulfinpyrazone and phenylbutazone interact with warfarin to cause enhanced decrease in prothrombin, increased inhibition of platelets, and increased risk of peptic ulcer. The following drugs can have adverse effects when co-administered with warfarin: antibiotics such as metronidazole, azithromycin, clarithromycin, dirithromycin, erythromycin, roxithromycin, and telithromycin; broad-spectrum antibiotics such as amoxicillin, imipenem, levofloxacin; antifungal agents such as fluconazole, miconazole, and ketoconazole; barbiturates; and trimethoprim-sulfamethoxazole, amiodarone, cimetidine, and disulfiram. Aspirin inhibits metabolism of the warfarin and nonsteroidal anti-inflammatory drugs (NSAIDs) inhibit the clotting of platelets. The third-generation cephalosporins increase the risk of bleeding with warfarin because these drugs destroy the intestinal bacteria that produce vitamin K. Always check on possible drug-drug interactions when administering warfarin and monitor patients who might be at risk.

Review Video: Warfarin - Uses and Side Effects
Visit mometrix.com/academy and enter code: 844117

THROMBOLYTICS

Thrombolytics are drugs used to dissolve clots in myocardial infarction, ischemic stroke, DVT, and pulmonary embolism. **Thrombolytics** may be given in combination with heparin or low-weight heparin to increase anticoagulation effect. Thrombolytics should be administered within 90 minutes but may be given up to 6 hours after an event. They may increase the danger of hemorrhage and are contraindicated with hemorrhagic strokes, recent surgery, or bleeding. Thrombolytics include:

- **Alteplase tissue-type plasminogen activator** (t-PA) (Activase) is an enzyme that converts plasminogen to plasmin, which is a fibrinolytic enzyme. t-PA is used for ischemic stroke, MI, and pulmonary embolism and must be given IV within 3–4.5 hours or by catheter directly to the site of occlusion within 6 hours.
- **Reteplase** (Retavase) is a plasminogen activator used after MI to prevent CHF (contraindicated for ischemic strokes). It is given in 2 doses, a 10-unit bolus over 2 minutes and then repeated in 30 minutes.
- **Tenecteplase** (TNKase) is used to treat acute MI with large ST elevation. It is administered in a one-time bolus over 5 seconds and should be administered within 30 minutes of the event.

Contraindications to thrombolytic therapy include:

- Evidence of cerebral or subarachnoid hemorrhage or other internal bleeding or history of intracranial hemorrhage, recent stroke, head trauma, or surgery (ruled out by CT scan before administration for ischemic stroke)
- Uncontrolled hypertension, seizures
- Intracranial AVM, neoplasm, or aneurysm
- Current anticoagulation therapy
- Low platelet count (<100,000 mm^3)

Review Video: Antiplatelets and Thrombolytics
Visit mometrix.com/academy and enter code: 711284

Review Video: Thrombolytics
Visit mometrix.com/academy and enter code: 832357

Anticonvulsants

Carbamazepine (Tegretol)

Use: Partial, tonic-clonic, and absence seizures; analgesia for trigeminal neuralgia

Side effects: Dizziness, drowsiness, nausea, and vomiting. Toxic reactions include severe skin rash, agranulocytosis, aplastic anemia, and hepatitis

Clonazepam (Klonopin)

Use: Akinetic, absence, and myoclonic seizures; Lennox-Gastaut syndrome

Side effects: Behavioral changes, hirsutism or alopecia, headaches, and drowsiness. Toxic reactions include hepatotoxicity, thrombocytopenia, ataxia, and bone marrow failure.

Ethosuximide (Zarontin)

Use: Absence seizures

Side effects: Headaches and gastrointestinal disorders. Toxic reactions include skin rash, blood dyscrasias (sometimes fatal), hepatitis, and lupus erythematosus.

Felbamate (Felbatol)

Use: Lennox-Gastaut syndrome

Side effects: Headache, fatigue, insomnia, and cognitive impairment. Toxic reactions include aplastic anemia and hepatic failure. It is recommended only if other medications have failed.

Fosphenytoin (Cerebyx)

Use: Status epilepticus prevention and treatment during neurosurgery

Side effects: CNS depression, hypotension, cardiovascular collapse, dizziness, nystagmus, and pruritus.

Gabapentin (Neurontin)

Use: Partial seizures; post-herpetic neuralgia

Side effects: Dizziness, somnolence, drowsiness, ataxia, weight gain, and nausea. Toxic reactions include hepatotoxicity and leukopenia.

Lamotrigine (Lamictal)

Use: Partial and primary generalized tonic-clonic seizures; Lennox-Gastaut syndrome

Side effects: Tremor, ataxia, weight gain, dizziness, headache, and drowsiness. Toxic reactions include severe rash, which may require hospitalization.

Levetiracetam (Keppra)

Use: Partial onset, myoclonic, and generalized tonic-clonic seizures

Side effects: Idiopathic generalized epilepsy, dizziness, somnolence, irritability, alopecia, double vision, sore throat, and fatigue. Toxic reactions include bone marrow suppression and liver failure.

Oxcarbazepine (Trileptal)

Use: Partial seizures

Side effects: Double or abnormal vision, tremor, abnormal gait, GI disorders, dizziness, and fatigue. A toxic reaction is hepatotoxicity.

Phenobarbital (Sezaby)

Use: Tonic-clonic and cortical local seizures; acute convulsive episodes; insomnia

Side effects: Sedation, double vision, agitation, and ataxia. Toxic reactions include anemia and skin rash.

Phenytoin (Dilantin)

Use: Tonic-clonic and complex partial seizures

Side effects: Nystagmus, vision disorders, gingival hyperplasia, hirsutism, dysrhythmias, and dysarthria. Toxic reactions include collapse of cardiovascular system and CNS depression.

Primidone (Mysoline)

Use: Grand mal, psychomotor, and focal seizures

Side effects: Double vision, ataxia, impotence, lethargy, and irritability. Toxic reactions include skin rash.

Tiagabine

Use: Partial seizures

Side effects: Concentration problems, weak knees, dysarthria, abdominal pain, tremor, dizziness, fatigue, and agitation.

Topiramate (Topamax)

Use: Partial and tonic-clonic seizures; migraines

Side effects: Anorexia, weight loss, somnolence, confusion, ataxia, and confusion. Toxic reactions include kidney stones.

Valproate/Valproic acid (Depakote, Depakene)

Use: Complex partial, simple, and complex absence seizures; bipolar disorder

Side effects: Weight gain, alopecia, tremor, menstrual disorders, nausea, and vomiting. Toxic reactions include hepatotoxicity, severe pancreatitis, rash, blood dyscrasias, and nephritis.

Zonisamide (Zonegran)

Use: Partial seizures

Side effects: Anorexia, nausea, agitation, rash, headache, dizziness, and somnolence. Toxic reactions include leukopenia and hepatotoxicity.

Hypertonic Saline Solution

Hypertonic saline solution (HSS) has a sodium concentration higher than 0.9% (NS) and is used to reduce intracranial pressure/cerebral edema and treat traumatic brain injury. Concentrations usually range from 2.0–23.4%. The hypertonic solution draws fluid from the tissue through osmosis. As edema decreases, circulation improves. HSS also expands plasma, increasing CPP, and counteracts hyponatremia that occurs in the brain after injury.

Administration:

- Peripheral lines: HSS <3% only
- Central lines: HSS ≥3%

HSS can be administered continuously at rates varying from 30–150 mL/hr. Rate must be carefully controlled. Fluid status must be monitored to prevent hypovolemia, which increases risk of renal failure. Boluses (typically 30 mL of 23.4%) may be administered over 15 minutes for acute increased ICP or transtentorial herniation.

Laboratory monitoring includes:

- Sodium (every 6 hours): Maintain at 145–155 mmol/L. Higher levels can cause heart/respiratory/renal failure.
- Serum osmolality (every 12 hours): Maintain at 320 mOsm/L. Higher levels can cause renal failure.

Mannitol

Mannitol is an osmotic diuretic that increases excretion of both sodium and water and reduces intracranial pressure and brain mass, especially after traumatic brain injury. Mannitol may also be used to shrink the cells of the blood-brain barrier in order to help other medications breach this barrier. Mannitol is administered per intravenous infusion:

- 0.5–2.0 g/kg in a 15–25% solution over 30–60 minutes
- A repeated dose of 0.25–1.0 g/kg every 4–6 hours based on patient response

Cerebral spinal fluid pressure should show decrease within 15 minutes. Fluid and electrolyte balances must be carefully monitored as well as intake and output and body weight. Concentrations of 20–25% require a filter. Crystals may form if the mannitol solution is too cold and the mannitol container may require heating (in 80 °C water) and shaking to dissolve crystals, but the solution should be cooled to below body temperature prior to administration. Mannitol cannot be administered in polyvinylchloride bags as precipitates form. Side effects include fluid and electrolyte imbalance, nausea, vomiting, hypotension, tachycardia, fever, and urticaria.

Histamine Receptor Antagonists

Histamine (H) receptor antagonists (actually reverse agonists) are used to treat conditions in which excessive stomach acid causes heartburn and GERD. They block histamine 2 (H_2) (parietal) cell receptors in the stomach, thereby decreasing acid production. These drugs are used less commonly now than proton-pump inhibitors. **Common H_2 antagonists** include:

- **Cimetidine**: The first H_2 antagonist, it is used less frequently than others because of inhibition of enzymes that results in drug interactions, especially with contraceptive agents and estrogen.
- **Famotidine (Pepcid)**: This may be combined with an antacid to increase the speed of effects as it has a slow onset. It may be used pre-surgically to reduce post-operative nausea.
- **Nizatidine**: The last H_2 antagonist developed, it is used to treat ulcers and GERD. It is about equal in potency and action to ranitidine, which was discontinued due to the presence of NDMA, a cancer-causing contaminant, when stored in high temperatures.

Antacids

Antacids are medications used to reduce stomach acids by raising the pH and neutralizing the acids present. They are commonly used to treat heartburn or indigestion. Adverse reactions are relatively rare unless taken to excess or with renal impairment. Drugs include:

- **Aluminum hydroxide** may cause constipation and with renal impairment, hypophosphatemia and osteomalacia.
- **Magnesium hydroxide** (Milk of Magnesia) may cause diarrhea and with renal impairment can cause hypermagnesemia.
- **Aluminum hydroxide with magnesium hydroxide** may cause nausea, vomiting and diarrhea, yeast infection (thrush), or hypophosphatemia.
- **Calcium carbonate** (TUMS, Titralac) may cause gastric distention. Excess calcium intake may cause toxic reactions, including kidney stones and renal failure, so excess intake should be avoided.
- **Alka-Seltzer** combines sodium bicarbonate with aspirin and citric acid so this compound may cause gastric irritation, nausea and vomiting, and tarry stools.
- **Bismuth subsalicylate** (Pepto-Bismol). Pepto-Bismol may react with sulfur in the body to create a black tongue and black stools, but this is temporary. Pepto-Bismol has been associated with Reye's syndrome in children with influenza or chickenpox.

Proton Pump Inhibitors

Proton pump inhibitors (PPIs) are now used more frequently than histamine receptor antagonists. PPIs interfere with an acid-producing enzyme in the stomach wall, reducing stomach acid. PPIs are used to treat GERD, stomach ulcers, and *H. pylori* (with antibiotics). PPIs are similar in action and include:

- Esomeprazole (Nexium)
- Lansoprazole (Prevacid)
- Omeprazole (Prilosec)
- Pantoprazole (Protonix)
- Rabeprazole (Aciphex)
- Omeprazole/sodium bicarbonate (Long-acting form of omeprazole)

Common side effects include gastrointestinal upset (nausea, diarrhea, and constipation), headache, and rash. In rare instances, PPIs may cause severe muscle pain; however, they are usually well-tolerated with few adverse effects. PPIs may interfere with the absorption of some drugs, such as those that are affected by stomach acid. Absorption of ketoconazole is impaired, and absorption of digoxin is increased, sometimes leading to toxicity. Omeprazole impacts the hepatic breakdown of drugs more than other PPIs and may cause increased levels of diazepam, phenytoin, and warfarin.

Anti-Lipids

Anti-lipid medications are frequently used to **lower cholesterol levels** if dietary modifications are unsuccessful in order to decrease coronary artery disease. There are several **types** of medications aimed at lowering cholesterol levels, with the most common being :

- **Statins** (3-hydroxy-3-methylglutaryl coenzyme A reductase inhibitors), such as atorvastatin (Lipitor), rosuvastatin (Crestor), fluvastatin (Lescol), lovastatin (Altoprev), pravastatin, and simvastatin (Zocor), inhibit the liver enzyme that produces cholesterol, but different statins vary in the ability to reduce cholesterol and in drug/other interactions (protease inhibitors, erythromycin, grapefruit juice, niacin, and fibric acids). Adverse effects include rhabdomyolysis (which causes severe muscle pain and weakness), headache, rash, weakness, and gastrointestinal disorders.
- **Nicotinic acid** (Niacor) decreases synthesis of lipoprotein, lowers low-density lipoprotein (LDL) and triglycerides, and increases high-density lipoprotein (HDL). It is used for low elevations of cholesterol and may be combined with statins. Adverse effects include flushing, hyperglycemia, gout, upper gastrointestinal disorders, and hepatotoxicity. Liver function must be monitored.
- **Bile acid sequestrants,** such as cholestyramine (Questran, Prevalite), colesevelam (WelChol), and colestipol HCL (Colestid), decrease LDL, increase HDL, and do not affect triglyceride levels. They bind to bile acids in the intestines so that more are excreted in the stool rather than returned to the liver, so the liver has to produce bile acids by converting cholesterol. Adverse effects include gastrointestinal disorders and decrease in absorption of other drugs.

Additional anti-lipid drugs include cholesterol absorption inhibitors (ezetimibe), fibric acid derivatives, and omega-3-acid ethyl esters.

Serotonin Antagonists

Serotonin antagonists block 5-HT_2 receptors of serotonin in the central and peripheral nervous systems and gastrointestinal system. An open channel can result in agitation, nausea, and vomiting, but antagonists close the channel and reduce these symptoms. Serotonin antagonists are frequently used to prevent and treat nausea associated with chemotherapy and anesthesia. Medications include:

- **Metoclopramide** (Reglan) is used to reduce nausea and vomiting from a wide range of causes. It is also a prokinetic drug that increases gastrointestinal contractions and promotes faster gastric emptying, so it is used for heartburn, GERD, and diabetic gastroparesis.
- **Ondansetron** (Zofran) reduces vagal stimulation of the medulla oblongata (vomiting center) and is used for nausea related to chemotherapy.
- **Granisetron** (Sancuso) is used to reduce nausea related to chemotherapy, surgery, and radiation.

Serotonin antagonists have fewer side effects than other antiemetics, but they may cause muscle cramping, agitation, diarrhea/constipation, dizziness, and headache.

Laxatives

The following are different types of laxatives:

- **Bulk formers** have high fiber content and both soften stool and create more formed stools. These include products such as Metamucil, Citrucel, and FiberCon, which are usually added to liquids because without adequate fluids, they can increase constipation.
- **Lubricants** include both oral mineral oil and glycerin suppositories. They coat the stool, preventing fluid absorption and keeping the stool soft. Mineral oil absorbs fat soluble vitamins and should be used only temporarily
- **Saline**, such as Milk of Magnesia and Epsom Salt, contain ions, such as magnesium phosphate, magnesium hydroxide, and citrate, which are not absorbed through the intestines and draw more fluid into the stool. The magnesium in the preparations also stimulates the bowel. People with impairment of kidney function should avoid magnesium products, and saline laxatives should be used infrequently to avoid dependence. Epsom Salt often has a purging effect and is rarely used.
- **Stool softeners** (emollients, such as Colace) use wetting agents, such as docusate sodium, to increase liquid in the stool, thereby softening it. They should not be used with mineral oil because of increased absorption of the oil through the intestines.
- **Hyperosmotics** (available by prescription) contain materials that are not digestible and serve to retain fluid in the stool. Products, such as Kristalose and MiraLAX soften the stool but may result in increased abdominal distension and flatus, especially initially. There are three types of hyperosmolar laxatives: lactulose, polymer, and saline. Lactulose types use a form of sugar and work similarly to saline laxatives, but more slowly, and may be used for long-term treatment. The salines empty the bowels quickly and are used short-term. The polymers contain polyethylene glycol, which retains fluid in the stool and is used short-term.
- **Combinations** use two or more types, such as stool softener with stimulant, and should be used only short-term.

Stimulants

Stimulants increase intestinal motility, moving the stool through the bowel faster and reducing the absorption of fluids so that the stool remains softer. Common ingredients include cascara in Castor oil and senna in Senokot. Stimulants work quickly and are effective but can result in electrolyte imbalance, Abdominal distension, and cramping. Chronic use may cause a cycle of constipation and diarrhea. Stimulant suppositories, such as Dulcolax, are also available.

Review Video: Gastrointestinal Drugs
Visit mometrix.com/academy and enter code: 455152

Pharmacologic Treatment of Wound Pain

Topical Anesthetics

There are numerous different types of pain medications that may be used to control pain from wounds, including **topical anesthetics**:

- **Lidocaine 2–4%** is frequently used during debridement or dressing changes. Lidocaine is useful only superficially and may take 15–30 minutes before it is effective.
- **Eutectic Mixture of Local Anesthetics (EMLA Cream)** provides good pain control. The wound is first cleansed and then the cream is applied thickly (1/4 inch) extending about 1/2 inch past the wound to the periwound tissue. The wound is then covered with plastic wrap, which is secured and left in place for about 20 minutes. The wrapped time may be extended to 45–60 minutes if necessary, to completely numb the tissue. The tissue should remain numb for about 1 hour after the plastic wrap is removed, allowing time for the wound to be cleansed, debrided, and/or redressed.

Review Video: Dermatology Drugs List
Visit mometrix.com/academy and enter code: 886820

Regional Anesthesia

Regional anesthesia (injectable subcutaneous and perineural medications) is administered locally about the wound or as nerve blocks. Medications include lidocaine, bupivacaine, and tetracaine in solution. Epinephrine is sometimes added to increase vasoconstriction and reduce bleeding, although it is avoided in distal areas of the limbs (hands and feet) to prevent ischemia.

- **Field blockade** involves injecting the anesthetic into the periwound tissue or into the wound margins. The effect may be decreased by inflammation. The effects last for limited periods of time.
- **Regional nerve blocks** may involve single injections, the effects of which are limited in duration but can provide pain relief for treatments. Techniques that use continuous catheter infusions are longer lasting and can be controlled more precisely. Blocks may involve nerves proximal to affected areas, such as peripheral nerve blocks, or large nerve blocks near the spinal cord, such as percutaneous lumbar sympathetic blocks (LSB). Long-term blocks may use alcohol-based medications to permanently inactivate the nerves.

WHO Pain Ladder

The WHO pain ladder was developed as an algorithm for treating pain through medications with progressively increasing potency. The approach can be used effectively with both adult and pediatric patients. Beginning with the least potent medication option, each step adds a stronger analgesic until optimum pain relief is reached.

The **WHO pain ladder** has three steps.

- **Step 1**: The patient is given a non-opioid medication which may be used alone or in conjunction with other adjuvant therapies.
- **Step 2**: If the patient reports no change in the pain level, mild- to moderate-level pain-relieving opioids are introduced along with adjuvants if they have not been previously introduced.
- **Step 3**: Uncontrolled pain is then treated with opioids for moderate to severe pain. Adjuvants may also be continued.

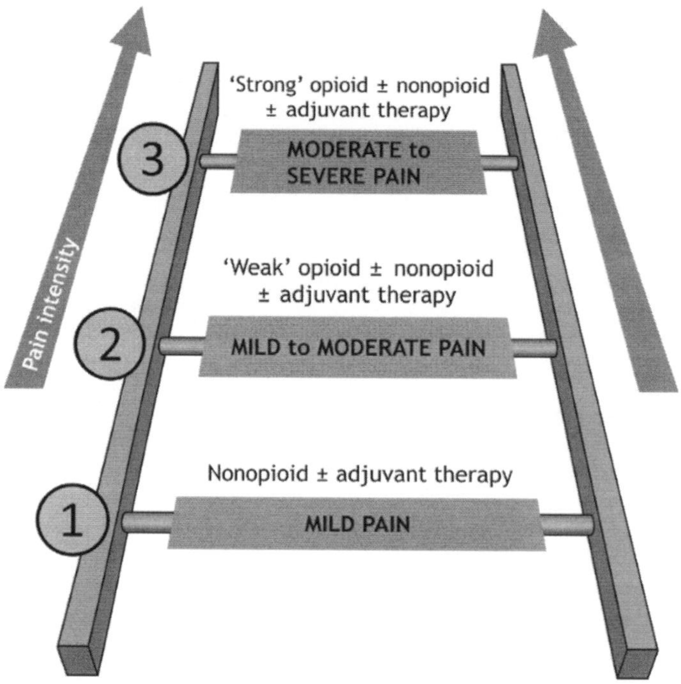

Review Video: Adjuvants
Visit mometrix.com/academy and enter code: 178200

Scheduling of Pain Medications

For mild to moderate pain, patients may take **acetaminophen** alternating with an **NSAID** such as ibuprofen on a regularly scheduled basis or as needed (PRN) at the onset of pain or when pain is anticipated (such as before a dressing change). However, for severe chronic pain, long-acting **opioid pain medications**, such as time-released morphine, fentanyl, and oxycodone, should be given regularly around the clock, because these medications help not only control but also prevent pain. The patient should not skip a dose when free of pain, because this makes control more difficult when the pain recurs. In addition to **time-scheduled medications**, the patient may need **short-acting supplementary medications**, such as Percocet, to take on a PRN basis. When taking short-acting medications, the patient should take the medication at the onset of pain, before anticipated pain, or at the onset of increased pain, rather than waiting until the pain is severe, because the goal should always be to keep the pain under control.

Acetaminophen

Acetaminophen remains one of the safest analgesics for **long-term use**. It can be used to treat mild pain or as an adjuvant with other analgesics for more severe pain. Nonspecific musculoskeletal pain and osteoarthritis are particularly responsive to acetaminophen therapy. Acetaminophen also has a limited **anti-inflammatory nature**.

Acetaminophen should, however, be used cautiously in persons with altered liver or kidney function, as well as those with a history of significant alcohol use, regardless of liver function compromise. It should be dosed separately from any opioid analgesic, which should be given separately as well. This allows for individual titration of each drug to assess the individual needs and side effects separately.

NSAIDs

NSAIDs act by inhibiting the cyclooxygenase (COX) enzyme, which controls prostaglandin formation. COX-1 affects platelet clumping, gastric blood flow, and mucosal integrity. COX-2 affects pain, inflammation, and fever. COX-1 and 2 inhibitors include aspirin and ibuprofen. Ibuprofen has a lower occurrence of side effects, such as gastric bleeding, than aspirin does. A COX-2 inhibitor, such as Celebrex, must be used with caution due to increased cardiovascular risks when used for over 18 months. NSAIDs are useful for both arthritis and bone cancer pain and work well with opioids for relief of postoperative and other severe pain. NSAIDs may increase the effects of antiseizure drugs and warfarin. Smaller doses are needed if kidney function is impaired.

Review Video: NSAID Side Effects
Visit mometrix.com/academy and enter code: 569064

Local Anesthetic Pain Relief

Local anesthetics block neural conduction of pain through the application of the anesthetic directly to the nerve endings in the area of pain. It can be injected prior to minor surgery or suturing. It can be injected intercostally for thoracic or high abdominal surgeries. The addition of a vasoconstrictor prolongs effectiveness of the anesthetic. A cream containing local anesthetics (EMLA) can be rubbed on the skin to decrease pain from IV starts or lumbar punctures. It should be applied 60–90 minutes prior to the procedure. A lidocaine 5% patch is approved to relieve pain from postherpetic neuralgia. The patient applies up to 3 patches for 12 hours at a time. Local anesthetics can be applied via the use of an epidural catheter to provide pain control for surgery, childbirth, or postoperative pain control. Opioids can be infused along with the anesthetic agent. Patients using an epidural catheter for postoperative pain tend to ambulate sooner, suffer fewer complications as a result, and go home more quickly.

Opioids

Guidelines for Opioid Use

Opioid analgesic therapy is a widely used method of chronic pain control. By adhering to clinical guidelines, pain control can be safely optimized. **Intramuscular administration** should be used as a last resort except in the presence of a "pain emergency" when no other treatment is readily available. Such cases are rare since subcutaneous delivery is almost always an alternative. Noninvasive routes such as **transdermal** and **transmucosal**, which bypass the enteral route, are optimal for continuous pain control and are often effective in eliminating breakthrough pain as well. Changing from one opioid to another, or altering the delivery method, may become necessary under the assumption that incomplete cross-tolerance among opioids occurs. Changing analgesics or method of delivery may result in a decreased drug requirement. When altering opioid delivery regimens, use **morphine equivalents** as the common factor for all dose conversions. This method will help reduce medication errors. Side effects such as sedation, constipation, nausea, and myoclonus should be anticipated in every care plan, and require both prevention and treatment methods.

Side Effects of Opioid Analgesics

Examples of **opioid analgesics** are numerous and include morphine, hydromorphone, oxymorphone, methadone, meperidine, fentanyl, sufentanil, levorphanol, codeine, oxycodone, hydrocodone, nalbuphine, and buprenorphine. Opioid analgesics have multiple effects on most of the organ systems of the body. Central nervous system (CNS) effects include respiratory depression, analgesia, euphoria, sedation, miosis, cough suppression, truncal rigidity, nausea, and vomiting. Cardiovascular effects are usually slight and include bradycardia, hypotension, reduced blood volume, and increased cerebral blood flow. Gastrointestinal effects can include constipation, decreased gastric motility, and decreased hydrochloric acid. Genitourinary effects are urinary retention and decreased renal function. Other effects are sweating, flushing, and histamine release with itching.

Opioid Use During Last Few Hours of Life

Assessment of pain continues in the **last hours of life**, and medication is adjusted according to assessment. Pain does not necessarily increase as death approaches. It can be assumed that if pain was present prior to loss of consciousness it will continue in the patient's unconscious state. It should be assessed for and treated accordingly. Research has confirmed that administering opioids at the end of life does not hasten nor prolong the dying process. The patient's **prior medication regimen** should be continued. However, adjustments may be made in consideration of reduced renal or hepatic clearance. The **route of administration** should also be assessed for appropriateness and adjusted as needed (e.g., loss of consciousness, inability to swallow).

Oral Transmucosal Fentanyl Citrate

Oral transmucosal fentanyl citrate consists of **fentanyl** on an oral applicator. The patient applies the dosage (starting at 200 mcg) to the **buccal mucosa** between the cheek and gum for rapid absorption and subsequent pain relief. This makes transmucosal fentanyl particularly useful for managing **breakthrough pain**. Pain relief generally begins within 5 minutes, but the patient should be instructed to wait 15 minutes after the previous dose has been completed before taking another dose. Swallowing even part of the dose rather than having it completely absorbed through the oral mucosa can affect the timing of pain relief onset. **Peak effect** occurs in 20–40 minutes with the total pain relief duration lasting 2–3 hours. Side effects can include somnolence, nausea, and dizziness. Consuming drinks such as coffee, tea, and juices that alter the oral secretion pH can also alter the absorption rate of transmucosal fentanyl.

Methadone

Methadone is useful for treating **severe or chronic pain** and may be particularly helpful in the presence of **neuropathic pain**. It has a long-acting pain relief factor for a lower cost than many comparable medications. However, the exact dosing ratios with morphine remain unclear within the available research. Metabolism of methadone can also be swayed (either increased or decreased) by many other medications normally taken by patients with chronic conditions. Methadone can also be used to treat opioid addiction. US law for the prescription of methadone for addiction in detoxification or maintenance programs requires a special license and patient enrollment. The words "for pain" need to be clearly stated in the prescription. Methadone can cause drowsiness, weakness, headache, nausea, vomiting, constipation, sweating, and flushing, as well as sedation, decreased respirations, or an irregular heart rate.

Oxycodone

Oxycodone, a synthetic formulation, is a long-acting opioid for **moderate to severe pain relief**. Side effects are similar to those of morphine. It has a similar pain relief ratio, with the possibility of less nausea and vomiting. Because of its extended-release nature, the medication cannot be cut or crushed for administration. Oxycodone does not carry any greater addiction risk than other types of opioids; however, public sensationalism related to this formulation may create hesitation for use among patients. Pharmacies may also limit the amount of this medication they will make available to an individual. Oxycodone should be used cautiously in patients with a history of hypothyroidism, Addison disease, urethral stricture, prostatic hypertrophy, or lung or liver disease.

Hydromorphone

Hydromorphone is available as tablets, liquid, suppository, and parenteral formulations. It offers the advantage of being synthetic, allowing for its use in the presence of a true **morphine allergy**. It is also helpful when significant side effects have occurred in the past or pain has been inadequately controlled with other medications. It may also be useful for controlling cough. However, neurotoxicity may occur, particularly myoclonus, hyperalgesia, and seizures. It should also be used cautiously in the presence of kidney, liver, heart, and thyroid disease, seizure disorders, respiratory disease, prostatic hypertrophy, or urinary problems. Common *side effects* include dizziness, lightheadedness, drowsiness, upset stomach if taken without food, vomiting, and constipation.

Titration of Morphine for Pain Control

Morphine titration protocols vary according to the type of morphine used, the severity of pain, and the patient's tolerance:

Type	Peak	Duration (hours)
Short-acting	60 minutes	4–5
Long-acting	3–4 hours	8–24
IM	30–60 minutes	4–5
SQ	50–90 minutes	4–5
IV	20 minutes	4–5
Rectal	20–60 minutes	3–7

For example, **optimal dosage** is usually calculated by starting with short-acting oral morphine at 30 mg every 3–4 hours with doses increased by 25–50% for moderate pain or 50–100% for severe pain each time until the patient has at least 50% reduction in pain on a scale of 1–10 or a behavior scale. The dose may need to be reduced if excessive sedation occurs. Once the patient's pain is controlled on short-acting morphine and 24-hour dosage needs are calculated, the patient could be switched to extended-release. **Breakthrough pain** is usually treated with dosages that are 10% of the 24-hour dose. Dosages may be repeated or increased if there is inadequate relief of pain at the peak time. Increasing the dose prior to peak time will result in increased drowsiness.

Morphine Use for Chronic Cancer Pain

One advantage of morphine for chronic cancer pain is that it has no **ceiling dose**. As tolerance to the medication increases or the disease progresses in severity, the dose can be gradually increased to an infinite level. It is also available in many different forms for administration, including intravenous, intramuscular, immediate release, sustained release, long-acting, liquid oral preparations, and suppositories. Morphine is often used as the **equivalency standard** for other opioid analgesics. Common *side effects* of morphine include sedation, respiratory depression, itching, nausea, chronic spasms or twitching of muscle groups, and constipation. Constipation is experienced by all patients receiving opioids. This inevitability should be planned for and treated aggressively. Hallucinations are common when morphine is initiated. After the first few days, most patients will overcome the respiratory depression, nausea, itching, and extreme sedation as tolerance for the medication is developed.

Dosages for Morphine, Codeine, Hydromorphone, and Levorphanol

The dosages for both the enteral and parenteral routes of morphine, codeine, hydromorphone, and levorphanol are as follows:

- **Morphine**: Enteral dosage is 30 mg (available as continuous and sustained-release formulations to last 12–24 hours); parenteral dosage is 10 mg.
- **Codeine**: Enteral dosage is 200 mg (not generally recommended); parenteral dosage is 130 mg.
- **Hydromorphone**: Enteral dosage is 7.5 mg (available as a continuous-release formula lasting 24 hours); parenteral dosage is 1.5 mg.
- **Levorphanol**: In acute pain episodes, enteral dosage is 4 mg; parenteral dosage is 2 mg. For chronic pain, dosage is equivalent for both enteral and parenteral at 1 mg. Levorphanol has a long half-life, increasing the chances of dosage accumulation over time.

Adhering to the statement "If the gut works, use it," as much as 90 percent of all patients will at least start out able to use oral medications instead of other routes.

Calculation for Converting Medication Regimen Between Two Opioids

Calculate the current 24-hour drug dose, or the total amount given in a 24-hour period. Multiply the current 24-hour dose times the ratio of the 24-hour equivalent dose for the new drug over the 24-hour equivalent of the old drug. This calculation provides the **equivalent 24-hour dose** for the new drug. Divide the new dose amount by the number of doses to be provided during the day. This amount equals the new **target dosage**.

$$\text{current 24 hr dose} \times \frac{\text{new drug 24 hr equiv dose}}{\text{current drug 24 hr equiv dose}} = \text{new 24 hr dose}$$

$$\frac{\text{new 24 hr dose}}{\text{doses per day}} = \text{new target dosage}$$

Ketamine

Ketamine is a dissociative anesthetic that can provide pain relief as an alternate or complement to an opioid. The dissociative quality is an effective way to help the patient separate from the sensation of pain. Ketamine treatment begins with an initial bolus of 0.1 mg/kg IV. If there is no improvement, a second bolus with double the dosage is provided in 5 minutes. This can be repeated as needed. Boluses should be followed by a decrease in the patient's current opioid dose by 50% and an infusion of ketamine. **Infusion dosing** for ketamine is 0.015 mg/kg/min, or about 1 mg/min for a 70 kg person. If IV access cannot be attained, subcutaneous infusion is a possibility with dosing of 0.3–0.5 mg/kg. Consider concurrent treatment with a **benzodiazepine** to prevent hallucinations or frightful dreams and observe for increased secretions, as these are all possible side effects of ketamine. The secretions may be treated with glycopyrrolate, scopolamine, or atropine as needed.

Treating Breakthrough Pain

The three basic types of breakthrough pain, and their treatment measures are as follows:

- **Incident pain**: Pain that can be specifically tied to an activity or event, such as a dressing change or physical therapy. These events can be anticipated and treated with a rapid-onset, short-acting analgesic just prior to the painful event.

- **Spontaneous pain**: This type of pain is unpredictable and cannot be pinpointed to a relationship with any certain time or event. There is no way to anticipate spontaneous pain. In the presence of neuropathic pain, adjuvant therapy may be useful. Otherwise, a rapid-onset, short-acting analgesic is used.
- **End-of-dose failure**: Pain that specifically occurs at the end of a routine analgesic dosing cycle when medication blood levels begin to taper off. Careful evaluation of end-of-dose failure can help prevent it sooner. It may indicate an increased dose tolerance and the need for medication dose alterations.

Treating Neuropathic Pain

Treatment options for neuropathic pain are often different from the methods used to treat other types of pain. The three drug classes most commonly used and proven effective for treating neuropathic pain are **anticonvulsants**, **anesthetics**, and **antidepressants**. Some are given on an as-needed basis, but most require consistent dosing with **24-hour symptom control**. Examples of the most common medications include amitriptyline, nortriptyline, duloxetine, gabapentin, topical lidocaine, opioids, and pregabalin. Medication choice is dependent on factors such as the type and progression of the disorder and the associated physical and emotional problems, such as nerve injury, muscle weakness or spasms, anxiety, depression, or sleep disturbances.

Review Video: Neuropathic Pain
Visit mometrix.com/academy and enter code: 780523

Treating Bone Pain

Treatment options for bone pain may depend on the causative agent related to the pain, such as the primary cancer site, severely weakened bones, or fractures. **Systemic treatment choices** include chemotherapy, radiation, and hormone therapy. **Hormone therapy** is used in the presence of estrogen and androgen receptors within the cancer cells. **Bisphosphonates**, such as ibandronate, zoledronate, and alendronate, may help strengthen the bones, slow damage, and prevent fractures; they can also help reduce pain. However, side effects can include fatigue, fever, nausea, vomiting, and anemia. **Surgery** may also be considered to remove cancerous cells or reinforce weakened areas of bone. **Opioids** and **NSAIDs/COX-2 inhibitors** are most often used for pain relief and need to be provided on a consistent basis.

Morphine combined with ibuprofen provides the benefit of a centrally acting opioid with a peripherally acting NSAID. Ibuprofen also acts as an effective adjuvant analgesic agent to enhance the relief provided by the opioid without increasing opioid side effects.

Measures Taken During Pain Crisis

During a pain crisis, assess for a change in the mechanism or location of the pain and attempt to differentiate between **terminal anxiety** or agitation and the **physical causes** of pain. Begin with a rapid increase in **opioid treatment**. If the pain is unresponsive to opioid titration, switching to **benzodiazepines**, such as diazepam and lorazepam, may produce a more effective response. If terminal symptoms remain unresponsive, assess for **drug absorption**. While invasive routes of medication delivery are generally avoided unless necessary, the only guaranteed route of drug delivery is the IV route. If there is any question about absorption, it is appropriate to establish parenteral access. IM delivery should be considered as a last resort. When all accessible resources have been exhausted, seek a pain management consultation as quickly as possible. Alternative methods of terminal pain control include radiotherapy, anesthetic, or neuroablative procedures.

Concerns Surrounding Use of Pain Medications with End-of-Life Patients

Common concerns surrounding the use of pain medications with end-of-life patients include:

- **Adequacy**: Patients are often concerned that medication may not be adequate to control pain and that chronic or breakthrough pain will occur. Patients may be concerned that if they take adequate pain medication, it will be less effective later when pain may be worse.
- **Sedation/addiction**: Some patients and family members are concerned about the risks of addiction, and others may be concerned about the effects of the medication on the patient's cognition, as some patients may become confused, disoriented, or sedated, depending on the medication or dosage.
- **Adverse effects**: Nausea and vomiting may be almost as debilitating to a patient as the pain it is intended to alleviate. Constipation, a common adverse effect, may be very uncomfortable for a patient. Some medications may result in itching and others may cause myoclonus, both of which are uncomfortable for the patient.

Addiction Challenges

In the presence of **addiction challenges**, it becomes important to choose a **long-acting opioid** that can facilitate around-the-clock dosing and minimize the need for short-term medications used for breakthrough doses. **Short-term medication** use should be very limited or eliminated entirely if possible. Whenever possible, **nondrug adjuvants** such as relaxation techniques, distraction, biofeedback, TNS, and therapeutic communication should be used in place of short-term medications. When short-term medication therapy is needed, a **nonopioid** is best. Limit the amount of medication available to the patient at any given time and monitor for compliance with pill counts and urine toxicology screens as necessary. In some instances, a referral to an addictions specialist is recommended.

Tolerance and Pseudotolerance

Tolerance is the adaptation of the body to continued exposure to a drug or chemical. The effects of the drug at the same level of exposure are minimized over time. Additional dosing is required to maintain the same outcomes.

Pseudotolerance is the misguided perception of the health care provider that a patient's need for increasing doses of a drug is due to the development of tolerance, when the reality is that disease progression or other factors are responsible for the increase in dosing needs.

Addiction and Pseudoaddiction

Addiction is a primary and constant neurobiologic disease with genetic, psychosocial, and environmental factors that create an obsessive and irrational need or preoccupation with a substance. Addictive behaviors include unrestricted, continued cravings, as well as compulsive and persistent use of a drug despite harmful experiences and side effects.

Pseudoaddiction is an assumption that the patient is addicted to a substance when in actuality the patient is not experiencing relief from the medication. It is prolonged, unrelieved pain that may be the result of undertreatment. This situation may lead the patient to become more aggressive in seeking medicated relief, thus resulting in the inappropriate "drug seeker" label.

Review Video: Addiction
Visit mometrix.com/academy and enter code: 460412

PHYSICAL DEPENDENCE

Physical dependence occurs when the body adapts to a drug, requiring increasing dosages over time to gain the same effect, and withdrawal of that drug then will result in an **abstinence syndrome** (withdrawal). Physical dependence can be described as a form of **addiction**. While physical dependence was commonly thought of as being related to narcotic drugs (such as morphine, methadone, fentanyl), many different types of drugs may cause some degree of physical dependence. For example, abruptly stopping a beta-blocker may result in cardiac arrhythmias or cardiac arrest. Abruptly stopping SSRIs may result in severe depression and anxiety. Thus, when considering stopping a patient's drugs near the end of life, physical dependence must be considered as many drugs should be **tapered** to avoid withdrawal effects. Drugs that affect the **central nervous system**, such as ethanol, barbiturates, and benzodiazepines, pose considerable risk of dependence and may result in severe withdrawal symptoms.

ANTIPSYCHOTIC MEDICATIONS

FIRST-GENERATION

There are a variety of first-generation antipsychotics available, though their use is becoming less prominent now that atypical antipsychotic agents are available. Some **first-generation antipsychotics** include:

- Chlorpromazine
- Thioridazine hydrochloride
- Haloperidol
- Pimozide
- Fluphenazine hydrochloride
- Molindone hydrochloride
- Trifluoperazine hydrochloride

Possible side effects include photosensitivity, sexual dysfunction, dry mouth, dry eyes, nasal congestion, blurred vision, constipation, urinary retention, exacerbation of narrow-angle glaucoma, various cardiac effects, extrapyramidal effects, dyskinesia, sedation, cognitive dulling, amenorrhea, menstrual irregularities, hyperglycemia or hypoglycemia, increased appetite, and weight gain. The most common extrapyramidal symptom caused by antipsychotic agents is tardive dyskinesia, in which clients are unable to control their movements, such as tics, lip-smacking, and eye blinking. The extrapyramidal system is a group of neural connections outside of the medulla that control movement. **Extrapyramidal effects** are the result of drug influence on the extrapyramidal system and include:

- Akinesia (inability to start movement)
- Akathisia (inability to stop movement)
- Dystonia (extreme and uncontrolled muscle contraction, torticollis, flexing, and twisting)

SECOND-GENERATION

Second-generation antipsychotics (SGAs), also called atypical antipsychotics, are used for bipolar disorders, schizophrenia, and psychosis, and include aripiprazole (Abilify), clozapine (Clozaril), olanzapine (Zyprexa), quetiapine (Seroquel), risperidone (Risperdal), and ziprasidone (Geodon). Females report more side effects than males, but the recommended doses for males and females are identical. Women were underrepresented when SGAs were clinically tested, because researchers feared teratogenic effects on fetuses:

- Side effects include constipation, increased appetite, weight gain, urinary retention, various sexual side effects, increased prolactin, menstrual irregularities, increased risk of diabetes mellitus, decreased blood pressure, dizziness, agranulocytosis, and leucopenia.
- Atypical antipsychotics may interact with fluvoxamine, phenytoin, carbamazepine, barbiturates, nicotine, ketoconazole, phenytoin, rifampin, and glucocorticoids.
- The use of atypical antipsychotic agents correlates with significant weight gain. Overweight and obese clients are likely to develop insulin resistance and glucose intolerance, which may lead to diabetes mellitus. Data show clozapine and olanzapine as the greatest offenders. Ziprasidone seems to present the lowest risk.

Review Video: Antipsychotic Drugs
Visit mometrix.com/academy and enter code: 369601

ANTIDEPRESSANTS

INDICATIONS FOR TREATMENT WITH ANTIDEPRESSANT

The main **indicator** for use of an antidepressant is simply **depression**. This can be further expanded to include major depression, atypical depression, and anxiety disorders. Depression-type symptoms commonly include loss of interest in usual or pleasurable activities, decreased levels of energy, having a depressed mood, decreased ability to concentrate, loss of appetite, or suicidal thoughts. Antidepressants are also commonly used to treat **anxiety disorders** that include panic attacks, obsessive-compulsive disorder (OCD), social phobias, and post-traumatic stress disorder. They may also be beneficial in treating chronic pain syndromes, premenstrual syndrome, insomnia, attention deficit hyperactivity disorder, or bed-wetting.

SSRIs

Selective serotonin reuptake inhibitors (SSRIs) prevent the reuptake of serotonin at the presynaptic membrane. This increases the amount of serotonin in the synapse for neurotransmission. This class of antidepressants has been shown to reduce depression and anxiety symptoms. Common side effects are usually short in duration and include headache, GI upset, and sexual dysfunction. They do not cause significant anticholinergic, cardiovascular, or significant patient sedation side effects. Examples of SSRIs include citalopram (Celexa), escitalopram (Lexapro), fluoxetine (Prozac), fluvoxamine (Luvox), paroxetine (Paxil), and sertraline (Zoloft). These drugs are not highly lethal in overdose.

MONITORING

SSRI monitoring includes the following:

- Monitor for increased depression and suicidal ideation, especially in adolescents.
- Inform patients of the following:
  - Smoking decreases effectiveness.
  - Fatal reactions may occur with monoamine oxidase inhibitors.
  - Taking SSRIs with benzodiazepines or alcohol has an additive effect.
  - Some drugs, such as citalopram, may increase the effects of β-blockers and warfarin.
- Avoid cimetidine, which is prescribed for ulcers and gastroesophageal reflux disease, and St. John's wort.

- Inform patients of possible decreased libido and sexual functioning.
- Monitor for insomnia and gastrointestinal upset.

Tricyclic Antidepressants

Tricyclic antidepressants not only block the reuptake of serotonin and norepinephrine, they also act to block muscarinic cholinergic receptors, histamine H1 receptors, and alpha1 noradrenergic receptors. These receptors do not affect depression symptoms, but their blockade is implicated in some of the side effects associated with tricyclics. The blockade of the muscarinic receptors produces anticholinergic side effects such as dry mouth, blurred vision, constipation, urinary retention, and tachycardia. The blockade of the histamine receptors is associated with drowsiness, low blood pressure, and weight gain. The alpha1 noradrenergic receptor blocking action produces the side effects associated with orthostatic hypotension, vertigo, and some memory disturbances.

Mechanism of Action and Necessary Evaluations

Most of the tricyclic antidepressants have very similar mechanisms of action and side effects. Although their exact **mechanism of action** is unknown, they are believed to act to inhibit the reuptake of both serotonin and norepinephrine. These drugs have a high **first-pass rate of metabolism** and are excreted by the kidneys. A complete **physical and history** should be obtained before starting a patient on tricyclic drugs. Because this class of antidepressants can cause death with an overdose, an initial **suicide risk assessment** must be obtained, and continued assessments for this risk are necessary. This class of drug can cause a prolongation in the electrical conduction of the heart. Therefore, a **baseline ECG** should be performed in children, young teenagers, anyone with cardiac electrical conduction problems, and adults over age 40.

Monitoring

Tricyclics monitoring includes the following:

- Observe for toxicity.
- Inform patients not to take with monoamine oxidase inhibitors.
- Observe for decreased therapeutic response to hypertensives (e.g., clonidine, guanethidine).
- Monitor other medications; the patient should avoid other central nervous system depressants, including alcohol. Some medications potentiate the effects of tricyclics, including bupropion, cimetidine, haloperidol, selective serotonin reuptake inhibitors, and valproic acid.
- Inform the patient to avoid prolonged exposure to sunlight or sunlamps.
- Administer major dosage of the drug at bedtime if the patient experiences drowsiness.
- Monitor for sedation, cardiac arrhythmias, insomnia, gastrointestinal upset, and weight gain.

MAOIs

The **mechanism of action** for monoamine oxidase inhibitors (MAOIs) is exactly what their name indicates. These drugs act to inhibit the enzyme **monoamine oxidase (MAO)**. There are actually two of these enzymes, **MAO-A** and **MAO-B**, and this class of medication inhibits both. These enzymes act to metabolize serotonin and norepinephrine. By inhibiting the production of these enzymes, there are increased levels of **serotonin** and **norepinephrine** available for neurotransmission. Medications that selectively inhibit MAO-B have no antidepressant effects and can be used to treat disease processes such as Parkinson's.

Side Effects

Side effects associated with the use of monoamine oxidase inhibitors (MAOIs) are similar to antipsychotic medications. They can include symptoms such as GI upset, vertigo, headaches, sleep disturbances, sexual dysfunction, dry mouth, visual disturbances, constipation, peripheral edema, urinary hesitancy, weakness, increased weight, or orthostatic hypotension. The elderly population is at greatest risk for problems with **orthostatic hypotension** and should have lying, sitting, and standing blood pressure checks to monitor for this side effect. Orthostatic hypotension can lead to injuries related to falls, such as fractures. The most dangerous side effect can be an extreme **elevation in blood pressure** or **hypertensive crisis**. Hypertension can develop due to the presence of increased levels of **tyramine**. These levels increase because **monoamine oxidase**, which normally metabolizes tyramine, is inhibited. Increased levels of tyramine produce a vasoconstrictive response by the body that leads to increased blood pressure. Symptoms associated with hypertensive crisis can include severe occipital headache, palpitations, chest pain, diaphoresis, nausea and vomiting, flushed face, or dilated pupils. Complications associated with hypertensive crisis include hemorrhagic stroke, severe headache, or death. It is vital that patients receive in-depth education about the symptoms of hypertension, the need for close monitoring of blood pressure, and methods for sustaining a low-tyramine diet.

Diet Restrictions

Monoamine oxidase inhibitors can lead to increased levels of **tyramine** in the nerve cell. These increased levels can lead to a dangerous and possibly fatal increase in **blood pressure**. Certain **foods that contain tyramine** should be avoided to help prevent hypertensive episodes. Foods high in tyramine include strong or aged cheeses, cured meats, smoked or processed meats, pickled or fermented foods, sauces, such as soy or teriyaki sauce, soybeans, snow peas or broad beans, dried or overripe fruits, meat tenderizers, products containing monosodium glutamate, yeast-extract spreads, alcoholic beverages, and improperly stored foods or spoiled foods.

Anti-Anxiety Medications

Benzodiazepines

Benzodiazepines are the most commonly prescribed medications for **anxiety**. Some of the more commonly prescribed include chlordiazepoxide, lorazepam, diazepam, flurazepam, and triazolam. Benzodiazepines act to enhance the neurotransmitter **GABA**. This neurotransmitter inhibits the firing rate of neurons and therefore leads to a decline in anxiety symptoms. Indications for their use can include anxiety, insomnia disorders, alcohol withdrawal, seizure control, skeletal muscle spasticity, or agitation. They can also be utilized to reduce the anxiety symptoms preoperatively or before any other type of medical procedure such as cardiac catheterization or colonoscopy. This class of drug is also the treatment of choice for alcohol withdrawal.

Side Effects

There are several common side effects associated with the use of benzodiazepines. One of the most common is the effect of **drowsiness**. Patients should be advised to use caution when operating motor vehicles or machinery. Activity will help decrease this effect. Other side effects include feelings of detachment, irritability, emotional lability, GI upset, dependency, or development of tolerance. The elderly population is at high risk for the development of **dizziness** or **cognitive impairment**, which places them at high risk for falls with associated injuries. When discontinuing a benzodiazepine after long-term use, the drug should be weaned off to prevent withdrawal side effects.

Treatment of Insomnia

Benzodiazepines are used to treat **insomnia** because of their **sedative-hypnotic effects**. There are three different types of insomnia, which include the inability to fall asleep, inability to stay asleep, or the combination of both. Many times, insomnia can be helped by a change in habits or talking about worries or stress the patient may be experiencing. When using a sedative-hypnotic to treat sleep disturbances, the medication should have rapid onset and allow the patient to wake up feeling refreshed instead of tired and groggy. When administered at bedtime, most benzodiazepines will produce a sleep-inducing effect and should be used on a short-term basis.

Review Video: Sedatives, Hypnotics, and Insomnia Management
Visit mometrix.com/academy and enter code: 666132

Review Video: Chronic Insomnia
Visit mometrix.com/academy and enter code: 293232

Use of Buspirone for Treatment of Anxiety

Due to the addictive potential of benzodiazepines, the use of **nonbenzodiazepines** to treat anxiety has increased. One of the most commonly used nonbenzodiazepine medications is the drug **buspirone**. This medication is highly effective in treating anxiety and its associated symptoms such as insomnia, poor concentration, tension, restlessness, irritability, and fatigue. Buspirone has no addiction potential, is not useful in alcohol withdrawal and seizures, and is not known to interact with other CNS depressants. Because it may take several weeks of continual use for the effects of this drug to be realized by the patient, it cannot be used on an as-needed basis. Buspirone does not increase depression symptoms and therefore is useful in treating anxiety associated with depression. Side effects associated with medication can include GI upset, dizziness, sleepiness, excitement, or headache.

Medication Considerations for Elderly Patients

An elderly patient has an increased chance of adverse effects from medications. Approximately 1/3 of hospitalizations that are related to side effects of drugs and 1/2 of drug-associated fatalities happen in patients that are at least 60 years of age. In the United States, expenses for prescriptions for elderly patients make up 30% of every prescription filled and 40–50% of non-prescription drugs. Elderly patients spend more than $3 billion annually on these medications. Most elderly individuals have at least one ongoing health condition, including arthritis, high blood pressure, heart problems, diabetes, or other conditions, often requiring more than one drug for treatment. There are more adverse drug reactions (ADR) amongst elderly patients, 10% of whom require hospitalization for treatment for the side effects. Frequently seen adverse reactions include edema, queasiness, vomiting, anorexia, vertigo, loose stools, infrequent and difficult stools, bewilderment, and urinary retention. Be careful not to misidentify these as another condition or symptom of aging.

Pharmacokinetics of Older Adults

Pharmacokinetics involves four steps: Absorption, distribution, metabolism, and elimination. All of these steps are affected by the age of the patient as the organs involved degenerate from wear and tear:

1. **Absorption** of most drugs occurs in the small intestine. Drug absorption in older adults may be delayed or decreased due to decreased blood flow to the small intestine. This could change the blood levels of drugs achieved in the geriatric patient.

2. **Distribution** of the drug is altered due to a change in body composition. Elderly patients have decreased total body water and lean muscle mass. This relative increase in total body fat may increase the duration of action of lipid-soluble drugs.
3. Most drugs are **metabolized** by either the liver or the kidneys. Decreased function of these organs leads to delayed metabolism and elimination of certain medications.
4. **Renal function** and **elimination effectiveness** diminish with age, often decreasing the kidney's ability to remove toxins and medications from the body. For this reason, drugs may remain in the body longer, therefore requiring smaller doses among the elderly.

Beers Criteria

The Beers Criteria, also called the Beers List, identifies inappropriate medication use among older adults. The list is used to determine which medications are beneficial compared to those that impose risks for older adults. Because older adults are at risk of polypharmacy and inappropriate medication use, the Beers Criteria helps healthcare providers identify which medications are truly necessary and are in the patient's best interests to use. All medications that the patient takes are identified, and indications are given as to whether the medications should be avoided among those older than age 65. The recommendations are then rated for strength, and the quality of the research supporting the recommendations is identified.

Difficulties the Elderly Population May Encounter with Medication Use

Common difficulties with medication use amongst the elderly include:

- Overuse of prescription medications
- Medication adherence and compliance issues (e.g., providing incorrect or incomplete past medical history to the professional, or using medicine that is out of date, changing dose without practitioner's orders to do so)
- Misunderstanding of how the medicine is supposed to be used due to problems with comprehension, hearing, or proper education style
- Not remembering the reason, amount, or how often the drug should be used (may result in repeating the medicine when it has already been taken)
- Difficulty affording the medication
- Vision issues resulting in misreading the label and taking the wrong dosage
- Problems getting the bottle open, dealing with small pills, cutting pills in half, and using inhalers
- More than one medical worker or more than one pharmacy can lead to inadvertent redundancy of the same medication, as can using the generic and brand name of the same thing at the same time

Common Adverse Outcomes of Frequently Used Prescription Medications

Certain physical and psychological states may be an adverse outcome resulting from a prescribed medication:

- **Bewilderment:** Digoxin, cimetidine, dopamine agent, antihistamine, hypnotic, sedative, anticholinergic, anticonvulsant
- **Anorexia**: Digoxin
- **Low energy or weakness:** Diuretic, antidepressant, antihypertensive
- **Absentmindedness**: Barbiturate
- **Difficult bowel movements**: Anticholinergic
- **Loose stool:** Oral antacid

- **GI upset:** Iron, NSAID, salicylate, corticosteroid, estrogen, alcohol
- **Ringing in the ears (tinnitus)**: Analgesic
- **Urinary retention:** Anticholinergic, alpha-agonist
- **Orthostatic low blood pressure:** Antihypertensive, sedative, diuretic, antidepressant
- **Depression:** Benzodiazepine
- **Vertigo:** Sedative, antihypertensive, anticonvulsant, diuretic

Adverse Outcomes of Histamine Blockers, Ibuprofen, and Beta-Blockers

Histamine blockers in the elderly can cause paradoxical central nervous system provocation that has an outcome of ataxia in this population. Antihistamines may cause problems with vision and walking, leading to falls, which may cause unforeseen hospital visits or require a nursing home. Antihistamines can also interfere with the effectiveness of other medications or enhance other medications' negative side effects.

Some elderly patients are already dealing with decreased renal functioning. **Ibuprofen** has the ability to worsen these issues leading to nephrosis, cirrhosis, and congestive heart failure.

If the patient is older, a **beta-blocker** is not a good option for treating hypertension due to their decreased beta-adrenergic receptor sensitivity for the elderly patient. Elderly patients need smaller amounts of calcium entry antagonists, ACE inhibitors, or diuretics. Too high a dose (in the elderly) will cause moodiness, impotence, weariness, and lessened ability to think clearly. Elderly patients are particularly prone to congestive heart failure and peripheral vascular insufficiency due to beta-adrenergic toxins.

Polypharmacy

Polypharmacy is a term used to describe inappropriate use of multiple medications at one time. It occurs when medications are taken that are not indicated, medications that have adverse interactions with one another are taken together, and patients take contraindicated medications. Polypharmacy is a common problem in the geriatric population. Most office visits result in new prescriptions being written and patients may accumulate many different medications in their home. Polypharmacy greatly increases the patient's risk of having an adverse drug reaction.

To manage polypharmacy and prevent complications, obtain a detailed drug history at each visit. This should include nonprescription medications and herbal remedies. Educating patients about the problem of polypharmacy is very important. This can occur in the clinician's office or with a community education program. Assist elderly patients with medication identification, recommending pill boxes to help the patient divide medications and minimize risks for medication misuse.

MASTER Rules for Rational Drug Therapy

Although drugs are often very useful and effective in treating illnesses, there is a point when it becomes dangerous to the patient. Drug resistance, drug interactions, and drug intolerances are all common problems, especially among elderly patients, because an iatrogenic illness can develop. For these reasons, it is important to limit drugs to only those that are absolutely necessary. To help the practitioner decide whether a drug should be used or not, they must remember the **MASTER rules**.

- **M** is for **minimizing** the number of drugs a patient is taking.
- **A** is for considering **alternate** treatments that may be as or more effective than using a drug.

- **S** is for **start** low and increase slowly. Only give the patient the minimum amount, and be careful when increasing doses.
- **T** is for **titration** of drugs; tailor the amount given over time to the individual patient.
- **E** is for **education** of the patient about the drugs he or she is taking.
- **R** is for **regular** reviewing of drugs and doses.

Physiological Integrity: Reduction of Risk Potential

Specimen Collection for Glucose Monitoring

Glucose Laboratory Test

Glucose is manufactured by the liver from ingested carbohydrates and is stored as glycogen for use by the cells. If intake is inadequate, glucose can be produced from muscle and fat tissue, leading to increased wasting. High levels of glucose are indicative of diabetes mellitus, which predisposes people to skin injuries, slow healing, and infection. **Fasting blood glucose levels** are used to diagnose and monitor this condition:

- Normal values: 70–99 mg/dL
- Impaired: 100–125 mg/dL
- Diabetes: ≥126 mg/dL

There are a number of different conditions that can increase glucose levels, including stress, renal failure, Cushing syndrome, hyperthyroidism, and pancreatic disorders. Medications, such as steroids, estrogens, lithium, phenytoin, diuretics, tricyclic antidepressants, may increase glucose levels. Other conditions, such as adrenal insufficiency, liver disease, hypothyroidism, and starvation can decrease glucose levels.

Collecting a Point-of-Care Glucose Test

Conducting a point-of-care blood glucose test includes:

- **Precautions**: Ask if the patient is taking medications that might interfere with readings (Sodium-glucose inhibitors, fluoroquinolones, hormones, cholesterol-lowering drugs). Use the device for only one patient or follow manufacturer's guidelines for cleaning and disinfection between patients. Use standard precautions. Check the expiration dates on test-strip vials.
- **Components**: Devices may vary by manufacturer, but generally include the testing device, test strips, and a control solution to check the accuracy of the readings. The control solution should be used to check test strips before initial use of the system, when opening a new container of test strips, and when results seem abnormally high or low.
- **Procedure**: Use the lancet on the side of the fingertip or the forearm (depending on the device). Note that a sample from the fingertip may be more accurate. The first drop is typically discarded and the second drop applied to the test strip. If obtaining a venous blood sample for testing, only test tubes containing sodium heparin should be used. The test strip is inserted into the device for the recommended time until the reading is displayed. Then, the strip is removed and discarded as biohazardous waste.

Hemoglobin A1c Laboratory Test

Hemoglobin A1c comprises hemoglobin A with a glucose molecule because hemoglobin holds onto excess blood glucose, so it shows the average blood glucose levels over a 3-month period and is used primarily to monitor long-term diabetic therapy:

- Normal value: <6%

Airway Management

Non-Invasive Ventilation

Nasal Cannula

A nasal cannula can be used to deliver supplemental oxygen to a patient, but it is only useful for flow rates ≤6 L/min as higher rates are drying of the nasal passages. As it is not an airtight system, some ambient air is breathed in as well so oxygen concentration ranges from about 24–44%. The nasal cannula does not allow for control of respiratory rate, so the patient must be able to breathe independently.

Non-Rebreather Mask

A non-rebreather mask can be used to deliver higher concentrations (60–90%) of oxygen to those patients who are able to breathe independently. The mask fits over the nose and mouth and is secured by an elastic strap. A 1.5 L reservoir bag is attached and connects to an oxygen source. The bag is inflated to about 1 liter at a rate of 8–15 L/min before the mask is applied as the patient breathes from this reservoir. A one-way exhalation valve prevents most exhaled air from being rebreathed.

Non-Invasive Positive Pressure Ventilators

Non-invasive positive pressure ventilators provide air through a tight-fitting nasal or face mask, usually pressure cycled, avoiding the need for intubation and reducing the danger of hospital-acquired infection and mortality rates. It can be used for acute respiratory failure and pulmonary edema. There are 2 types of non-invasive positive pressure ventilators:

- **CPAP (Continuous positive airway pressure)** provides a steady stream of pressurized air throughout both inspiration and expiration. CPAP improves breathing by decreasing preload for patients with congestive heart failure. It reduces the effort required for breathing by increasing residual volume and improving gas exchange.
- **Bi-PAP (Bi-level positive airway pressure)** provides a steady stream of pressurized air as CPAP but it senses inspiratory effort and increases pressure during inspiration. Bi-PAP pressures for inspiration and expiration can be set independently. Machines can be programmed with a backup rate to ensure a set number of respirations per minute.

**NEVER place a patient in wrist restraints while wearing these devices. If the patient vomits, they need to be able to remove the mask to prevent aspiration.*

Face Mask

Ensuring that a face mask (Ambu bag) is the correct fit and type is important for adequate ventilation, oxygenation, and prevention of aspiration. Difficulties in management of face mask ventilation relate to risk factors: >55 years, obesity, beard, edentulous, and history of snoring. In some cases, if dentures are adhered well, they may be left in place during induction. The face mask is applied by lifting the mandible (jaw thrust) to the mask and avoiding pressure on soft tissue. Oral or nasal airways may be used, ensuring that the distal end is at the angle of the mandible. There are a number of steps to prevent mask airway leaks:

- Increasing or decreasing the amount of air to the mask to allow better seal
- Securing the mask with both hands while another person ventilates
- Accommodating a large nose by using the mask upside down
- Utilizing a laryngeal mask airway if excessive beard prevents seal

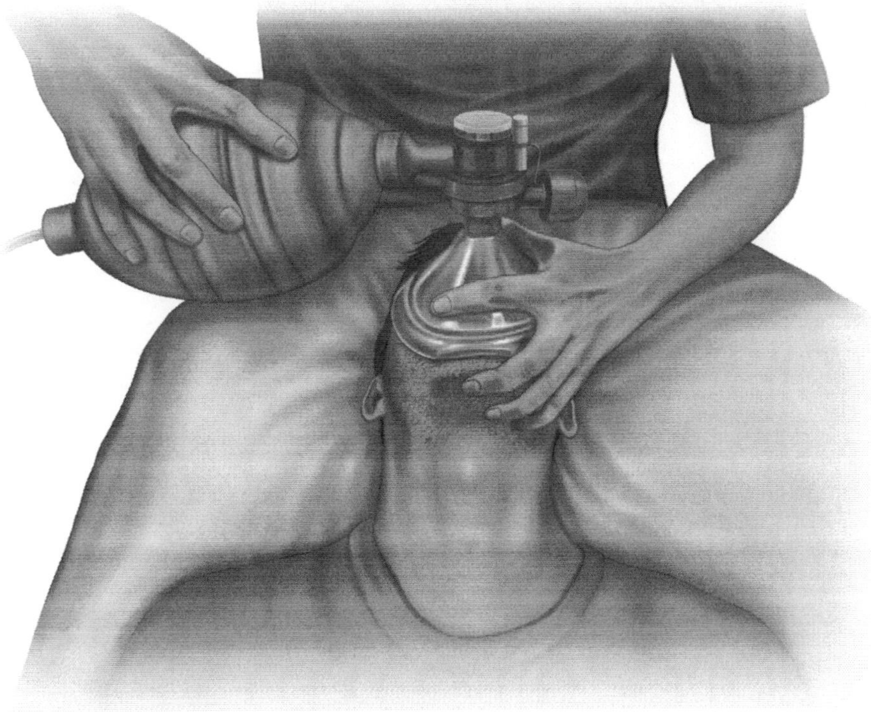

High and Low Flow Oxygen Delivery

High flow oxygen delivery devices provide oxygen at flow rates higher than the patient's inspiratory flow rate at specific medium to high FiO_2, up to 100%. However, a flow of 100% oxygen actually provides only 60–80% FiO_2 to the patient because the patient also breathes in some room air, diluting the oxygen. The actual amount of oxygen received depends on the type of interface or mask. Additionally, the flow rate is actually less than the inspiratory flow rate upon actual delivery. High flow oxygen delivery is usually not used in the sleep center. Humidification is usually required because the high flow is drying.

Low flow oxygen delivery devices provide 100% oxygen at flow rates lower than the patient's inspiratory flow rate, but the oxygen mixes with room air, so the FiO_2 varies. Humidification is usually only required if flow rate is >3L/min. Much oxygen is wasted with exhalation, so a number of different devices to conserve oxygen are available. Interfaces include transtracheal catheters and cannulae with reservoirs.

Airway Devices

Oropharyngeal, Nasopharyngeal, and Tracheostomy Tubes

Airways are used to establish a patent airway and facilitate respirations:

- **Oropharyngeal**: This plastic airway curves over the tongue and creates space between the mouth and the posterior pharynx. It is used for anesthetized or unconscious patients to keep tongue and epiglottis from blocking the airway.

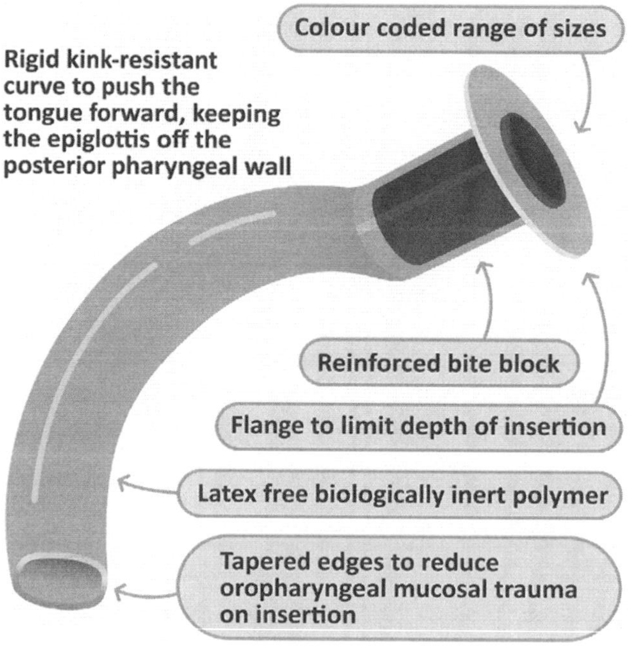

- **Nasopharyngeal** (trumpet): This smaller flexible airway is more commonly used in conscious patients and is inserted through one nostril, extending to the nasopharynx. It is commonly utilized in patients who need frequent suctioning.

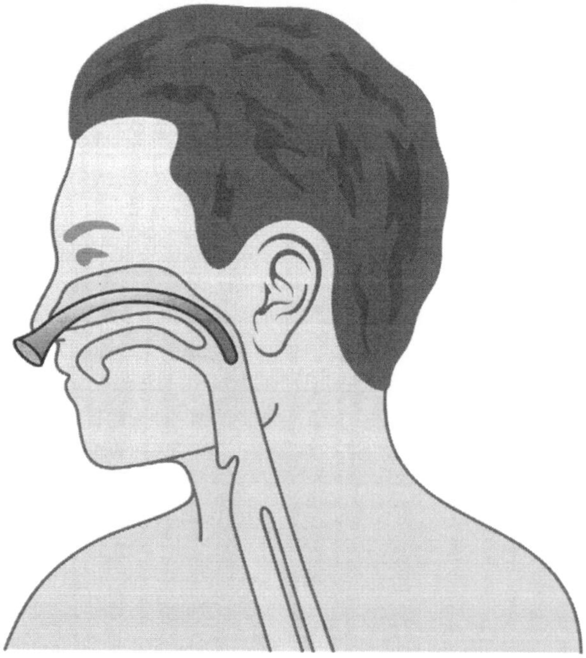

- **Tracheostomy tubes**: Tracheostomy may be utilized for mechanical ventilation. Tubes are inserted into the opening in the trachea to provide a conduit and maintain the opening. The tube is secured with ties around the neck. Because the air entering the lungs through the tracheostomy bypasses the warming and moistening effects of the upper airway, air is humidified through a room humidifier or through the delivery of humidified air through a special mask or mechanical ventilation. If the tracheostomy is going to be long-term, eventually a stoma will form at the site, and the tube can be removed.

Laryngeal Mask Airway

The laryngeal-mask airway (LMA) is an intermediate airway allowing ventilation but not complete respiratory control. The LMA consists of an inflatable cuff (the mask) with a connecting tube. It may be used temporarily before tracheal intubation or when tracheal intubation can't be done. It can also be a conduit for later blind insertion of an endotracheal tube. The head and neck must be in neutral position for insertion of the LMA. If the patient has a gag reflex, conscious sedation or topical anesthesia (deep oropharyngeal) is required. The LMA is inserted by sliding along the hard palate, using the finger as a guide, into the pharynx, and the ring is inflated to create a seal about the opening to the larynx, allowing ventilation with mild positive-pressure. The ProSeal LMA has a modified cuff that extends onto the back of the mask to improve seal. LMA is contraindicated in morbid obesity, obstructions or abnormalities of oropharynx, and non-fasting patients, as some aspiration is possible even with the cuff seal inflated.

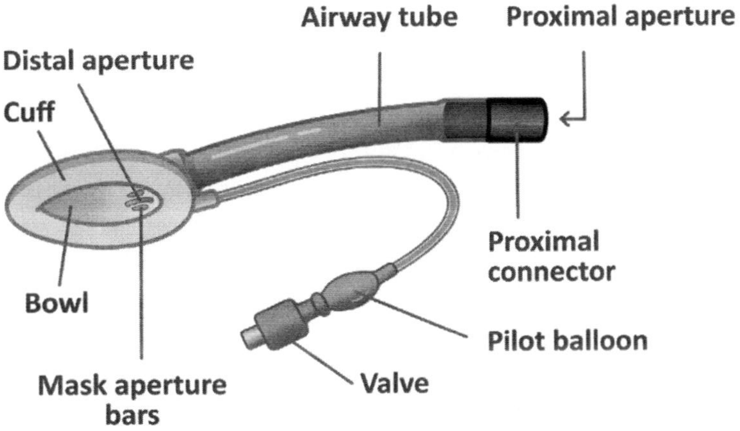

Esophageal-Tracheal Combitube

The esophageal tracheal Combitube (ETC) is an intermediate airway that contains two lumens and can be inserted into either the trachea or the esophagus (≤91%). The twin-lumen tube has a proximal cuff providing a seal of the oropharynx and a distal cuff providing a seal about the distal tube. Prior to insertion, the Combitube cuffs should be checked for leaks (15 mL of air into distal and 85 mL of air into proximal). The patient should be non-responsive and with absent gag reflex with head in neutral position. The tube is passed along the tongue and into the pharynx, utilizing markings on the tube (black guidelines) to determine depth by aligning the ETC with the upper incisors or alveolar ridge. Once in place the distal cuff is inflated (10–15 mL) and then placement in the trachea or esophagus should be determined, so the proper lumen for ventilation can be used. The proximal cuff is inflated (usually to 50–75 mL) and ventilation begun. A capnogram should be used to confirm ventilation.

Mechanical Ventilation

Endotracheal Intubation

Endotracheal intubation is often necessary with respiratory failure for control of hypoxemia, hypercapnia, hypoventilation, and/or obstructed airway. Equipment should be assembled and tubes and connections checked for air leaks with a 10 mL syringe. The mouth and/or nose should be cleaned of secretions and suctioned if necessary. The patient should be supine with the patient's head level with the lower sternum of the clinician. With orotracheal/endotracheal intubation, the clinician holds the laryngoscope (in left hand) and inserts it into right corner of mouth, the epiglottis is lifted and the larynx exposed. A thin flexible intubation stylet may be used and the endotracheal tube (ETT) (in right hand) is inserted through the vocal cords and into the trachea, cuff inflated to minimal air leak (10 mL initially until patient stabilizes), and placement confirmed through capnometry or esophageal detection devices. While insertion depths vary, the generally accepted depth for males is 23 cm and for females is 21 cm. This acts as a starting point from which minor adjustments can be made. After insertion, the tube is secured.

Review Video: Mechanical Ventilation
Visit mometrix.com/academy and enter code: 679637

Rapid Sequence Intubation (RSI)

Rapid sequence intubation (RSI) is the simultaneous giving of a sedative and a paralytic in order to facilitate emergency intubation and is considered to be the standard of care for emergency airway management (except in patients with anticipated difficult intubation or in those with contraindications to sedatives/paralytics).

Initial preparation includes inserting 2 IV lines and establishing cardiac monitoring, oximetry, and capnography. The patient should be preoxygenated (100%) for at least 3 minutes, but without pressure ventilation that may cause aspiration of stomach contents. Procedure includes:

- **Induction agent**: Ketamine, etomidate, propofol
- **Paralysis**: Succinylcholine, rocuronium, other NMBAs
- **Sellick's maneuver** (pressure applied externally with thumb and index finger to cricoid) to close off the esophagus and prevent aspiration
- **Suction** to clear mouth if necessary
- **Laryngoscopy** to visual vocal cords
- **EET** inserted, cuff inflated, and ETT secured

Proper placement verified by capnometer or capnograph. Breath sounds should be auscultated. Post intubation chest x-ray to assess depth of tube and check for any trauma or issue. Induction agents and use of additional sedation may vary from one institution to another, but the primary goal is to safely anesthetize and intubate while preventing regurgitation of stomach contents.

Confirming Correct Placement of Endotracheal Tubes

There are a number of methods to **confirm correct placement** of endotracheal tubes. Clinical assessment alone is not adequate.

- **Capnometry** utilizes an end-tidal CO_2 ($ETCO_2$) detector that measures the concentration of CO_2 in expired air, usually through pH sensitive paper that changes color (commonly purple to yellow). The capnometer is attached to the ETT and a bag-valve-mask (BVM) ventilator is also attached. The patient is provided 6 ventilations and the CO_2 concentration is checked.
- **Capnography** is attached to the ETT and provides a waveform graph, showing the varying concentrations of CO_2 in real time throughout each ventilation (with increased CO_2 on expiration) and can indicate changes in respiratory status.
- **Esophageal detection devices** fit over the end of the ETT so that a large syringe can be used to attempt to aspirate. If the ETT is in the esophagus, the walls collapse on aspiration and resistance occurs, whereas the syringe fills with air if the ETT is in the trachea. A self-inflating bulb (Ellik device) may also be used.
- **Chest x-ray** provides visual confirmation of placement.

Ventilator Management

There are many types of ventilators now in use, and the specific directions for each type must be followed carefully, but there are general principles that apply to all **ventilator management**. The following should be monitored:

- **Type of ventilation:** Volume-cycled, pressure-cycled, negative-pressure, HFJV, HFOV, CPAP, Bi-PAP
- **Control mode**: Controlled ventilation, assisted ventilation, synchronized intermittent mandatory (allows spontaneous breaths between ventilator-controlled inhalation/exhalation), positive end-expiratory pressure (PEEP), CPAP, Bi-PAP
- **Tidal volume** (TV) range should be set in relation to respiratory rate
- **Inspiratory-expiratory ratio** (I:E) usually ranges from 1:2–1:5, but may vary
- **Respiratory rate** will depend upon TV and $PaCO_2$ target
- **Fraction of inspired oxygen** (FiO_2) [percentage of oxygen in the inspired air], usually ranging from 21–100%, usually maintained <40% to avoid toxicity
- **Sensitivity** determines the effort needed to trigger inspiration
- **Pressure** controls the pressure exerted in delivering TV
- **Rate of flow** controls the L/min speed of TV

Tracheostomy

Tracheostomy, surgical tracheal opening, may be utilized for mechanical ventilation. Tracheostomy tubes are inserted directly into an opening in the trachea to provide a conduit and maintain the opening. Tracheostomy tubes are usually silastic or plastic, and may have permanent or disposable inner cannulas. The tube is secured with ties around the neck. Because the air entering the lungs through the tracheostomy bypasses the warming and moistening effects of the upper airway, air is humidified through a room humidifier or through delivery of humidified air through a special mask or mechanical ventilation. The patient with a tracheostomy must have continuous monitoring of vital signs and respiratory status to ensure patency of tracheostomy. The inner cannula should be cleaned/replaced regularly (every 8–24 hours and PRN). Regular suctioning is needed, especially initially, to remove secretions:

- Suction catheter should be 50% the size of the tracheostomy tube to allow ventilation during suctioning
- Vacuum pressure: 80–100 mmHg
- Catheter should only be inserted ≤0.5 cm beyond tube to avoid damage to tissues or perforation
- Catheter should be inserted without suction and intermittent suction on withdrawal

Ventilation-Induced Lung Injury

Ventilation-induced lung injury (VILI) is damage caused by mechanical ventilation. It is common in acute distress syndrome (ARDS) but can affect any mechanically ventilated patient. VILI comprises four interrelated elements:

- **Barotrauma**: Damage to the lung caused by excessive pressure
- **Volutrauma**: Alveolar damage related to high tidal volume ventilation
- **Atelectotrauma**: Injury caused by repetitive forced opening and closing of alveoli
- **Biotrauma**: Inflammatory response

In VILI, essentially the increased pressure and tidal volume over-distends the alveoli, which rupture, and air moves into the interstitial tissue resulting in pulmonary interstitial emphysema. With continued ventilation, the air in the interstitium moves into the subcutaneous tissue and may result in pneumopericardium and pneumomediastinum, or rupture the pleural sac which can cause tension pneumothorax and mediastinal shift, which can cause respiratory failure and cardiac arrest. VILI has caused a change in ventilation procedures with lower tidal volumes and pressures used as well as newer forms of ventilation, HFJV and HFOV, preferred to traditional mechanical ventilation for many patients.

Preventing Complications from Ventilators

Methods to prevent complications from mechanical ventilation ("ventilator bundle") include:

- Elevate patient's head and chest to 30° to prevent aspiration and ventilation-associated pneumonia.
- Reposition patient every 2 hours.
- Provide DVT prophylaxis, such as external compression support and/or heparin (5000 u sq 2–3 times daily).
- Administer famotidine or pantoprazole PO/IV daily to prevent gastrointestinal stress-ulcers/bleeding.
- Decrease and eliminate sedation/analgesia as soon as possible—regular sedation vacations to assess neurological status.
- Follow careful protocols for pressure settings to prevent barotrauma. Tidal volumes are usually maintained at 8–12 mL/kg PBW (per AACN guidelines), but in incidences of high probability of ARDS, volumes should be less (6 mL/kg) to avoid lung injury.
- Monitor for pneumothorax or evidence of barotrauma.
- Conduct nutritional assessment (including lab tests) to prevent malnutrition.
- Monitor intake and output carefully and administer IV fluids to prevent dehydration.
- Do daily spontaneous breathing trials and discontinue ventilation as soon as possible.

Ventilator Weaning

Ventilator weaning has three phases: Changing settings of the ventilator to allow the patient to demonstrate the ability to breath on their own (standby mode), extubation, and finally removal of supportive oxygen. Criteria for ventilator weaning may include some or all of the following, depending on facility guidelines:

- Vital capacity 10–15 mL/kg
- Maximum (negative) inspiratory pressure of at least -20 cmH_2O
- Tidal volume (TV) of 7–9 mL/kg
- Minute ventilation of about 6L/min (Respiratory rate x TV)
- Rapid shallow breathing index <100 breaths/min/L
- PaO_2 >60 mmHg
- FiO_2 <40%
- pH >7.25
- Hemodynamic stability (minimal to no dependence on vasopressors for blood pressure maintenance)

If these criteria are met and the patient passes a spontaneous breathing trial (SBT), then extubation can be done. Various protocols are followed in weaning patients off of ventilators, including the use of intermittent mandatory ventilation (IMV) and synchronized intermittent mandatory ventilation (SIMV), which can be used with pressure support ventilation (PSV).

Criteria for oxygen weaning:

- FiO_2 reduced until PaO_2 70–100 mmHg on room air
- Supplemental O_2 necessary with PaO_2<70 mmHg (Medicare requires PaO_2 55 mmHg for reimbursement for home oxygen use)

Spontaneous Breathing Trial as Preparation for Extubation

A spontaneous breathing trial (SBT) is when a patient is taken off mechanical ventilation while remaining intubated (usually by changing the ventilator settings to CPAP) for a short period of time (30–120 minutes) to assess readiness to extubate. SBTs are often performed daily to ensure extubation possibility is identified as early as possible. SBT should be used prior to extubating a patient if the patient is not agitated and has no evidence of myocardial ischemia or increased ICP. The patient should exhibit some spontaneous triggering of respirations and should not be receiving large doses of vasopressor or inotropic agent. SpO_2 should be ≥88% with FiO_2 of 0.50 and PEEP at 7.5 cmH_2O prior to the SBT. The SBT should be done in the morning for a prescribed period (usually 30–120 minutes). The ventilator rate is adjusted to 0 and pressure support decreased to 0–7. The SBT should be discontinued if the following occur:

- Respiratory rate >35 or <8 for at least 5 minutes
- Mental status changes
- SpO_2 <88% for >15 minutes
- Respiratory distress (HR >130 BPM or <60 BPM, marked dyspnea, diaphoresis, increased use of accessory respiratory muscles, respiratory arrest)

Patients who pass the SBT have an 85–90% chance of breathing successfully after extubation. Patients who repeatedly fail daily SBT may require tracheostomy.

FAILURE TO WEAN FROM MECHANICAL VENTILATION

Failure to wean from mechanical ventilation can occur in approximately 20–30% of ventilated patients. Many factors affect a patient's ability to wean from mechanical ventilation including physical, psychological, and situational factors. Before discontinuation of ventilation can be considered, the patient must be able to protect his/her airway, be hemodynamically stable and have resolution of the clinical problem that initiated the need for mechanical ventilation. Weaning protocols use clinical criteria such as oxygen saturation, blood pressure, respiratory rate, and tidal volume to determine the patient's tolerance of lessening mechanical ventilator support. Failure to wean is demonstrated by multiple daily spontaneous breathing trial failures or the need for reintubation within 48 hours of extubation. Failure to resolve the clinical problem(s) that initiated mechanical ventilation, insufficient ventilator drive, respiratory muscle weakness, co-morbidities, and/or the development of new clinical problems (e.g., infection) may contribute to the inability to wean.

Signs/symptoms: Decreased tidal volume, increased respiratory rate, increased $PaCO_2$, oxygen desaturation, anxiety, diaphoresis, fatigue, changes in blood pressure or heart rate, mental status changes, and hemodynamic changes.

Treatment: The initial treatment strategy for patients who experience a dysfunctional ventilator weaning response is identification and treatment of the underlying cause(s) of the weaning failure. In addition, other treatment strategies may include psychological preparation of the patient for further weaning attempts, readiness testing and respiratory muscle training.

SEDATION/ANALGESIA WITH MECHANICAL VENTILATION

Patients intubated for mechanical ventilation are usually given **sedation and/or analgesia** initially, but medications should be reduced and given in boluses rather than with continuous IV drip with a goal of stopping sedation as it prolongs ventilation time. Typical sedatives include midazolam, propofol, and lorazepam. Narcotic analgesics include fentanyl and morphine sulfate. Uses of sedation include:

- Controlling agitation and excessive movement that may interfere with ventilation
- Reduce pain and discomfort associated with ventilation
- Control respiratory distress

Triglyceride levels must be checked periodically if propofol is administered for more than 24–48 hours. Neuromuscular blocking agents are rarely used because they may cause long-term weakness and increase length of ventilation although they may be indicated in some cases, such as with excessive shivering or cardiac arrest. Many patients are able to tolerate mechanical ventilation without sedation, and sedation should always be decreased to the minimal amount necessary as excess sedation may delay extubation. An ideal level of sedation will keep the patient calm and compliant with the ventilator but still alert and able to follow commands.

Conscious Sedation

Conscious sedation is used to decrease sensations of pain and awareness caused by a surgical or invasive procedure, such a biopsy, chest tube insertion, fracture repair, and endoscopy. It is also used during presurgical preparations, such as insertion of central lines, catheters, and use of cooling blankets. Conscious sedation uses a combination of analgesia and sedation so that patients can remain responsive and follow verbal cues but have a brief amnesia preventing recall of the procedures. The patient must be monitored carefully, including pulse oximetry, during this type of sedation. The most commonly used drugs include:

- Midazolam (Versed): This is a short-acting water-soluble sedative, with onset of 1–5 minutes, peaking in 30, and duration usually about 1 hour (up to 6 hours).
- Fentanyl: This is a short-acting opioid with immediate onset, peaking in 10–15 minutes and with a duration of about 20–45 minutes. Monitor respiratory function.

The fentanyl/midazolam combination provides both sedation and pain control. Conscious sedation usually requires 6 hours fasting prior to administration.

Therapeutic Gases

Carbon dioxide is a potent stimulator of respirations, but it is rarely used therapeutically because it can depress respirations if hypercarbia or respiratory acidosis is present. CO_2 may be administered at times as part of anesthesia, but it is most commonly used for insufflation for laparoscopic/endoscopic procedures.

Nitric oxide (NO) is used as a pulmonary vessel dilator to improve oxygenation by decreasing pulmonary artery pressure and pulmonary vascular resistance. NO is FDA-approved for use for neonatal PPH but is sometimes used for adults with pulmonary arterial hypertension (PAH) who require acute vasodilator testing prior to initiating additional therapies. NO is an effective drug to use when testing acute vasoreactivity. During acute vasodilator testing, inhaled NO is administered at 10–80 ppm for 5–10 minutes during which hemodynamics are measured and monitored. Studies have not shown it to be an effective treatment for ARDS. Toxic reactions include methemoglobinemia and platelet inhibition with resultant bleeding.

Heliox is helium mixed with oxygen that is used to reduce airway resistance during mechanical ventilation and for pulmonary function tests. Heliox may also be used to treat respiratory obstruction and is used during laser surgery on the airway because it readily conducts heat away from the surgical site, reducing tissue damage. Heliox is sometimes used for COPD patients as it increases hyperventilation and reduces carbon dioxide levels.

Nasogastric Intubation and Enteral Feedings

NG Tubes, Sump Tubes, and Levin Tubes

Nasogastric **(NG) tubes** are plastic or vinyl tubes inserted through the nose, down the esophagus, and into the stomach. **Sump tubes** are radiopaque with a vent lumen to prevent a vacuum from forming with high suction. **Levin tubes** have no vent lumen and are used only with low suction. NG tubes drain gastric secretions, allow sampling of secretions, or provide access to the stomach and upper GI tract. They are used for lavage after medication overdose, for decompression, and for instillation of medications or fluids. NG tubes are contraindicated with obstruction proximal to the stomach or gastric pathology, such as hemorrhage.

Levin Tube

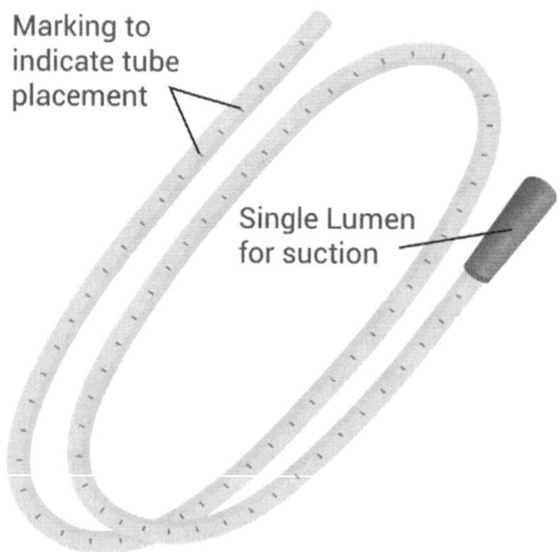

NG Tube Insertion

Insertion of a nasogastric tube includes:

- **Examination**: Review the patient's medical history for possible contraindications. Assess the size and patency of the nares and select the most patent side. Assess mental status.
- **Select and measure tube**: For decompression, 14–16 Fr is most common; for enteral feeding, 8–12 Fr. Adult insertion length is about 55 cm. To estimate, measure from the tip of the nose to the earlobe and then to the xiphoid process; mark the desired length (permanent marker, tape).
- **Preparation**: Drape the patient's chest and provide an emesis basin. Prepare tape and an anchoring device. Inject 10 mL of water into the tube to check patency. Lubricate 2–3 inches of the tube (with a water-soluble lubricant). For decompression, connect the tube to the suction machine to prevent aspiration of emesis, but leave the machine off.
- **Insertion**: Place the patient in high Fowler's position (at least 60°). Gently insert the tube posteriorly into the nasopharynx, which usually triggers gag reflex. Ask the patient to flex their head forward and take sips of water or suck on ice chips so swallowing will help guide tube. At 25–30 cm, listen for air exchange at distal end of tube and watch carefully for signs of pulmonary placement (cough, cyanosis, abnormal breathing). Continue inserting tube to desired length. Anchor tube. Verify correct placement (x-ray, pH testing).

PEG TUBE

Percutaneous endoscopic gastrostomy (PEG), used for tube feedings, involves intubation of the esophagus with the endoscope and insertion of a sheathed needle with a guidewire through the abdomen and stomach wall so that a catheter can be fed down the esophagus, snared, and pulled out through the opening where the needle was inserted and secured. The PEG tube should not be secured to the abdomen until the PEG is fully healed, which usually takes 2–4 weeks, because tension caused by taping the tube against the abdomen may cause the tract to change shape and direction. The tract should be straight to facilitate insertion and removal of catheters. Once the tract has healed, the original PEG tube can generally be replaced with a balloon gastrostomy tube. External stabilizing devices can be applied to the skin to hold the tube in place but should be placed 1–2 cm above the skin surface to prevent excessive tension that may result in buried bumper syndrome (BBS) in which the internal fixation device becomes lodged in the mucosal lining of the gastric wall, resulting in ulceration.

DRAINS

The following are different types of drains a patient may have, including pertinent nursing considerations:

- **Simple drains** are latex or vinyl tubes of varying sizes/lengths. They are usually placed through a stab wound near the area of involvement.
- **Penrose drains** are flat, soft rubber/latex tubes placed in surgical wounds to drain fluid by gravity and capillary action.

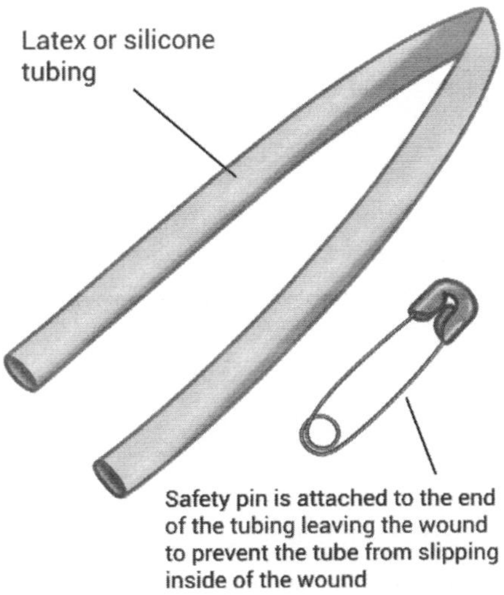

- **Sump drains** are double-lumen or tri-lumen tubes (with a third lumen for infusions). The multiple lumens produce venting when air enters the inflow lumen and forces drainage out of the large lumen.

- **A percutaneous drainage catheter** is inserted into the wound to provide continuous drainage for infection/fluid collection. Irrigation of the catheter may be required to maintain patency. Skin barriers and pouching systems may also be necessary.

SAFE PERCUTANEOUS DRAINAGE KIT

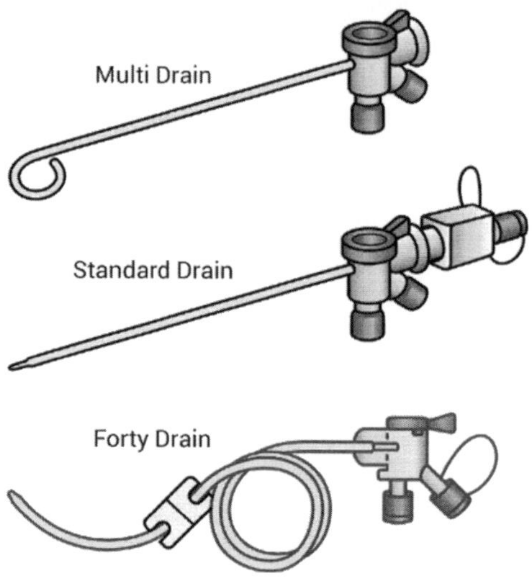

- **Closed drainage systems** use low-pressure suction to provide continuous gravity drainage of wounds. Drains are attached to collapsible suction reservoirs that provide negative pressure. The nurse must remember to always re-establish negative pressure after emptying these drains. There are two types in frequent use:
    - *Jackson-Pratt is* a bulb-type drain that is about the size of a lemon. A thin plastic drain from the wound extends to a squeeze bulb that can hold about 100 mL of drainage.

JACKSON PRATT DRAIN

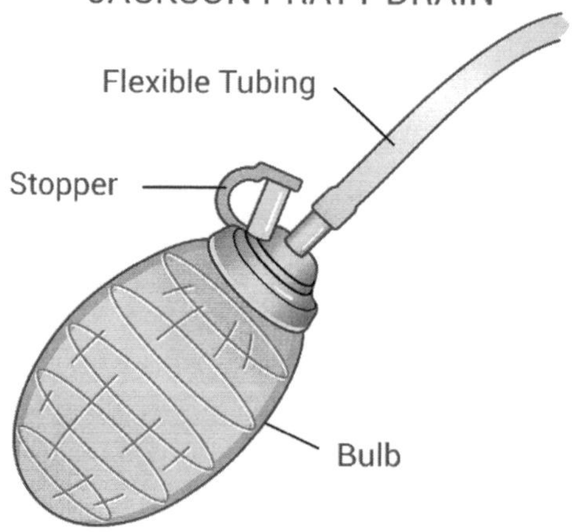

    - *Hemovac* is a round drain with coiled springs inside that are compressed after emptying to create suction. The device can hold up to 500 mL of drainage.

Enteral Support and Parenteral Support

Enteral nutrition is a method of providing nutrition to a patient through a tube; the tube may be placed in either the nose (a nasogastric tube), the stomach (a percutaneous endoscopic gastrostomy [PEG] tube), or the small bowel (a percutaneous endoscopic jejunal [J] tube). When the tube has been placed, nutrition can be administered through the tube and absorbed by the patient's digestive system. Various **enteric formulas** exist, and the choice is dependent on the nutritional requirements of the patient.

Parenteral nutrition (also called total parenteral nutrition [**TPN**]) is a method of providing nutrition that completely bypasses the digestive system by administering nutrition through an intravenous line. Enteral support is the preferred method of providing nutrition, although in patients suffering from some compromise of the gastrointestinal tract, parenteral nutrition is the only option.

Trouble-Shooting Problems Related to Enteral Feedings

Feeding tubes are commonly found in the critical care setting, as many patients are intubated and unable to take oral nutrition or medication. General maintenance involves checking placement before flushing anything into the tube (prevents aspiration), flushing the tubes with at least 30 mL of water before and after use, and every 4 hours. Never crush enteric-coated medications, and keep the HOB inclined at least 30° at all times during feeding. **Complications** include:

- **Vomiting/aspiration:** Caused by incorrect placement, gastric emptying, and/or formula intolerance.
    - Treatment: Confirm placement by checking pH (preferred to air bolus); delay feeding one hour and check residual volume before resuming. Refrigerate formula, check expiration, and use only for 24 hours.
- **Diarrhea:** Caused by rapid feeding, antibiotics/medications, intolerance of formula or hypertonic formula, and/or tube migration.
    - Treatment: Reduce rate of feeding, evaluate medications, avoid hanging feedings longer than 8 hours, and add fiber or decrease sodium in the feed.
- **Displacement of tube:**
    - Treatment: For NG tube, replace using the other nostril, only if not surgically placed. For G-tube or J-tube, cover the site and notify the physician.
    - Prevention: secure all tubes with the appropriate device and mark placement to identify migration.
- **Tube occlusion:**
    - Treatment: Check for kinks and obvious problems. Aspirate fluid, instill warm water, and aspirate to loosen occlusion. The physician may order an enzyme or sodium bicarb solution.

Physiological Integrity: Physiological Adaptation

Pressure Injury, Wounds, and Wound Management

Assessing Etiologic Factors

Wounds should be evaluated for **etiology** (the origin of the wound) during the initial assessment to ensure proper treatment. Wounds can arise from a number of different etiologies:

- **Pressure**: Wounds that occur over bony prominences, such as the heels and coccyx, may be related to pressure, shear, or friction. The skin should be carefully examined for discolorations or changes in texture that might indicate compromise.
- **Arterial**: Arterial insufficiency is associated with a decrease in pedal pulses, and cool atrophic (shiny, dry) skin. It may result in small punctate-type ulcers, frequently on the dorsum of foot.
- **Venous stasis**: A decrease in venous circulation often results in hemoglobin leaking into the tissues of the lower leg, causing a brown discoloration. Tissue is often edematous, and ulcers are most common near the medial malleolus.
- **Diabetic neuropathy/ischemia**: Neuropathy can result in a lack of sensation to pain so that injuries to the feet may go unnoticed. Diabetes may also cause damage to small vessels, resulting in ischemia that can lead to ulcerations.
- **Trauma**: Injuries resulting from accidents or other types of trauma may vary considerably with some resulting in extensive damage to bones, tissues, organs, and circulation. Additionally, the wounds may be contaminated. Each wound must be assessed individually for multiple factors.
- **Burns**: Burn wounds may be chemical, thermal, or electric and should be assessed according to the area, the percentage of the body burned, and the depth of the burn.
- **Infection**: An infected surgical or wound site can result in pain, edema, cellulitis, drainage, erosion of the sutures and ulceration of the tissue. Surgical sites must be assessed carefully and laboratory findings reviewed.

Assessing Oxygenation

Assessment of oxygenation includes:

- **Color**: Impaired oxygenation may cause a change in the color of the skin, including pallor and cyanosis, especially in the extremities and about the mouth and nose. Individuals with darker skin may take on a gray, ashy appearance.
- **Respiratory rate**: As oxygenation falls, air hunger may occur with the patient becoming increasingly dyspneic.
- **Oxygen saturation**: While normal oxygen saturation is greater than 95%, as oxygenation is impaired, the level may fall below 92%. Oxygen saturation loses accuracy if the level falls below 80%, so blood gas analysis should be done in those cases.
- **Blood gas analysis**: PO_2 should be greater than 80 mmHg but may fall below 60 mmHg (indicating hypoxemia).
- **Altered mental status**: As oxygen levels fall, the patient may exhibit confusion.
- **Blood lactate level**: Results higher than 2 mEq/L indicate impaired tissue oxygenation.

Neurological/Neurovascular Assessment

Neurological/neurovascular assessment includes:

- **Cranial nerve assessment**: Assess cranial nerves I through VII.
- **Inspection of muscles**: Determine if they are of normal size, strength, and tone and equal bilaterally. Note any involuntary movements (twitches, tremors).
- **Balance assessment**: Assess gait, Romberg test (feet together, eyes closed for 20 seconds), rapid alternating movements, finger-to-finger or finger-to-nose, and heel-to-shin test.
- **Sensory assessment**: Assess spinothalamic tracts for perception of pain, temperature, and light touch. Assess posterior column tract with vibration, position, fine touch, stereognosis, graphesthesia, two-point discrimination, extinction, and point location testing.
- **Reflexes**: Assess deep tendon reflexes (biceps reflex, triceps reflex, brachioradialis reflex, quadriceps reflex, Achilles reflex, and clonus) and superficial cutaneous reflexes (abdominal reflexes, cremasteric reflex, and plantar reflex).
- **Developmental status**: An age-appropriate assessment should determine if the patient's development is within normal parameters. Older adults may exhibit slower response times than younger adults and may exhibit tremors and unsteady gait related to age changes.

Elements of Wound Assessment

Location and Size

Wound location should be described in terms of anatomic position using landmarks (such as sternal notch, umbilicus, lateral malleolus), correct medical terminology, and directional terms:

- Anterior (in front)
- Posterior (behind)
- Superior (above)
- Inferior (below)

Wound size should be carefully described through actual measurement rather than association (the size of a dime). Measurements should be done with a disposable ruler in millimeters or centimeters. The current standard for measurement:

$$\text{length} \times \text{width} \times \text{depth} = \text{dimension}$$

However, a clear description requires more detail. The measurement should be done at the greatest width and greatest length. More than two measurements may be needed if the wound is very irregularly shaped. The depth of the wound should be measured by inserting a sterile applicator and grasping or marking the applicator at skin level and then measuring the length below. Ideally, the wound should be photographed as well, following protocols for photography.

WOUND BED TISSUE

Wound bed tissue should be described as completely as possible, including color and general appearance:

- **Granulation tissue** is slightly granular in appearance and deep pink to bright red and moist, bleeding easily if disturbed.
- **Clean non-granular tissue** is smooth and deep pink or red and is not healing.
- **Hypergranulation** is excessive, soft, flaccid granulating tissue that is raised above the level of the periwound tissue, preventing proper epithelization, and may reflect excess moisture in the wound.
- **Epithelization** should appear at wound edges first and then eventually cover the wound. It is dry and light pink or violet in color.
- **Slough** is necrotic tissue that is viscous, soft, and yellow-gray in appearance and adheres to the wound.
- **Eschar** is hard dark brown or black leathery necrotic tissue that accumulates with death of the tissue.

WOUND MARGINS

Wound margins and the tissue surrounding the wound should be described carefully and with correct terminology:

- **Color** should be described using color descriptions and such terms as blanched, erythematous (red), or ecchymosed (purple, green, yellow).
- **Skin texture** may be normal, indurated (hardened), or edematous (swollen). Note if there is cellulitis or maceration evident.
- **Wound edges** may be diffuse (without clear margins), well defined, or rolled. A healing ridge may be evident if granulation has begun. Note if the wound is closed (as with a surgical incision) or open (as with dehiscence or ulcerations). Note if wound edges are attached or unattached (indicating undermining or tunneling).
- **Tunneling or undermining** should be assessed by probing the wound margins with a moist sterile cotton applicator, using clock face locators (toward the head is 12 o'clock, for example). Tunneling may be described as extending from 3 o'clock to 4 o'clock. A large area is usually described as undermining. The size should be measured or estimated as closely as possible.

DISTRIBUTION, DRAINAGE, AND ODOR

Distribution of lesions should be clearly delineated if there is more than one lesion over an area. The arrangement of the lesions can be helpful for diagnosis and treatments.

- Linear (in a line)
- Satellites (small lesions around a larger one)
- Diffuse (scattered freely over an area)

Drainage may vary considerably from nothing at all to copious outpourings of discharge.

- Serous drainage is usually clear to slightly yellow.
- Serosanguineous drainage is a combination of serous drainage and blood.
- Sanguineous drainage is bloody.
- Purulent discharge may be thick and milky, yellow, brownish, or green, depending upon the infective agent.

Odor requires more subjective assessment, but the odor and type of discharge together can provide useful information. Some infective agents, such as *Pseudomonas*, produce distinctive odors, which may be described in various ways: musty, foul, sweet.

Wound Exudate

Wound exudate is fluid found in the wound, consisting of blood serum, debris from cells, bacteria, and white blood cells (leukocytes). **Wound exudate** can occur in small to large amounts and, depending on the presence of an organism, may be colored clear or pale yellow (serous), pink or blood tinged (serosanguineous), red (sanguineous), or white/yellow (purulent pus). Consistency can range from thin to milky to thick, and odor may occur. When fluid covers less than one-third of the dressing, it is termed small in amount. Fluid covering one-third to two-thirds of the dressing is considered moderate, and fluid covering over two-thirds of the surface of the dressing is considered large. The presence of exudate can occur when the wound is left untreated or when venous insufficiency, congestive heart failure, malnutrition, kidney or liver disease, or infection is present. One must remember that some odors may be caused by the reaction of the wound fluid on the dressing. Odor can also be caused when the dressing is not changed often enough.

Wound Measurement

Wound measurement determines the progress of healing and must be done accurately and consistently each time. When the wound is a surgical one, it is sufficient to measure length and width, but depth is important for pressure injuries:

- One should use millimeters or centimeters, not inches, in measurement.
- Linear measurement utilizes a plastic or paper ruler marked in centimeters, measuring the greatest length and the greatest width or making the measurements perpendicular to each other. This is the most common method, but it doesn't take into account the shape of the wound and can overestimate the surface area involved when the measurement is multiplied length by width.
- The outline of the wound may also be traced onto an acetate sheet marked in centimeters and the surface area determined by counting the squares.
- Depth is then determined by inserting a sterile moist cotton applicator into the deepest part of the wound.
- Undermining and tunneling tracts are measured in the same manner.

Measuring Wounds

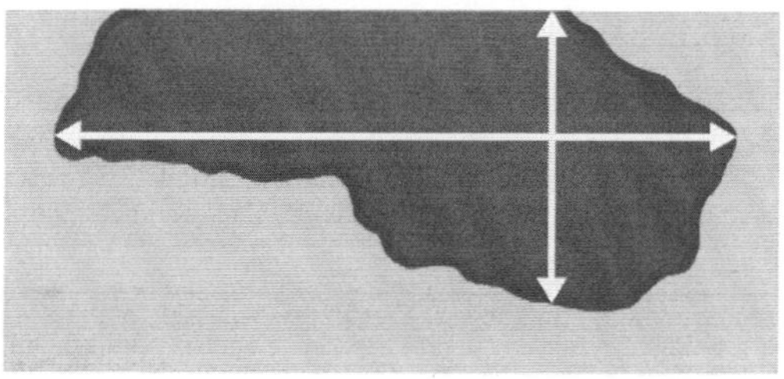

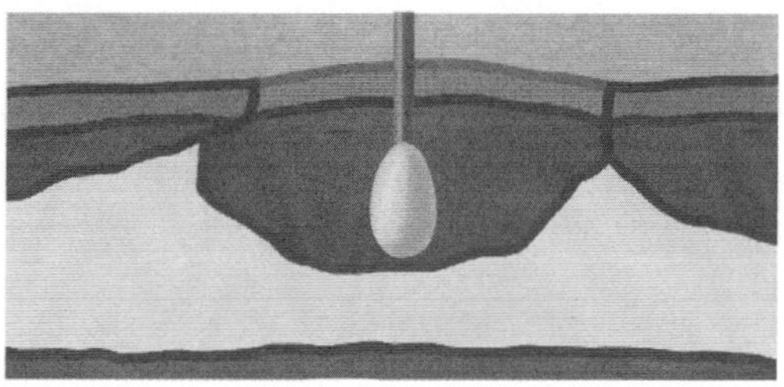

Digital Methods of Wound Measurement

A number of different tools are available for measuring and monitoring wounds using digital equipment. These tools are often more accurate than manual measurements and maintain a historical record that can be easily accessed to track changes. Most tools are software applications that can be loaded onto a smartphone (camera-enabled) or iPad, requiring only that the healthcare provider position the device and take photos. Some programs, such as WoundDesk (Digital

MedLab) are primarily management software to improve documentation, but others, such as Scout (WoundVision) provide visual and infrared imaging and both physical and physiological (blood flow, metabolic activity) monitoring. Another program, WoundZoom, contains a 3D sensor and can provide an image of the wound that includes the length, depth, and breadth. Swift Skin and Wound, a widely-used program, offers a wound management system (Swift App for measurement, Swift HealX to calibrate size, color, lighting, and Swift dashboard to display data) that includes wound measurement, imaging, and tracking.

Assessment of Periwound Environment

The periwound environment includes the area around the wound and is an important part of wound assessment:

- Note signs of inflammation such as warmth, erythema, and edema.
- Palpate the skin for firmness and fluctuation that may indicate a subcutaneous abscess.
- Look for signs of breakdown from tape.
- Observe for signs of pale, moist, soft skin that may be maceration caused by exudate from the wound.
- Check the skin for flakiness or evidence of dryness, as the surrounding skin may be too dry if the dressing wicks the moisture out of the skin.
- Examine the skin for signs of circulatory impairment, such as abnormal hair distribution, rubor, or pallor.
- Note evidence of undermining or tunneling that extends under the tissue.

Documentation of the Wound Assessment

The care provider can use the acronym **ASSESSMENT** to help document the thorough assessment of a wound:

- **A**natomically locate the wound on the body and include the age of the wound
- **S**ize of the wound in centimeters: length, width, and depth, including shape and stage of the wound
- **S**inus tracts, tunneling, fistulas, and undermining at the edges
- **E**xudate color, amount, and consistency
- **S**epsis present in the wound or systemically
- **S**urrounding skin color, edema, status
- **M**argins of the wound, attachment to the wound bed, rolling, presence of maceration
- **E**rythema, presence of epithelialization or eschar
- **N**ecrotic tissue presence, odor of wound, visible blood vessels
- **T**issue of wound bed, amount of granulation present, wound tenderness, tension, and temperature

Assessment Characteristics of Arterial, Neuropathic, and Venous Ulcers

The assessment process is important in delineating between the arterial, neuropathic, or venous origin of the ulcer. Characteristics of each must be known and closely examined:

Location

- **Arterial**: Ends of toes, pressure points, traumatic nonhealing wounds
- **Neuropathic**: Plantar surface, metatarsal heads, toes, and sides of feet
- **Venous**: Between knees and ankles, medial malleolus

Wound Bed

- **Arterial**: Pale, necrotic
- **Neuropathic**: Red (or ischemic)
- **Venous**: Dark red, fibrinous slough

Exudate

- **Arterial**: Slight amount, infection common
- **Neuropathic**: Moderate to large amounts, infection common
- **Venous**: Moderate to large amounts

Wound Perimeter

- **Arterial**: Circular, well-defined
- **Neuropathic**: Circular, well-defined, often with callous formation
- **Venous**: Irregular, poorly-defined

Pain

- **Arterial**: Very painful
- **Neuropathic**: Pain often absent because of reduced sensation
- **Venous**: Pain varies

Skin

- **Arterial**: Pale, friable, shiny, and hairless, with dependent rubor and elevational pallor
- **Neuropathic**: Ischemic signs (as in arterial) may be evident with co-morbidity
- **Venous**: Brownish discoloration of ankles and shin, edema common

Pulses

- **Arterial**: Weak or absent
- **Neuropathic**: Present and palpable, diminished in neuroischemic ulcers
- **Venous**: Present and palpable

ASSESSING FOR WOUND COMPLICATIONS

CHRONIC INFLAMMATION

Chronic inflammation of a wound can last for months, delaying wound healing. The immune system may fail to adequately phagocytose debris and dead tissue in the wound and fight infection, and wound care may be inadequate, such as failure to debride the wound or clear infection. Chronic inflammation is caused by debris, necrotic tissue, repeated injury to the wound, and continued effects of histamine release from mast cells. The blood vessels stay dilated, causing warmth, redness, and swelling. The wound-encircling erythema is a ring of redness in light skin or a ring of darkness in dark skin. Pain may be absent or intense if there is infection or arterial vascular disease present. Necrotic tissue may extend over all or part of the wound bed and may be light or dark in color and hard, soft, or stringy. Exudate may be thick, yellow, brown, or green with an odor. The exudate should be cleansed from the wound so that the odor of the wound bed itself can be determined.

UNDERMINING

Undermining occurs at the edges of a wound and may result from shear injuries. The tissues pull away from the base of the wound and a cavity occurs under the intact skin of the wound periphery. The opening of the wound is thus smaller than the area of tissue damage beneath the surface of the skin surrounding the wound. The degree of undermining should be documented by using the face of the clock to describe the location of the undermining in relation to the opening and by recording the depth of the undermining into surrounding tissues by gently probing with a moist sterile cotton applicator. There are two basic **types of undermining**:

- **Initial**: This is related to discharge of liquefied necrotic tissue, leaving undermining that circles the wound. The wound usually lacks signs of epithelialization.
- **Late**: This is related to external pressure (after discharge undermining), and leaves more localized undermining, often in the direction of a bony prominence. The wound shows signs of epithelialization in non-undermined areas.

Undermining

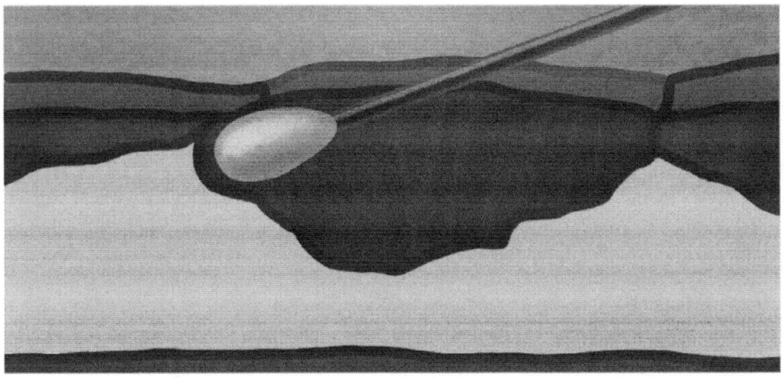

Wound Tunneling

Wound tunneling is a form of undermining that creates a tract that leads away from the wound through subcutaneous tissues between muscles. Tunneling occurs when the fascia that holds muscles together in bundles is cut. Tunneling must be measured with a sterile moist cotton applicator and documented as to depth and width, using the clock face to describe location (3 to 4 o'clock) and then packed loosely to stimulate the healing process. If tunneling ends in a dead space, infection of the wound can progress through the tunnel to cause development of abscess. Tunneling may be caused by infection, pressure that causes tissue necrosis (over bony prominences), or foreign bodies, such as a suture or dressing material left in the wound. It is important for tunnels to heal prior to wound closure to prevent abscess formation, necessitating surgical drainage later. Tunnels are common in surgical wounds in which dehiscence occurs, and the tunnels can join together to form sinus tracts.

Tunneling

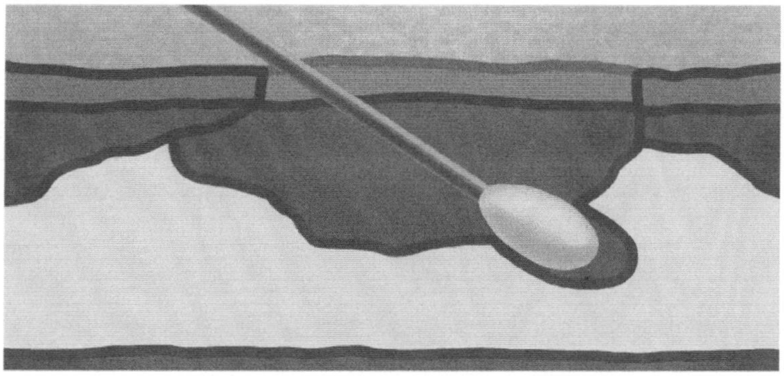

Classification of Wounds by Cause

Wounds can be classified in various ways. The most common classification of wounds is that according to cause:

- **Vascular wounds:** Vascular changes can result in wounds that occur most commonly in the lower extremities, such as those that result from arterial insufficiency and ischemia, those that relate to changes in the lymphatic system, and those related to venous insufficiency.
- **Neuropathic wounds:** Neuropathic changes that occur with chronic diseases, such as diabetes, and chronic alcoholism can decrease sensation and circulation, resulting in ulcerations.
- **Pressure injuries:** Shear friction and pressure, especially over bony prominences such as the sacral area and heels, causes erosion of the tissue.
- **Traumatic wounds:** Trauma often results in contaminated wounds.
- **Surgical wounds:** Surgery can result in wounds that are originally contaminated or originally clean, depending upon the type of surgery and the reason.
- **Infected wounds:** Inflammation and infection may result in deteriorating wounds or fistulas.
- **Self-inflicted wounds:** Vary widely, from minor cuts to traumatic gunshot wounds.
- **Dysfunctional healing wounds:** Hypergranulation/keloid formation can change the character of a wound and prevent adequate healing.

Modified Wagner Ulcer Classification System for Foot Ulcers

The modified Wagner Ulcer Classification System divides foot ulcers into six grades, based on lesion depth, osteomyelitis or gangrene, infection, ischemia, and neuropathy:

- **Grade 0**: At risk but no open ulcers
- **Grade 1**: Superficial ulcer, extending into subcutaneous tissue; superficial infection with or without cellulitis
- **Grade 2**: Full-thickness ulcer to tendon or joint with no abscess or osteomyelitis
- **Grade 3**: Full-thickness ulcer that may extend to bone with abscess, osteomyelitis, or sepsis of joint and may include deep plantar infections, abscesses, fasciitis, or infections of tendon sheath
- **Grade 4**: Gangrene in one area of foot, but the foot is salvageable
- **Grade 5**: Gangrene of entire foot, requiring amputation

While this classification system is useful in predicting outcomes, it does not contain information about the size of the ulcer or the type of infection, so it should be only one part of an assessment, as more detailed information is needed to fully evaluate an ulcer.

University of Texas Diabetic Foot Wound Classification System

The University of Texas created a wound classification system to account for the shortcomings of the Wagner classification system. Although the Wagner system is still used today, it has limitations at predicting outcome after grade 3 and lacks certain aspects of the wound assessment, making it less comprehensive in nature. The University of Texas wound classification system considers the wound's depth and infection status, as well as the presence of peripheral arterial occlusive disease, and evaluates the wound by both grade (0 through 3) and Stage (A, B, C, or D), which are defined as follows:

Stage	Grade 0	Grade 1	Grade 2	Grade 3
A	Lesion (pre- or post-ulcerative) is completely epithelialized	Ulcer is superficial and does not involve tendon or bone	Ulcer penetrates to the tendon	Ulcer penetrates to the bone/joint space
B	Infection present	Infection present	Infection present	Infection present
C	Ischemia present	Ischemia present	Ischemia present	Ischemia present
D	Both infection and ischemia present	Both infection and ischemia present	Both infection and ischemia present	Both infection and ischemia present

S(AD) SAD Classification System

S(AD) SAD stands for Size (Area and Depth), Sepsis, Arteriopathy, and Denervation. The S(AD) SAD classification system for lower-extremity neuropathic disease is one of many that builds upon the original or modified Wagner classification system and assigns a 0-3 grade based on 5 categories: area, depth, sepsis, arteriopathy, and denervation.

- **Grade 0**: No pathology is evident.
- **Grade 1**: Ulcer is <10 mm^2, involving subcutaneous tissue with superficial slough or exudate, diminution or absence of pulses, and reduced sensation.
- **Grade 2**: Ulcer is 10-30 mm^2, extending to tendon, joint, capsule, or periosteum with cellulitis, absence of pulses except for neuropathy dominant ulcers that have palpable pedal pulses.
- **Grade 3**: Ulcer is >30 mm^2, extending to bones and/or joints; seen with osteomyelitis, gangrene, and Charcot's foot.

This grading system is useful, but as with most other classification systems, it doesn't provide a simple way to distinguish those wounds that follow an atypical pattern or may be consistent with the grade in some areas and inconsistent in others.

CEAP Classification for Chronic Venous Disorders

Clinical (C0-C6)

- 0: No apparent venous disease
- 1: Telangiectasia/reticular veins
- 2: Varicose veins
- 3: Edema
- 4: Skin changes
- 5: Healed ulcer
- 6: Active ulcer

Etiologic

- E_C: Congenital
- E_P: Primary
- E_S: Secondary
- E_N: No cause identified

Anatomic distribution

- A_S: Superficial veins
- A_D: Deep veins
- A_P: Perforating veins
- A_N: No location identified

Pathophysiological classification

- P_R: Reflux
- P_O: Obstruction
- $P_{R,O}$: Reflux and obstruction
- P_N: No pathophysiology identified

Staging System for Pressure Injuries

Pressure-related injuries result from pressure with or without shear and/or friction over bony prominences. The National Pressure Injury Advisory Panel developed a staging system to ensure that definitions for pressure injuries were standardized:

- **Suspected deep tissue injury**: Skin discolored, intact or blood blister
- **Stage I**: Intact skin with non-blanching reddened area
- **Stage II**: Abrasion or blistered area without slough but with partial-thickness skin loss
- **Stage III**: Deep tissue injury with exposed subcutaneous tissue; tunneling or undermining may be evident with or without slough or epibole (rolling inward of wound edge)
- **Stage IV**: Deep tissue injury, full thickness, with necrosis into muscle, bone, tendons, and/or joints
- **Unstageable**: Eschar and/or slough prevents staging prior to debridement

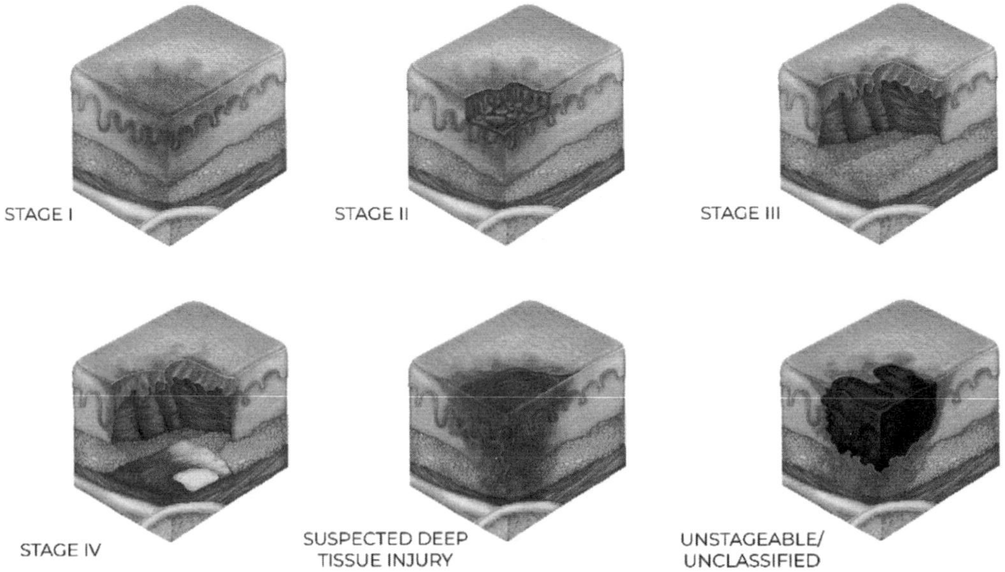

Assessment of Pressure Injuries

When assessing a tissue injury, it is necessary to determine whether it is a pressure injury or non-pressure injury because the treatment protocol may vary depending upon whether the injury is caused by pressure, venous or arterial insufficiency, or neuropathic disorders. The clinical basis for this determination should be clearly outlined.

- The pressure injury should be classified according to the stage and the characteristics, including size (length, width, and depth).
- Pain associated with the pressure injury should be described.
- Photographs should be taken if a protocol is in place.
- Pressure injuries should be monitored daily and any changes carefully documented.
- The injury should be evaluated for signs of infection.

It is important to differentiate between colonization, which is very common, and infection, which usually presents with symptoms such as periwound erythema, induration, and increased pain as well as delayed healing of the wound. Wound culture and blood tests should be done if there are indications of infection. Treatment should be determined according to the characteristics of the wound.

Causes of Pressure Injuries

Pressure Intensity, Pressure Duration, and Tissue Tolerance

Pressure injuries are caused primarily by pressure, but there are numerous additional considerations:

- **Pressure intensity***:* Capillary closing pressure (10–32 mmHg) is the minimal pressure needed to collapse capillaries, reducing tissue perfusion. This pressure can be easily exceeded in the sitting or supine position if weight is not shifted.
- **Duration of pressure**: Low pressure for long periods and high pressure for short periods can both result in pressure injuries.
- **Tissue tolerance***:* The tissue tolerance is the ability of the skin to tolerate and redistribute pressure, preventing anoxia. Both extrinsic and intrinsic factors can affect tissue tolerance. Extrinsic factors include shear (the skin stays in place but the underlying tissue slides), friction (moving the skin against bedding or other objects), and moisture. Intrinsic factors include poor nutrition, advanced age, low blood pressure, stress, smoking, and low body temperature.

Shear and Friction

Shear occurs when the skin stays in place and the underlying tissue in the deep fascia over the bony prominences stretches and slides, damaging vessels and tissue and often resulting in undermining. Shear is one of the most common causes of pressure injuries, which are often described as pressure ulcers but are technically somewhat different, although the effects of shearing are often combined with pressure. The most common cause of shear is elevation of the head of the bed over 30°. Friction against the sheets holds the skin in place while the body slides down the bed, resulting in pressure and damage in the sacrococcygeal area. The underlying vessels are damaged and thrombosed, leading to undermining and deep ulceration.

Friction is a significant cause of pressure injuries because it acts with gravity to cause shear. Friction by itself results only in damage to the epidermis and dermis, such as abrasions or denudement referred to as "sheet burn." Friction and pressure can combine, however, to form tissue injury.

Measures to Control Shear and Friction

Because **shear** and **friction** are primary factors in the development of pressure injuries, measures to reduce them are essential:

- The head of the bed should never be elevated more than 30°; however, bed-bound patients may not be able to feed themselves at this angle. If the bed is elevated higher, the patient should be carefully positioned, using a pull sheet or overhead trapeze to make sure the patient is at the right position. The bed should be lowered as soon as possible.

Note: Elevating the foot of the bed to prevent sliding and shear simply increases pressure to the sacrococcygeal area, solving one problem by creating another.

- Making sure that the skin is dry; using fine cornstarch-based powders may help prevent the skin from "sticking" to the sheets.
- Pull sheets or mechanical lifting devices should be used to lift, move, or transfer the patient.
- Medical treatments may reduce restlessness.
- Heel and elbow protectors provide protection.

Management of Pressure Injuries

Measures to Promote Mobility

Mobility is a problem for many patients with pressure injuries because their restricted mobility is often the cause of the injury in the first place. However, promoting mobility to the extent possible improves circulation, aids healing, and decreases risk of developing further pressure injury:

- Bed-bound patients must be repositioned on a scheduled basis and should receive passive ROM exercises and active bed exercises if tolerated daily. The patient's head should be elevated only to 30° for short periods of time.
- Patients with limited mobility should be evaluated by physical and occupational therapists in order to develop an individualized plan for activities. Patients may need assistive devices, such as walkers, canes, or wheelchairs. Because the wound must be protected without compromise to circulation, the amount and type of mobility or exercises must be designed with respect to the area and stage of the pressure injury as well as underlying pathology or co-morbid conditions.

Measures to Control Fecal Incontinence

Control of fecal incontinence is necessary to prevent deterioration of tissue that can increase the risk of pressure injuries and to prevent contamination of existing pressure injuries:

- Assess incontinence to determine cause and whether it is temporary, related to health problems, or chronic.
- Determine the type of incontinence:
  - Passive, in which the person is unaware.
  - Urge, which is the inability to retain stool.
  - Seepage, after a bowel movement or around a blockage.
- Use medications as indicated to control diarrhea or constipation.
- Place on a bowel-training regimen with scheduled bowel movements, using suppositories, stool softeners, and bulk formers as indicated, according to cause of incontinence. Use skin moisture barriers and absorbent pads or adult briefs as needed.
- Modify diet as needed with foods to control diarrhea or constipation.
- Ensure adequate fluid intake.
- Consider fecal pouches or fecal containment devices if incontinence cannot be otherwise controlled.

Measures to Control Urinary Incontinence

Control of urinary incontinence is necessary to prevent deterioration of the tissue that can increase the risk of pressure injuries:

- Assess incontinence to determine cause and whether it is temporary, related to health problems, or chronic.
- A temporary Foley catheter may be used in some cases while tissue heals, but long-term use is contraindicated because of the danger of infections.
- Medications may be indicated to treat urinary infections or frequency. Scheduled toileting with reinforcement may help to decrease incidence.
- Use absorbent pads or adult briefs that wick liquid away from the body, and establish a regular schedule for changing.
- Cleanse soiled skin with no-rinse wipes, as they are less drying to skin than soap and water.
- Use skin moisture barrier ointments to protect skin from urine.

- Use protective and support devices as needed.
- Avoid positioning on existing pressure injuries.

Tissue Interface Pressures

Tissue interface pressure is the amount of pressure exerted on the body by a surface that the body is lying or sitting on. Small sensors are placed between the patient and the surface to measure pressures in localized areas. The measurement is important to assess whether the pressure is great enough to occlude the capillaries in the area, increasing the risk of tissue ischemia and injury formation. The force that closes capillaries is 12-32 mmHg. This range is used as a comparison along with patient condition, skin condition, nutrition, and other factors to decide whether a support surface relieves enough pressure in a specific location on that particular patient. However, research has not demonstrated that there is a specific threshold at which pressure will cause harm, so the tissue interface pressure should only be used as a guide and not a substitute for observation.

Pressure Injury Prevention

Every patient should be assessed for **risk factors** for pressure injuries. These include immobility, inactivity, moisture and incontinence, poor nutritional state and intake, friction and shear, decreased sensation, mental status changes, fragile skin condition, and certain medications. Tools are available for assessing patient risk for pressure injuries, including the Gosnell Scale and the Braden Scale. Use of these scales provides consistency in assessment from patient to patient and can be used to assess changes in risk level as a result of interventions. Once the risk factors are defined, prevention can concentrate on alleviating these factors. Interventions are designed, and patient and family teaching is performed. Interventions are specific for each patient, disease status, and individual situation. Several solutions for risk factors are possible, and solutions must be individualized for the patient.

Turning and Repositioning to Reduce Pressure

Measures to reduce pressure include turning and repositioning.

- Goals for repositioning and a turning schedule of at least every 2 hours should be established for each individual, with documentation required.
- Devices, such as pillows or foam, should be used to correctly position patients so that bony prominences are protected and not in direct contact with each other.
- Re-position patients carefully to avoid friction or shear.
- Assistive devices should be used if necessary to move patients.
- Use chairs of correct size and height and use pressure relieving devices for the seats.
- Limit chair time for those who are acutely ill to no more than 2 hours.
- Patients should be taught or reminded to redistribute weight every 15 minutes. A timer may be used to remind patients.
- Use the 30° lateral position rather than the 90° side-lying position.

Positioning Strategies in the Bed and Chair

Passive repositioning should be performed on the patient in both the bed and the chair:

- **Bed**: When positioned on his or her side, the patient should be turned to a 30° laterally-inclined position rather than a 90° side-lying position, which puts pressure on the trochanter. Two people should use a turn sheet, draw sheet, and pillows to pull up in bed, turn, and position the patient. Pillows should be placed under the head, under the legs to keep heels off the bed, behind the back, and between the ankles and knees.
- **Chair**: Patients in chairs need repositioning hourly as well. The patient should be assisted to stand and sit down again. Small changes in seated patients include changing leg position from dependent to elevated. The body should be in proper alignment, using pillows or cushions if needed. Patients who are cognizant and able to shift position should be instructed to do so every 15 minutes while seated.

Use of Support Surfaces to Prevent Pressure Injuries

A support surface redistributes pressure to prevent pressure injuries and reduce shear and friction. There are various types of support surfaces for beds, examining tables, operating tables, and chairs. General use guidelines include:

- Pressure redistribution support surfaces should be used in beds, operating tables, and examining tables for at-risk individuals.
- Patients with multiple injuries or with stage II to stage IV injuries require support surfaces.
- Chairs should have gel or air support surfaces to redistribute pressure for chair bound patients, critically ill patients, and those who cannot move independently.
- Support surface material should provide at least an inch of support under areas to be protected when in use to prevent bottoming out. (Check by placing hand palm-up under overlay below the pressure point.)
- Static support surfaces are appropriate for patients who can change position without increasing pressure to an injury.
- Dynamic support surfaces are needed for those who need assistance to move or when static pressure devices provide less than an inch of support.

Categories of Support Surfaces

There are five elements that are used to categorize support surfaces:

- **Pressure redistribution** may be preventive (≤32 mmHg, but not consistently) or therapeutic (≤32 mmHg, consistently). Preventive devices are used for those at risk or with stage I or II injuries. Therapeutic devices are used for those with stage III and IV pressure injuries.
- **Device forms** are varied and may supplement or replace existing equipment. Devices include chair cushions, mattress overlays, pressure-reducing mattresses, and specialty bed systems used in place of traditional hospital beds.
- **Active support surfaces** are powered, requiring attachment to an electrical motor for utilization, (dynamic) or non-powered (static).
- **Medium** may be different types of foam, water, gels, or air.
- **Medicare reimbursement group**:
    - Group 1: Used as a preventive measure and includes overlays and mattresses.
    - Group 2: Used as a therapeutic measure and includes non-powered and powered overlays and mattresses.
    - Group 3: Used as a therapeutic measure and includes air-fluidized beds.

Functions of Support Surfaces

Support surfaces are designed for a number of functions:

- **Pressure redistribution** occurs through *immersion* (spreading the pressure out) and *envelopment* (conforming to shape without increasing pressure). The aim is to reduce pressure on the skin to less than the capillary closing pressure (<32 mmHg), but lower pressures may be necessary for elderly patients. *Interface pressure measurement* is measurement of the pressure exerted between the body and the support surface. This measurement is currently used to evaluate the pressure redistribution efficiency of devices although it has not been demonstrated through research that this measurement can predict clinical performance. Thin, flexible sensors are placed under the support surface and the patient and computerized readings indicate if the support surface is adequate. A number of new measurement devices are now marketed that show colored-coded computerized pictures demonstrating different levels of pressure.
- **Temperature control** is important because temperature increases can lead to skin breakdown. Skin temperature relates to the specific heat of the material in the support surface. Specific heat (the ability to conduct heat) varies considerably from one type of material to another. Air has a low specific heat, and water has a high specific heat. Material with high specific heat may conduct heat away from the body, decreasing skin temperature.
- **Moisture control** prevents moisture damage to skin, but there are wide ranges of materials in use in support surfaces. Some materials, such as rubber or plastic, may increase perspiration and moisture, while some porous materials, such as some foams, may reduce perspiration.
- **Friction/shear control** is more difficult to achieve although some surface coverings, such as those with Gortex, are purposely slick to decrease friction. However, proper positioning, lifting, and repositioning still must be done.

Bacterial, Viral, Fungal, and Parasitic Infections

Viral Infections

Herpes Simplex Virus Infections

There are 2 types of the herpes simplex virus (HSV), human herpesvirus 1 and 2. **HSV-1** usually causes a **gingivostomatitis** (often referred to as "cold sores" or "fever blisters") and is transmitted through **close contact**. **HSV-2** usually causes painful **genital lesions** through **sexual contact**. Either may be found in other areas of the body.

- **Incubation** period is around 2–12 days.
- The primary infection is usually more severe (causes systemic **symptoms**) than the reactivated infection, but it may be asymptomatic. After the primary infection, the virus remains dormant in the nerve ganglia, and can be reactivated especially during times of stress, illness, immunosuppression, or sun exposure. While patients are most contagious during times of active lesions, the disease may be spread while asymptomatic. The frequency of the outbreaks usually decreases over time.
- HSV **lesions** are grouped vesicles with an erythematous base. They are usually painful, and a prodrome of tingling, pain, or burning sensations may be felt hours to a couple days before the eruption. Lesions last for approximately 2–3 weeks in primary infection (up to 4 weeks with genital HSV), and 1–2 weeks in recurrent infections.
- HSV is **diagnosed** clinically and confirmed with a + culture, PCR test, or HSV antibody tests (HSV-1 or HSV-2: IgM= active or recent infection; IgG= previous infection).
- Symptomatic **treatment**, proper wound care, and antivirals (acyclovir, valacyclovir, or famciclovir) may be given.
- **Complications** include perinatal infection, keratitis, herpetic whitlow, herpes gladiatorum, secondary infections, and encephalitis.

Epstein-Barr Infection

Epstein-Barr virus (EBV) is a **herpesvirus** (human herpesvirus 4) and is responsible for causing **infectious mononucleosis**. After the initial infection, it remains latent in B cells and epithelial cells. It has been linked to certain epithelial and lymphatic neoplasms (e.g., nasopharyngeal carcinoma, Burkitt lymphoma, Hodgkin lymphoma).

- EBV is **transmitted** through **body fluids** like saliva, so it is sometimes referred to as the kissing disease. It is most common in teenagers and college-age young adults
- **Incubation** period is typically 30–50 days.
- **Symptoms** of EBV infection range from being asymptomatic to swollen painful lymph nodes, pharyngitis (can mimic strep pharyngitis), extreme fatigue, fever, and possibly hepatosplenomegaly. The WBC count is elevated (~10,000–20,000 cells/mL) with 10–30% atypical lymphocytes in the differential.
- Confirm **diagnosis** with a Mono Spot test or EBV antibody serology tests.
- **Treatment** is supportive, and antibiotics are not helpful in treating this viral infection. Therefore, avoid unnecessary antibiotics in those with EBV, especially since administration of ampicillin or amoxicillin is often associated with a pruritic, maculopapular rash. Analgesics, warm salt water gargles, increased fluid intake, and rest will help to relieve some of the symptoms. Symptoms may last for several weeks and fatigue may last even longer. Patients should avoid contact sports for up to 2 months.
- **Complications** include hepatitis, cytopenias (e.g., thrombocytopenia), Guillain Barré syndrome, and splenic rupture.

Measles, Mumps, and Rubella

Measles (rubeola) virus is highly contagious, is spread through **respiratory secretions** (incubation is 7–14 days), and peaks in late winter to spring. It causes a prodrome of high fever (4–7 days), cough, congestion, conjunctivitis; then Koplik spots (pathognomonic), and finally a maculopapular rash (spreads cephalocaudally). Report suspected cases immediately to the health dept. **Diagnose** with a + IgM antibody test (collected after 3 days of rash), viral culture, or PCR. **Treatment** is supportive.

Mumps (parotitis) is a viral infection that is spread via **saliva** (incubation is 12–24 days), and often occurs during winter and spring. It causes painful swelling of the salivary glands (parotid). Report to health dept. Supportive **treatment**. Complications include orchitis (infertility), pancreatitis, and meningitis.

Rubella (German measles) is a virus that spreads via **respiratory droplets** (incubation is 2–3 weeks), and peaks in the spring. There is a mild prodrome (fever, aches, sore throat, conjunctivitis, swollen nodes [esp. suboccipital, postauricular, & posterior cervical]), then a maculopapular rash (face first, then down). Report to health dept. Confirm with rubella antibodies IgM or IgG. Symptomatic care.

Influenza

Influenza is a highly contagious viral infection that affects the entire **respiratory system** from the nose to the lungs. There are 3 types of **influenza virus**: **A** (causes epidemics), **B** (only in humans), and **C**. Types A and B are seen most often and are the strains that the annual flu vaccine is most effective against; and type C is not as common and much less severe.

- Prevention is key and annual, age-appropriate influenza **vaccines** should be given to those ≥6 months; 2 vaccines are required in first-time vaccine patients if 6 mo. through 8-year-olds (separated by 28 days).
- **Incubation** period is 1–4 days and it is spread via respiratory droplets.
- Though **symptoms** can be very similar, the flu and the common cold differ in that the flu has a very sudden onset. Symptoms of influenza include a high fever (may last up to 5 days), headache, myalgias, dry cough, rhinorrhea, and fatigue. There may also be vomiting and diarrhea, although children are more prone to this.
- Clinical judgment, community patterns, and rapid influenza tests (high specificity, but lower sensitivity) aid in **diagnosis**, but RT-PCR or viral culture definitively confirm the diagnosis; pulse oximetry and CXR as needed for pulmonary issues.
- Antibiotic **treatment** is not effective unless there is a secondary bacterial infection (e.g., pneumonia). Look for signs of secondary infections (e.g., dyspnea, cyanosis, fever that goes away and returns, confusion/lethargy). Supportive treatment with rest, fluids, and analgesics. Antivirals should be considered in those who are at high risk (<5 years old, elderly, pregnant, chronic conditions). These are most effective if initiated within 24–48 hours of symptom onset. The neuraminidase inhibitors (oseltamivir, zanamivir) treat type A, type B, and avian H5N1. There is extensive resistance to the adamantanes (amantadine, rimantadine) so they are rarely used.
- **Complications** include pneumonia, ARDS, and death.

CORONAVIRUS

A coronavirus is a common virus that causes cold-like symptoms, including a cough, runny nose, sore throat, and congestion. Most cases of coronavirus are not dangerous and are often given little attention or go entirely unnoticed. However, specific coronavirus strains have led to two worldwide pandemics. The first, **severe acute respiratory syndrome (SARS)**, appeared in China in 2002 and quickly spread worldwide. Presenting symptoms of SARS were fever, cough, dyspnea, and general malaise. It was extremely virulent, spreading easily from person to person through close contact by way of contaminated droplets produced by coughing or sneezing. SARS was also very deadly, with a case fatality rate of nearly 10%. High rates of infection occurred in health care workers and others in contact with infected patients, so prompt diagnosis and proper isolation were essential. By 2004, there were no longer any documented active cases of SARS.

The most recent coronavirus outbreak was the **COVID-19** strain, which first appeared in China in 2019 and quickly became a global pandemic. Presentation of COVID-19 was similar to that of SARS, with the notable additional symptom of acute loss of taste/smell as a unique identifier.

Precautions to take when treating patients with COVID-19 include the following:

- Contact and droplet precautions, including eye protection and appropriate personal protection equipment.
- Airborne precautions (recommended by the CDC), especially with aerosol-producing procedures (ventilators, nebulizers, intubation).
- Activity restrictions of exposed health care workers planned in coordination with public health officials.

CYTOMEGALOVIRUS

Cytomegalovirus (CMV) is a herpes virus, occurring in most people by the time they are adults.

- **Transmission** can occur through secretions during personal contact and from mother to baby before, during or after birth.
- Most cases have no **symptoms**, although a few infants will have fetal damage, such as jaundice, hepatitis, brain damage, or growth retardation.
- **Treatment** for those with severe infections is with ganciclovir, an antiviral drug.

RESPIRATORY SYNCYTIAL VIRUS

Respiratory syncytial virus (RSV) is a virus that infects the respiratory tract, causing symptoms of nasal congestion, cough, sore throat, and headache. Severe cases can lead to high fever, breathing difficulties, severe cough, and cyanosis.

- Respiratory syncytial virus may **manifest** as a cold in adults and older children; however, there are some children who are more at risk of developing complications.
- **Transmission** is through contact with droplets from an infected person's nose or throat, generally through coughing and sneezing.
- Infants born prematurely, children with chronic lung disease, children with cystic fibrosis, and children who are in an immunocompromised state because of surgery or illness are at **high risk** of breathing difficulties, poor oxygenation, and even death from RSV.

Vaccination for RSV is now recommended for at-risk populations, including pregnant women, infants who are less than 8 months old and entering into season of high RSV spread (fall to spring), adults ages 60–74 with increased risk for complications, and all adults ages 75 and older. Vaccination may not prevent the disease, but will lessen its severity.

Fifth Disease

Fifth disease, or **erythema infectiosum**, is a viral illness caused by parvovirus B19. It is most prevalent in the spring, with outbreaks in preschools, daycares, and elementary schools.

- The **incubation** period is 4-20 days, and it may be communicable for several days before the rash appears.
- **Transmission** occurs through oral and nasal secretions and possibly blood.
- **Symptoms** are possible fever, headache, nasal congestion, general unwell feeling, and rash starting on the cheeks (slapped cheek appearance). The rash typically spreads to the rest of the body as a lacy red rash that may come and go for up to a month.
- Use over-the-counter fever medications as needed and provide **supportive care**.
- The virus can cause fetal death if contracted during pregnancy. There is no vaccine for fifth disease, and because it is a viral infection, it is not treated with antibiotics.

Chickenpox

Chickenpox (Varicella) is a viral infection, most prevalent in the late winter and early spring in children under 10 years of age.

- It has an **incubation** period of 10-21 days and is communicable from 1-2 days before the rash appears to after all lesions have dried up.
- **Transmission** is through direct contact and contact with respiratory droplets.
- **Symptoms** are low fever and feeling unwell, followed by the itchy rash (raised red bumps that develop vesicles which then ooze and crust over).
- The patient should be isolated until all lesions are dry. Aveeno baths and Benadryl help with the itching. Ibuprofen or acetaminophen can be used for the fever, and acyclovir is indicated in some cases. Encourage the patient not to scratch the lesions to prevent secondary infections. Provide supportive care as indicated.

Roseola

Roseola is a viral illness, most prevalent in children 6-24 months of age.

- The **incubation** period is about 9 days.
- **Transmission** may be through oral and nasal.
- The illness begins with a high fever for 3-5 days; the patient appears well otherwise. The fever drops and then the rash appears. The rash is a light pink maculopapular rash which lasts 1-2 days.
- Parents should **treat the fever** as needed with anti-inflammatory medications.

Poliomyelitis

Poliomyelitis (commonly referred to as **polio**) is caused by an enterovirus and occurs most often in babies and young children.

- The **incubation** period is 3-14 days, and transmission occurs through direct contact with respiratory secretions and the oral-fecal route.
- The **symptoms** are slight fever, sore throat, general malaise, nausea and vomiting, headache, stomach ache, and constipation, but there can be severe pain, muscular weakness, and then paralysis.
- There are no drug therapies for polio. Observe for respiratory distress, provide general support measures, and provide for physical therapy.

Rotavirus

Rotavirus is a viral illness that causes diarrhea, fever, and vomiting in children.

- It can be extremely **contagious** within groups where large numbers of children are present, such as in daycare centers, preschools, pediatric offices, clinics, and children's units in hospitals.
- Rotavirus can be prevented through **immunization** with a vaccine, as recommended by the American Academy of Pediatrics. Immunization can prevent up to 98% of severe cases of the illness.
- Children should wash their hands before eating and after using the bathroom to avoid spreading the disease. Caregivers should wash their hands before preparing food, after changing diapers, and after using the bathroom; they should avoid letting small children place toys or other items in their mouths and should disinfect surfaces after use.

Bacterial Infections

Diphtheria

Diphtheria, caused by ***Corynebacterium diphtheriae***, is most prevalent in fall and winter.

- The **incubation** period is 2–7 days, possibly longer, and transmission is through direct contact with nasal, eye, and oral secretions.
- The **symptoms** are slight fever, nasal discharge, sore throat, feeling unwell, poor appetite, and swelling of the airway.
- If the disease is severe, death can result. The patient requires isolation, bed rest, fluids, antibiotics, medication for fever, and an antitoxin. The patient may also require oxygen therapy and tracheostomy if the airway is obstructed.

Tetanus

Tetanus, caused by ***Clostridium tetani***, occurs all over the world. The spores formed by the bacillus are present in soil, dust, and the GI tracts of animals and humans.

- The **incubation** period is 3–21 days.
- **Symptoms** start with headache, irritability, jaw muscle spasms, and inability to open the mouth. This is followed by severe back muscle spasms, seizures, incontinence, and fever.
- **Treatment** requires human tetanus immune globulin, penicillin G, Valium, and placement on a ventilator. The environment should be kept quiet because the spasms are initiated by stimuli.

Scarlet Fever

Scarlet fever, caused by **group A beta-hemolytic streptococci**, is most prevalent in school-age children during the fall, winter, and spring.

- The **incubation** period is 1-7 days, and transmission occurs through direct or indirect contact with oral and nasal secretions.
- The illness begins with a high fever, very sore throat, headache, malaise, chills and possibly vomiting and stomach pain. A rash appears in about 12 hours as sandpapery red pinpoints in creases of the skin, flushed face and then a strawberry tongue.
- Antibiotics will be prescribed, but patients should be isolated until taking the antibiotic for 24 hours. Analgesics are needed to bring down the fever and the patient should be encouraged to drink plenty of fluids.

Whooping Cough

Whooping cough, caused by ***Bordetella pertussis* bacillus**, is most prevalent in infants and children who were not immunized.

- The **incubation** period is 6-20 days, and transmission occurs through direct contact with oral and nasal secretions.
- The **symptoms** are cold symptoms for 1-2 weeks, when the cough will worsen and progress to a whoop sound, usually occurring at night. Vomiting will usually follow an episode of intense coughing. As the patient recovers, the coughing will subside. In babies, a mucus plug or apnea can result in death by respiratory arrest. Hospitalization is usually required for infants less than 6 months of age and those with a severe case of pertussis.
- The patient needs isolation and bed rest, with a calm, quiet environment to limit coughing spells. Fluid intake needs to be monitored and humidified air will help.
- Watch for signs of respiratory distress and give antibiotic and pertussis immune globulin as prescribed.

Impetigo

Impetigo is a skin infection that is most commonly seen in preschool children or those in young childhood.

- Impetigo causes blister-like sores on skin areas that may already be compromised, such as under the nose, on the hands or neck, or in the diaper area. It is caused by a bacterial infection, most commonly *Staphylococcus aureus* or group A *Streptococcus*. The sores may itch or the patient may already have irritation at the site, such as a diaper rash.
- To **prevent the spread of infection**, children and caregivers should wash their hands frequently and avoid scratching the sores and then touching items. Isolation by staying home from school or daycare may be necessary until the sores have crusted over. Treating skin irritations, such as poison ivy or eczema, can also prevent infection from spreading to impetigo.

Fungal Infections

Cryptococcosis

Cryptococcosis is an infection resulting from inhaling the **fungus** *Cryptococcus neoformans,* which is found worldwide in soil (can be associated with bird droppings), or *Cryptococcus gattii,* which is associated with certain trees in the Northwest.

- Cryptococcosis is most often due to *C. neoformans*. It is often found among those with compromised immune systems and is an **AIDS-defining opportunistic infection**.
- Healthy patients may be asymptomatic and the only finding may be pulmonary lesions on CXR that resolve spontaneously. The fungus can disseminate and cause meningitis, encephalitis, cutaneous lesions, and affect long bones and other tissues. **Symptoms** are based on the area of involvement. Patients may experience cough, pleuritic chest pain, weight loss, and fever if there is pulmonary involvement; headache, double vision, light sensitivity, N/V, and confusion if CNS involvement; cutaneous lesions (papules, pustules, nodules, ulcers) if the skin is involved.
- **Diagnosis** includes microscopic analysis, culture (gold standard), or an antigen test (highly sensitive; good for detecting early infection) for *Cryptococcus* using CSF, tissue, sputum, blood, or urine. Check CSF by India ink (limited sensitivity) or culture so meningitis can be ruled out. Confirm that no mass lesion is present by CT or MRI before LP is performed.

- Mild cases may only require monitoring to ensure that the infection does not spread. In more advanced cases, the infection is treated with different antifungal medications (e.g., fluconazole for pulmonary infections, amphotericin B ± flucytosine for meningitis). The patient should also be monitored for CNS infection and medication side effects. AIDS patients may need lifelong antifungals.
- **Complications** include cryptococcal meningitis, neural deficits, optic nerve damage, and hydrocephalus.

HISTOPLASMOSIS

Histoplasmosis is an infection caused by inhalation of **spores** from the fungus *Histoplasma capsulatum* that is found in soil and is associated with bird and bat droppings (e.g., chicken coops, caves).

- Healthy patients are usually asymptomatic and those with symptoms are typically immunocompromised or those who've had a heavy exposure to spores. The primary **pulmonary infection** occurs 3–17 days after exposure and can present with flu-like symptoms. It is typically self-limited but may become chronic. Histoplasmosis can also spread through the **blood** and can cause progressive disseminated disease in the immunocompromised (high mortality rate); this is an **AIDS-defining illness**.
- **Diagnose** through antigen tests (urine, serum), histopathology, or cultures; order a CXR. Mild and even moderate acute pulmonary histoplasmosis may resolve on its own.
- If needed, **treat** mild to moderate infections with itraconazole and severe illness with amphotericin B.

PNEUMOCYSTIS

Pneumocystis jiroveci is a **fungus** (previously known as *Pneumocystis* carinii) that causes **pneumonia** (PJP, previously PCP) in the immunocompromised. Most people have been exposed to this by the age of 3 or 4.

- **Symptoms** of PJP include a dry nonproductive cough, fever, dyspnea, and weight loss.
- CXR may show diffuse bilateral infiltrates or it may be normal; and pulse oximetry may be low, especially on exertion. **Diagnosis** is confirmed with sputum histopathology using sputum induction or bronchoalveolar lavage.
- **Treat** immediately with TMP-SMX (trimethoprim/sulfamethoxazole) for 21 days if HIV + and for 14 days in other cases. Steroids may be added for HIV patients with severe PJP. HIV/AIDS patients with CD4 counts <200/μL should receive PJP prophylaxis with TMP-SMX. Dapsone and pentamidine are alternatives.
- **Complications** include ARDS and death.

CANDIDAL INFECTIONS

Candida is a type of yeast that may cause a variety of infections:

- **Oral thrush** is commonly seen in diabetic patients and those who are immunosuppressed (HIV or underlying neoplasm). Patients often complain of burning on the tongue or in the mouth, associated with "curd-like" white patches that can be scraped away leaving reddish tissue underneath. Diagnosis is with KOH prep. Treatment is with oral or topical antifungals, including nystatin (swish and swallow or troches).
- **Candida esophagitis** also occurs in the immunosuppressed population, and patients may complain of dysphasia, odynophagia, and chest pain. This is diagnosed on EGD and may be treated with oral or IV antifungals (ketoconazole).

- **Candidal intertrigo**, or diaper rash, presents with beefy-red lesions at skin fold areas as well as satellite lesions. Treatment is with topical antifungals.
- **Candidemia** is diagnosed with fungal blood cultures and may lead to osteomyelitis, endocarditis, and other complications. Treatment is with IV antifungals.

Ringworm

Ringworm is caused by an infection from the ***Tinea* fungus**, which produces patches on the skin that have normal centers, giving the appearance of a ring.

- The fungus can cause hair loss and patches of scaly skin that may develop blisters that ooze or crust.
- It is **transmitted** by touching the affected skin or through objects that have touched the affected skin.
- Ringworm may be **diagnosed** by viewing the skin section under a Wood's lamp. Skin cultures may also be taken for examination to identify the fungus. A potassium hydroxide (KOH) exam involves scraping the affected skin and placing the skin sample in KOH to test for the presence of the fungus.

Vector-Borne and Parasitic Infections

Malaria

Malaria is a **blood-borne disease** caused by a **parasite** from the genus *Plasmodium and* found in tropical areas. There are 4 known to cause disease in humans (*P. malariae*, *P. vivax*, *P. ovale*, and *P. falciparum*). These protozoa are transmitted by the **female *Anopheles* mosquito**. They travel to the **liver** where they multiply, are released, and then infect the RBCs, where they continue to multiply. Incubation time can be as little as 9 days or as much as multiple years depending on the species of the infecting parasite.

- **Signs/symptoms** include headache, high fever with shaking chills and sweating (rigors; occurs when merozoites, an immature form of the parasite, are released from RBCs), jaundice, anemia, and hepatosplenomegaly. Take a thorough history including recent travel.
- **Diagnose** with 3 thin and thick blood smears (gold standard) stained with Giemsa (preferred) and obtained 12–24 hours apart. Labs typically show elevated LDH, thrombocytopenia, and atypical lymphocytes. Rapid antigen tests are also available as well as PCR.
- **Treat** with chloroquine. If travelling, chemoprophylaxis depends on the area of travel due to species and resistance patterns, and may include chloroquine, primaquine, mefloquine, Malarone, or doxycycline. Report infections to your local or state health department.
- **Complications** include severe anemia and hemolysis, organ failure (liver, spleen, kidneys), cerebral malaria, ARDS, and death.

Lyme Disease

Lyme disease occurs from a bite from a **deer tick** (blacklegged tick) infected with the **spirochete bacterium** *Borrelia burgdorferi*. It is the most common tick-borne disease in the U.S. and is more prevalent in heavily wooded areas. Adult ticks are more active during colder times whereas the nymphs (<2 mm in size) are more active in the warm, spring or summer months. Once the tick bites, it stays attached; however, it takes about 36–48 hours for nymphs and about 48–72 hours for adult ticks before the spirochete is transmitted to the person. **Incubation** period is 3–30 days. There are 3 stages to this disease: early localized, early disseminated, and chronic disseminated.

- At **Stage 1**, 75% have the characteristic expanding red rash (erythema migrans; can be large, ~30cm) which can progress to have central clearing (bull's eye), headache, fever, chills, myalgias, and fatigue.
- **Stage 2** occurs weeks to months after initial infection and involves systemic symptoms (flu-like), neck stiffness, headaches, migrating pain in muscles and joints, rashes, paresthesias, Bell's palsy, confusion, fatigue, myocarditis, and heart palpitations.
- **Stage 3** occurs months to years after initial infection and involves neurologic (e.g., encephalitis) and rheumatologic issues, especially arthritis of large joints (e.g., knee).

Review Video: Lyme Disease
Visit mometrix.com/academy and enter code: 505529

Diagnosis and Treatment of Lyme Disease

Diagnose Lyme disease using 2-tiered testing: antibodies (IgM, IgG), then Western blot. Antibiotic treatment for localized Lyme disease involves 2–3 weeks of doxycycline, amoxicillin, or cefuroxime axetil is started immediately after diagnosis. IV antibiotics may be needed for severe disease (e.g., IV ceftriaxone). Prevention is key by wearing clothes covering the skin, using tick repellents, showering soon after being outdoors in tick-prone areas, and thoroughly checking for ticks (especially in hard to see areas by using a mirror). The Lyme vaccine is no longer available and previous vaccine recipients are still at risk of contracting the disease as protection decreases over time. Complications are prevalent with untreated Lyme disease and include chronic arthritis, fatigue, chronic musculoskeletal issues, acrodermatitis chronica atrophicans, and memory and concentration issues. Report cases to the local health dept.

Rocky Mountain Spotted Fever

Rocky Mountain spotted fever is a tick-borne illness caused by **Rickettsia rickettsii**. It tends to occur in spring and summer throughout the United States.

- **Incubation** period is about one week.
- **Symptoms** include headache, fever, nausea, vomiting, loss of appetite, muscle pain, and rash on the ankles and wrists.
- **Treatment** requires an antibiotic, usually doxycycline.

Zika Virus in Pregnant Women

Zika virus is a **flavivirus** that is transmitted by the *Aedes* mosquito and through sexual contact. This virus can be passed on to an unborn baby causing severe congenital defects while causing mild or no disease in the mother. It is advised that all pregnant women avoid traveling to areas with the Zika virus (e.g., Central and South America, Mexico, Caribbean, Africa).

- **Incubation** period is 3–14 days and symptoms may last 4–7 days. The virus has been found to remain longer in semen than in other body fluids.
- If **symptoms** are present, they may include fever, headache, myalgias, arthralgias, a maculopapular rash, and conjunctivitis. Congenital defects include severe microcephaly, severe brain abnormalities, macular scarring, hearing loss, motor disabilities (e.g., hypertonia), and contractures. Women should be screened for Zika exposure at each prenatal visit.
- **Diagnostic** testing is recommended for all asymptomatic pregnant women who have continued exposure to Zika and for all symptomatic pregnant women who have possibly been exposed to the Zika virus. Testing includes RNA NAT testing on serum and urine, and serum IgM Zika antibody testing. Prenatal ultrasound helps determine if the effects of Zika are present. Report cases to the state health department; and the CDC can be consulted.
- There is **no treatment** or cure for the Zika virus.

Helminth Infestations

Helminth infestations (worms) include **roundworms** [nematodes: *Ascaris*, hookworms (cause anemia), **filariae** (cause elephantiasis)] and **flatworms** [tapeworms (cause weight loss); **flukes** (intestinal or liver)]. **Pinworms** are a type of roundworm that cause enterobiasis and is the most common helminth infestation. Pinworms are more prevalent in warmer areas of the country and infestations occur more frequently in children. The worms lay eggs within the digestive tract and then travel to the anal area where they are usually found. Pinworms are highly contagious. As a patient itches the anal area where the eggs are located, the eggs cling to the fingers and can easily be transmitted to other people either directly or through food or surfaces. The eggs can survive for 2–3 weeks on inanimate objects.

- Patients may be asymptomatic or have intense anal itching that is usually worse at night and can cause insomnia. Abdominal pain, nausea, and vomiting can also occur.
- **Diagnose** with the "tape test" which involves pressing cellophane tape over the perianal area to pick up eggs or worms and examine under the microscope. Most other helminth infestations can be diagnosed with a stool sample for ova and parasites; filariasis requires a blood smear or antigen test.
- Anthelmintic medications are given in a single dose and repeated in 2 weeks to kill the pinworms and their larvae (mebendazole, albendazole, or pyrantel pamoate). The entire family and close contacts should be treated simultaneously since pinworms are so contagious.

Giardia Lamblia

Giardia lamblia is a **protozoan** that infects water supplies and spreads to children through the fecal-oral route. It is the most common cause of non-bacterial diarrhea in the United States, causing about 20,000 cases of infection each year in all ages.

- Children often become infected after swallowing recreational waters (pools, lakes) while swimming or putting contaminated items into the mouth. *Giardia* live and multiply within the small intestine where cysts develop.
- **Symptoms** occur 7–14 days after ingestion of 1 or more cysts and include diarrhea with greasy floating stools (rarely bloody), stomach cramps, nausea, and flatulence, lasting 2–6 weeks. A chronic infection may develop that can last for months or years.
- **Treatment** includes furazolidone 5–8 mg/kg/day in 4 doses for 7–10 days or metronidazole 40 mg/kg/day in 3 doses for 7–10 days. Chronic infections are often very resistant to treatment.

Toxoplasmosis

Toxoplasmosis is an infection caused by the **parasite *Toxoplasma gondii***, which is commonly found in soil. It is widespread and transmitted through cat feces; however, it also may be contracted by eating undercooked meat (especially pork, lamb, or venison) or poorly washed vegetables. Toxoplasmosis can cause serious disease and can affect various organs; and immunocompromised and pregnant women and their unborn babies are especially likely to have side effects of the disease (the "T" in congenital TORCH infections).

- Healthy patients are usually asymptomatic; however, once infected the parasite can remain latent until the patient becomes immunocompromised and the parasite is reactivated causing **symptoms**. The disease can cause a flu-like illness with fever, myalgias, and lymphadenopathy. More serious effects include retinochoroiditis, brain lesions, and encephalitis. Congenital toxoplasmosis may cause retinochoroiditis, microcephaly, hydrocephalus, intellectual disability, and possibly miscarriage or stillbirth.
- **Diagnose** with serology for *Toxoplasma* antibodies IgM and IgG. Also, PCR may be used to test amniotic fluid, CSF, or tissue.
- **Treat** with pyrimethamine (preferred) plus folinic acid or sulfadiazine plus folinic acid. Pregnant women should avoid high-risk practices like changing the cat litter and should avoid sand boxes.

Fluid Imbalances

Fluid Shifts Associated with Cardiac Surgery

Fluid shifts between spaces are controlled by differences in hydrostatic and colloid osmotic pressure (COP). While water usually moves freely among intracellular, intravascular, and interstitial spaces, sodium moves freely only between the intravascular and interstitial spaces and does not move passively into the intracellular spaces unless serum osmolality and sodium concentration decrease, pulling fluid into the intracellular space. Cardiac surgery results in decreased COP by increasing capillary permeability, shifting fluid from intravascular to interstitial spaces. Cardiopulmonary bypass (CPB) results in a 20–30% increase in extracellular volume and increased sodium retention and potassium excretion. Each hour of CPB results in 800 mL fluid buildup; a 50% decrease is COP. Low levels of serum sodium postoperatively usually indicate total body fluid overload. Increased pulmonary capillary wedge pressure or decreased serum albumin pressures shifts fluid from the intravascular space to the interstitial space, resulting in pulmonary and tissue edema. Extracellular fluid (intravascular serum and interstitial fluid) is more easily lost than intracellular fluid. Electrolyte values reflect plasma levels and indicate the status of extracellular fluid.

Postoperative Fluid Management

Postoperative fluid management after cardiac surgery presents numerous challenges. Cardiopulmonary bypass (CPB) results in total body fluid and sodium overload, causing increased weight. This is not reflected in cardiac filling pressures because of capillary leak, decreased plasma and colloid osmotic pressure, and impaired myocardial function. Despite fluid overload, low-filling pressures are common with hypovolemia. Fluid administration is usually indicated to maintain intravascular volumes and adequate hemodynamics. Blood products and colloids are more effective in expanding intravascular volume than hypotonic solutions or crystalloids. If patients are well oxygenated, up to 1 L of crystalloid may be administered, followed by colloids if the response is not adequate. Colloids may include 5% albumin, which has less effect on coagulation than hydroxyethyl starches. Colloids with 5% albumin may increase interstitial fluid and cause decreased intracellular fluid. Hypertonic 25% albumin solutions reduce the amount of fluid necessary. Hydroxyethyl starch preparations are excellent volume expanders but may have adverse effects on renal function. Hypertonic saline solutions (3%) can increase intravascular volume but may cause hypernatremia.

Colloids

Colloids are solutions (usually isotonic saline but available with glucose and in hypertonic solutions) with dissolved, high-molecular-weight (large), non-crystalline molecules and electrolytes. Colloids stay in the intravascular space more readily than crystalloids, so they are effective volume expanders. They are used primarily for fluid replacement with severe intravascular deficits, such as from hemorrhage and in conditions with severe hypoalbuminemia or where protein loss is probable, such as severe burns. Colloids are derived from plasma proteins or synthetic glucose polymers. Colloids obtained from plasma contain albumin (5% or 25% solutions) and plasma protein fractions (5%). Jehovah's Witnesses may object to receiving these solutions. Colloids obtained from synthetic glucose contain hydroxyethyl starches and gelatin. Colloids have more safety concerns than crystalloids. Allergic reactions (including anaphylaxis) may be caused by dextran, hydroxyethyl, and (to a lesser degree) albumin. Bleeding may also result from a reduction in platelet aggregation, factor VII, von Willebrand factor, and prolonged partial thromboplastin time, so colloids should be avoided in patients with coagulopathies.

Crystalloid Solutions

Both colloids and crystalloid solutions (or a combination) are used as intravenous fluid therapy during surgery. Crystalloids are solutions of inorganic small molecules, glucose, or saline, dissolved in water. There are many **types of crystalloid solutions**:

- **Hypotonic solutions** are maintenance solutions used to replace water loss. Dextrose in water (D5W) is commonly used when patients have a water deficit and for those with sodium restriction.
- **Hypertonic solutions** are used for hyponatremia (3% saline) and severe hypovolemic shock (3–7.5% saline).
- **Isotonic solutions** are replacement solutions for loss of water and electrolytes. Isotonic crystalloids, such as normal saline (0.9%), Ringer's lactate (contains potassium), and Plasmalyte (contains potassium) are most commonly used. Different solutions contain different electrolytes (e.g., sodium, chloride, potassium, calcium, lactate, magnesium), so monitoring electrolytes is essential.

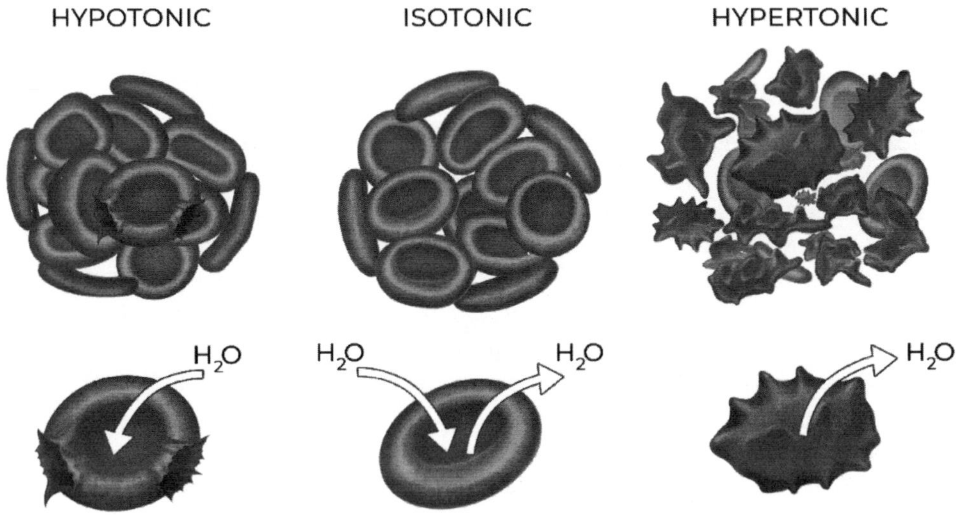

Crystalloids are effective in restoring fluid volume, but blood replacement requires 3:1 administration of crystalloids, while colloids are 1:1 replacement, and rapid crystalloid administration may result in tissue edema. Crystalloids are usually given as initial resuscitation fluid in emergencies. Glucose in some solutions may prevent ketosis and hypoglycemia.

Hypertonic Saline Solution

Hypertonic saline solution (HSS) has a sodium concentration higher than 0.9% (normal saline) and is used to reduce intracranial pressure/cerebral edema. Concentrations usually range from 2–23%, but 3% solutions may be used with cardiac surgery patients to treat total body fluid overload. HSS draws fluid from the tissue through osmosis. As edema decreases, circulation improves. HSS also expands plasma, increasing cerebral perfusion pressure, and counteracts hyponatremia that can occur in the brain after injury, causing increased intracranial pressure. Peripheral administration can only tolerate a concentration up to 3% of HSS in a large bore (18-gauge) catheter. Higher concentrations of HSS must be administered via central line.

HSS can be administered continuously at rates varying from 30–100 mL/hr. Rates must be carefully controlled. Fluid status must be monitored to prevent hypovolemia, which increases the risk of renal failure. **Laboratory monitoring** includes the following:

- Sodium (every 6 hours) is maintained at 135–155 mmol/L. Higher levels can cause heart, respiratory, and renal failure.
- Serum osmolality (every 12 hours) is maintained at 320 mOsm/L. Higher levels can cause renal failure.

Mannitol

Mannitol is an osmotic diuretic that increases excretion of both sodium and water and reduces intracranial pressure and brain mass. Mannitol may also be used to shrink the cells of the blood–brain barrier to help other medications breach this barrier. Mannitol is administered by intravenous infusion. It may be used during cardiopulmonary bypass to control blood pressure. Additionally, 20% mannitol at 5 mL/kg is given with furosemide, 1 g, and dopamine, 2–3 μg/kg/min, to produce diuresis within 6 hours of onset of oliguria. Fluid and electrolyte balances must be carefully monitored as well as intake, output, and body weight. Concentrations of 20–25% require a filter. Crystals may form if the mannitol solution is too cold, and the mannitol container may require heating (in 80 °C water) and shaking to dissolve crystals; the solution should be cooled to body temperature or less before administration. Mannitol cannot be administered in polyvinylchloride bags as precipitates form. Side effects include fluid and electrolyte imbalance, nausea, vomiting, hypotension, tachycardia, fever, and urticaria.

Intravenous Fluid Warmers

Intravenous fluid warmers warm fluids to body temperature to avoid inducing or worsening hypothermia, especially in geriatric patients. In cases of severe hypothermia, warmed fluids (104–108 °F) may be administered to raise core temperature. Also, medications are absorbed more effectively in warmed fluids. There are numerous types of fluid warmers. Simple warmers warm fluid in the tubing as the tubing passes through the warming device. Some units are disposable and battery powered, some are approved for both blood and fluids, and some units require special tubing or equipment. All must be monitored carefully. Special heating chambers may heat a number of IV fluid bags at one time in a cabinet-type structure. Intraoperative warming of IV fluids may prevent anesthesia-associated hypothermia.

Fluid Resuscitation for Burn Injuries

Burn victims are at risk for hypovolemia and electrolyte imbalances because of loss of body fluids through burned areas. **Fluid resuscitation** is indicated with burns of 20% or more of total body surface area (TBSA) burned. Lactated Ringers IV solution is used instead of NS, which can lead to hypernatremia and hyperchloremia. The Parkland/Baxter formula is used to calculate the volume of LR solution needed:

$$\text{24 hour volume} = (\text{body weight [kg]}) \times (\text{TBSA burned [\%]}) \times (4\text{ mL})$$

Example—70 kg adult with 36% TBSA burned:

$$\text{24 hour volume} = 70 \times 36 \times 4\text{ mL} = 10{,}080\text{ mL}$$

Half of the volume is administered over the first 8 hours and half over the next 16 hours. Using the preceding example, this patient will receive 5,040 mL each over the first 8 hours (rate = (5040/8) = 630 mL/hr), and over the following 16 hours (rate = (5040/16) = 315 mL/hr). Fluid intake should be sufficient to produce 30–50 mL of urine per hour. In the second 24 hours, fluid volume should be 1.5–2.0 times the normal maintenance values with crystalloid with appropriate electrolyte balance.

Maintenance Fluid Requirements and Fluid Replacement

Pediatric fluid deficit must be carefully estimated and managed. Fluid deficit should be replaced over 3 hours with half in the first hour and a quarter in the remaining 2 hours. Preoperative deficits usually are treated with lactated Ringer's or normal saline (which may cause hyperchloremic acidosis). Glucose containing fluids may contribute to hyperglycemia.

Weight in kg	24-hour fluid requirement	Hourly requirement
<10 kg	100 mL/kg	4 mL/kg
10-20 kg	1000 mL and 50 mL/kg for each kg above 10 kg	40 mL and 2 mL/kg for each kg above 10 kg
>20 kg	1500 mL and 20 mL/kg for each kg above 20 kg	60 mL and 1 mL/kg for each kg above 20 kg

Fluid replacement must account for both blood loss and third-space loss: Replacement may be with Lactated Ringers (3 mL per 1 mL blood loss) or 5% albumin colloid (1 mL per 1 mL blood loss) to maintain hematocrit at predetermined adequate minimal level:

- **Infants and neonates**: >30% (may be as high as 40-50%)
- **Older children**: 20-26%

Electrolyte Imbalances

Sodium Imbalance

Sodium (**Na**) regulates fluid volume, osmolality, acid-base balance, and activity in the muscles, nerves, and myocardium. It is the primary **cation** (positive ion) in extracellular fluid (ECF), necessary to maintain ECF levels that are needed for tissue perfusion:

- Normal range: 135–145 mEq/L
- Hyponatremia: <135 mEq/L
- Hypernatremia: >145 mEq/L

Hyponatremia may result from inadequate sodium intake, excess sodium loss through diarrhea, vomiting, or NG suctioning, or illness, such as severe burns, fever, SIADH, and ketoacidosis.

- **Symptoms**: Irritability to lethargy and alterations in consciousness, cerebral edema with seizures and coma, dyspnea to respiratory failure.
- **Treatment**: Identify and treat the underlying cause and provide Na replacement.

Hypernatremia may result from renal disease, diabetes insipidus, and fluid depletion.

- **Symptoms**: Irritability to lethargy to confusion to coma; seizures; flushing; muscle weakness and spasms; thirst.
- **Treatment**: Identify and treat the underlying cause, monitor Na levels carefully, and give IV fluid replacement.

Potassium Imbalance

Potassium (**K**) is the primary **electrolyte** in intracellular fluid (ICF), with about 98% inside cells and only 2% in ECF, although this small amount is important for neuromuscular activity. Potassium influences activity of the skeletal and cardiac muscles. Its level is dependent upon adequate renal functioning because 80% is excreted through the kidneys and 20% through the bowels and sweat:

- Normal range: 3.5–5.5 mEq/L
- Hypokalemia: <3.5 mEq/L. Critical value: <2.5 mEq/L
- Hyperkalemia: >5.5 mEq/L. Critical value: >6.5 mEq/L

A healthy NPO patient will need about 40 mEq of K per day to maintain serum K levels. Expect alterations in renal disease and other disease processes.

Hypokalemia is caused by alkalosis, decreased intake associated with starvation, nephritis, and loss of potassium through diarrhea, vomiting, gastric suction, and diuresis.

- **Symptoms**: Lethargy and weakness; nausea and vomiting; paresthesia and tetany; muscle cramps with hyporeflexia; hypotension; dysrhythmias with EKG changes: PVCs or flattened T-waves.
- **Treatment**: Treatment involves identifying and treating the underlying cause and replacing K. When possible, oral replacement is preferable to IV, as it allows slower adjustment of K levels. When given IV, K should be given no faster than 20 mEq/hour via central line if possible. If given peripherally, 10 mEq/hour is preferable for patient comfort.

Hyperkalemia is caused by renal disease, adrenal insufficiency, metabolic acidosis, severe dehydration, burns, hemolysis, and trauma. It rarely occurs without renal disease but may be induced by treatment (such as NSAIDs and potassium-sparing diuretics). Untreated renal failure results in reduced excretion. Those with Addison disease and deficient adrenal hormones suffer sodium loss that results in potassium retention.

- **Symptoms**: The primary symptoms relate to the effect on the cardiac muscle: ventricular arrhythmias with increasing changes in EKG lead to cardiac and respiratory arrest, weakness with ascending paralysis and hyperreflexia, diarrhea, and increasing confusion.
- **Treatment**: Treatment includes identifying the underlying cause and discontinuing sources of increased K. Calcium gluconate to decrease cardiac effects. Sodium bicarbonate, insulin, and hypertonic dextrose shift K into the cells temporarily. Cation exchange resin (Kayexalate) to decrease K. Peritoneal dialysis or hemodialysis to remove excess K.

Note: When a tourniquet is on, a patient opening and closing their hand can lead to falsely elevated K levels.

Calcium Imbalance

More than 99% of calcium (**Ca**) is in the skeletal system with 1% in serum, but it is important for transmitting nerve impulses and regulating muscle contraction and relaxation, including the myocardium. Calcium activates enzymes that stimulate chemical reactions and has a role in the coagulation of blood:

- Normal range: 8.2–10.2 mg/dL
- Hypocalcemia: <8.2. Critical value: <7 mg/dL
- Hypercalcemia: >10.2 mg/dL. Critical value: >12 mg/dL

Hypercalcemia may be caused by acidosis, kidney disease, hyperparathyroidism, prolonged immobilization, and malignancies. Crisis carries a 50% mortality rate.

- **Symptoms**: Increasing muscle weakness with hypotonicity; anorexia; nausea and vomiting; constipation; bradycardia and cardiac arrest.
- **Treatment**: Identify and treat underlying cause, loop diuretics, IV fluids, phosphate.

Hypocalcemia may be caused by damage to the parathyroid resulting in hypoparathyroidism (directly decreasing calcium production), vitamin D resistance or inadequacy, or liver/kidney disease.

- **Symptoms**: Muscle cramping or spasms; seizures; numbness or tingling of the feet, hands, or lips; tetany if severe.
- **Treatment**: Identify and treat underlying cause, replace calcium by administering IV calcium gluconate in acute circumstances or increasing oral Vitamin D and calcium in chronic cases.

Phosphorus Imbalance

Phosphorus, or phosphate, **(PO_4)** is necessary for neuromuscular and red blood cell function, the maintenance of acid-base balance, and provides structure for teeth and bones. About 85% is in the bones, 14% in soft tissue, and <1% in ECF.

- Normal range: 2.4–4.5 mEq/L
- Hypophosphatemia: <2.4mEq/L
- Hyperphosphatemia: >4.5 mEq/L

Hypophosphatemia occurs with severe protein-calorie malnutrition, hyperventilation, severe burns, diabetic ketoacidosis, and excess antacids with magnesium, calcium, or aluminum.

- **Symptoms**: Irritability, tremors, seizures to coma; hemolytic anemia; decreased myocardial function; respiratory failure.
- **Treatment**: Identify and treat underlying cause and replace phosphorus.

Hyperphosphatemia occurs with renal failure, hypoparathyroidism, excessive intake, neoplastic disease, diabetic ketoacidosis, muscle necrosis, and chemotherapy.

- **Symptoms**: Tachycardia; muscle cramping; hyperreflexia and tetany; nausea and diarrhea.
- **Treatment**: Identify and treat underlying cause, correct hypocalcemia, and provide antacids and dialysis.

Magnesium Imbalance

Magnesium (**Mg**) is the second most common intracellular electrolyte (after potassium) and activates many intracellular enzyme systems. Mg is important for carbohydrate and protein metabolism, neuromuscular function, and cardiovascular function, producing vasodilation and directly affecting the peripheral arterial system:

- Normal range: 1.7–2.2 mg/dL
- Hypomagnesemia critical value: <1.2 mg/dL
- Hypermagnesemia critical value: >4.9 mg/dL

Hypomagnesemia occurs with chronic diarrhea, chronic renal disease, chronic pancreatitis, excess diuretic or laxative use, hyperthyroidism, hypoparathyroidism, severe burns, and diaphoresis.

- **Symptoms**: Neuromuscular excitability or tetany; confusion, headaches, dizziness; seizure and coma; tachycardia with ventricular arrhythmias; respiratory depression.
- **Treatment**: Identify and treat underlying cause, provide magnesium replacement. IV magnesium is a vasodilator, 2 g over 60 mins.

Hypermagnesemia occurs with renal failure or inadequate renal function, diabetic ketoacidosis, hypothyroidism, and Addison disease.

- **Symptoms**: Muscle weakness, seizures, and dysphagia with decreased gag reflex; tachycardia with hypotension.
- **Treatment**: Identify and treat underlying cause, IV hydration with calcium, and dialysis.

Review Video: Fluid and Electrolyte Balance
Visit mometrix.com/academy and enter code: 384389

Metabolic and Respiratory Acidosis

Pathophysiology

- Metabolic acidosis
  - Increase in fixed acid and inability to excrete acid, or loss of base, with compensatory increase of CO_2 excretion by lungs
- Respiratory acidosis
  - Hypoventilation and CO_2 retention with renal compensatory retention of bicarbonate (HCO_3) and increased excretion of hydrogen

Laboratory

- Metabolic acidosis
  - Decreased serum pH (<7.35) and PCO_2 normal if uncompensated and decreased if compensated
  - Decreased HCO_3
- Respiratory acidosis
  - Decreased serum pH (< 7.35) and increased PCO_2
  - Increased HCO_3 if compensated and normal if uncompensated

Causes

- Metabolic acidosis
  - DKA, lactic acidosis, diarrhea, starvation, renal failure, shock, renal tubular acidosis, starvation
- Respiratory acidosis
  - COPD, overdose of sedative or barbiturate (leading to hypoventilation), obesity, severe pneumonia/atelectasis, muscle weakness (Guillain-Barré), mechanical hypoventilation

Symptoms

- Metabolic acidosis
  - Neuro/muscular: Drowsiness, confusion, headache, coma
  - Cardiac: Decreased BP, arrhythmias, flushed skin
  - GI: Nausea, vomiting, abdominal pain, diarrhea
  - Respiratory: Deep inspired tachypnea
- Respiratory acidosis
  - Neuro/muscular: Drowsiness, dizziness, headache, coma, disorientation, seizures
  - Cardiac: Flushed skin, VF, ↓BP
  - GI: Absent
  - Respiratory: Hypoventilation with hypoxia

Metabolic and Respiratory Alkalosis

Pathophysiology

- Metabolic alkalosis
  - Decreased strong acid or increased base with possible compensatory CO_2 retention by lungs
- Respiratory alkalosis
  - Hyperventilation and increased excretion of CO_2 with compensatory HCO_3 excretion by kidneys

Laboratory

- Metabolic alkalosis
  - Increased serum pH (>7.45)
  - PCO_2 normal if uncompensated and increased if compensated
  - Increased HCO_3
- Respiratory alkalosis
  - Increased serum pH (>7.45)
  - Decreased PCO_2
  - HCO_3 normal if uncompensated and decreased if compensated

Causes

- Metabolic alkalosis
  - Excessive vomiting, gastric suctioning, diuretics, potassium deficit, excessive mineralocorticoids and $NaHCO_3$ intake
- Respiratory alkalosis
  - Hyperventilation associated with hypoxia, pulmonary embolus, exercise, anxiety, pain, and fever
  - Encephalopathy, septicemia, brain injury, salicylate overdose, and mechanical hyperventilation

Symptoms

- Metabolic alkalosis
  - Neuromuscular: Dizziness, confusion, nervousness, anxiety, tremors, muscle cramping, tetany, tingling, seizures
  - Cardiac: Tachycardia and arrhythmias
  - GI: Nausea, vomiting, anorexia
  - Respiratory: Compensatory hypoventilation
- Respiratory alkalosis
  - Neuro/muscular: Light-headedness, confusion, lethargy
  - Cardiac: Tachycardia and arrhythmias
  - GI: Epigastric pain, nausea, and vomiting
  - Respiratory: Hyperventilation

Fundamentals of Nursing Practice Test #1

Want to take this practice test in an online interactive format?
Check out the online resources page, which includes interactive practice questions and much more: **mometrix.com/resources719/fundnursing**

1. What drip rate should the nurse set to deliver 1000 mL of intravenous D5W in 3 hours and 20 minutes if the drop factor is 15 drops per 1 mL? ***Record your answer as a whole number.***

_________ drops/min

2. A client is taking the loop diuretic furosemide for edema associated with heart failure. Which electrolyte imbalance resulting from the medication is of most concern?

1. Hypokalemia
2. Hyperkalemia
3. Hypercalcemia
4. Hypocalcemia

3. A client comes to a clinic with a severe cough and fever, but all of the exam rooms are full when the client arrives. Which of the following is the best action for the nurse to take?

1. Tell the client to reschedule an appointment for a less busy hour.
2. Ask the client to wait outside until an exam room becomes available.
3. Arovide the client a facemask and seat her in the waiting area with other clients.
4. Provide the client a facemask and seat the client in a separate area as far as possible from other clients.

4. A client has had a pacemaker inserted recently but complains that he is experiencing heart palpitations, generalized weakness, and slight pain in the chest and jaw. On examination, the nurse notes that the client appears quite anxious, and the nurse observes pulsations in the neck and abdomen. Which of the following is the most likely cause of these findings?

1. Pacemaker wiring has become dislodged
2. Infection
3. Coronary artery occlusion
4. Pacemaker syndrome

5. A client has experienced a cardiac arrest at an office visit and the nurse is going to administer defibrillation with an automated external defibrillator (AED). Which of the following should the nurse remove prior to administering a shock?

1. The client's watch
2. The client's bra with metal wires
3. The client's dentures
4. The client's nose ring

6. A client with terminal cancer states she is not afraid of death but is afraid of the process of dying. Which of the following is the best response?

1. "What aspects of the dying process are you most concerned about?"
2. "Those are normal feelings."
3. "What can I do to help?"
4. "I'm so sorry."

7. A 70-year-old female states that she has difficulty falling asleep and sleeps poorly, often lying awake much of the night. The nurse should anticipate which of the following as the initial intervention?

1. Assessment of sleep patterns
2. Nocturnal polysomnogram
3. Prescription for hypnotic
4. Dietary modifications

8. The mother of a 6-month-old child reports that she has a very good baby who is very quiet and sleeps well. The nurse notes that when the phone rings across the room, the child continues to look at the mother. Which of the following should the nurse suspect?

1. The child has a hearing deficit.
2. The child is anxious.
3. The child has cognitive impairment.
4. The child is exhibiting normal behavior for age.

9. A 38-year-old client with rheumatoid arthritis tells the nurse that she is having increasing difficulty dressing herself and managing activities of daily living at home because of her disabilities. Which referral may be most effective?

1. Physical therapist
2. Occupational therapist
3. Housekeeping service
4. Home health agency

10. A 60-kilogram adult is to receive a medication that is administered at 0.5 mg per kg per 24 hours. If the medication is given in 2 equal doses (every 12 hours), how many milligrams should be in each dose? *Record your answer as a whole number.*

_________ mg

11. The first-time mother of a 6-month old infant is concerned that the child's physical development is delayed because the child cannot crawl. Which of the following is the most appropriate response?

1. "Most infants can crawl by 9 months."
2. "Most infants can crawl by 6 months."
3. "Don't worry, infants vary widely in abilities."
4. "Look at all your child can do!"

12. A client has a colostomy in the following anatomic position (see diagram). When teaching the patient about colostomy care, which of the following information should the nurse include? *Select all that apply.*

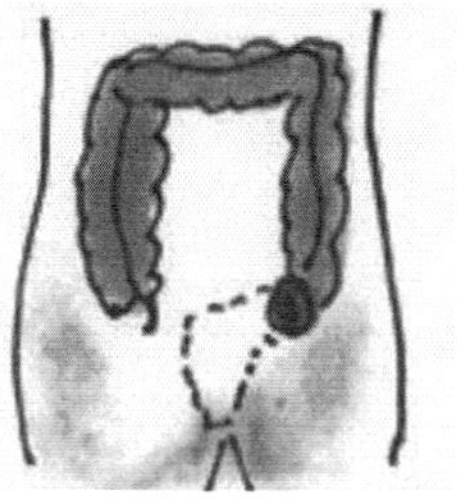

1. "You should expect to have a bowel movement every day."
2. "You may be able to regulate your bowel movements with diet or irrigations."
3. "Your stool may be soft to solid."
4. "There are different types of colostomy appliances available."
5. "Your stool will probably be semi-liquid."

13. Which of the following should never be delegated to unlicensed assistive personnel?

1. Monitoring and controlling blood therapy
2. Bathing a patient
3. Ambulating a patient
4. Monitoring urinary output

14. A client is receiving a liter of normal saline intravenously but must receive 150 mL of antibiotic solution by piggyback. Which of the following is the most correct procedure?

1. Clamp the primary tubing and adjust the flow rate of the piggyback unit.
2. Hang the piggyback unit 6 inches lower than the primary unit and adjust flow rate of the piggyback unit only.
3. Hang the piggyback unit 6 inches higher than the primary unit and adjust flow rate of the piggyback unit only.
4. Hang the piggyback unit at the same level as the primary unit, clamp the primary tubing, and adjust flow rate of the piggyback unit.

15. When conducting a physical examination of a 62-year-old female, the nurse notes nodules on the dorsolateral aspects of the distal interphalangeal joints (Heberden's nodes) of the right hand. Which of the following diseases does this finding suggest?

1. Acute tenosynovitis
2. Gout
3. Rheumatoid arthritis
4. Osteoarthritis

16. A client is scheduled to undergo a cholecystectomy. Which of the following is a required element of informed consent?

1. Duration of operation
2. Names of surgical staff
3. Risks and benefits
4. Insurance coverage

17. A client has been recovering well from a knee replacement but has a sudden onset of restlessness and anxiety. The client complains of chest pain, shortness of breath, and a cough with frothy, blood-tinged sputum. The client has a pulse of 110 bpm and a temperature of 101.2 °F (38.4 °C). The nurse notes rales in the right lung and tachypnea. Based on these findings, which of the following complications is most likely?

1. Pulmonary embolism
2. Atelectasis
3. Pneumonia
4. Pneumothorax

18. A nurse assesses a patient's IV site and notes slight swelling around the insertion site. The skin is cool to touch and the patient verbalizes discomfort. The nurse identifies this as most likely being:

1. Phlebitis
2. Infiltration
3. Extravasation
4. Infection

19. A client complains of blurred vision, fatigue, loss of appetite, weight loss, increased thirst, and frequent urination. Which of the following laboratory assessment(s) would be most indicated?

1. Blood glucose and HbA1c
2. Serum and urine osmolality
3. Complete blood count
4. Urinalysis

20. The nurse is serving on the performance improvement committee, which has agreed to some changes in procedures on the basis of evidence-based research. If the committee wants to convince staff members to comply with the changes, which of the following actions should the committee carry out first?

1. Identify and gain support of key staff.
2. Explain the consequences of failure to comply.
3. Determine a reward system for compliance.
4. Clearly outline expectations in written format.

21. A client with a large pressure injury is suffering from malnutrition and has had little protein in her diet. What effect does inadequate protein intake have on wound healing?

1. It has little or no effect.
2. It inhibits phagocytosis of white blood cells.
3. It slows the healing process because of the lack of amino acids.
4. It causes vasoconstriction that impairs circulation.

22. The nurse is discussing the use of a condom with a sexually active 17-year-old male client being treated for gonorrhea. Which of the following information should the nurse include? *Select all that apply.*

1. Use a condom every time for every sexual encounter.
2. Use natural membrane condoms, which provide better protection than latex.
3. Use only water-based lubricants.
4. Hold the condom in place when withdrawing the penis after ejaculation.
5. Apply the condom so it fits snugly against the glans of the penis.

23. A client is admitted to the hospital from a board-and-care facility with a coccygeal pressure injury that is 5 by 8 cm in size, involves partial thickness loss of dermis, and has a red/pink wound surface without slough. Based on these observations, what stage is the pressure injury?

1. Stage I
2. Stage II
3. Stage III
4. Stage IV

24. The nurse is completing a physical examination of a client and evaluating the client for peripheral arterial and venous insufficiency. Which of the following findings are consistent with peripheral arterial insufficiency? *Select all that apply.*

1. Brownish discoloration appears about the ankles and anterior tibial area.
2. The foot exhibits rubor on dependency and pallor on elevation.
3. Ulcers are evident on the end of the great toe and heel.
4. Peripheral edema is marked.
5. Ulcers are superficial and irregular, often on medial or lateral malleolus.

25. A pregnant woman admitted for preeclampsia experiences a seizure. In what position should the nurse place the client during the seizure?

1. Supine semi-Fowler's position
2. Right lateral
3. Supine flat position
4. Left lateral

26. The most common route of entry of microbial agents into the lungs is through:

1. Aspiration
2. Translocation from the GI tract
3. Inhalation
4. Vascular spread from a distant site

27. A train accident has resulted in many severe casualties, and the emergency department is inundated with clients, but few hospital beds are available. What is the best solution to this emergency situation?

1. Transfer incoming clients to other facilities as soon as they are stabilized.
2. Place newly admitted clients in the hallways.
3. Close the emergency room to further clients.
4. Carry out early discharge for low-risk, noncritical clients to free up some beds.

28. The nurse is irrigating a Foley urinary catheter using open intermittent irrigation and has instilled 30 mL of fluid, but the fluid does not drain back after the syringe is removed. What is the next step the nurse should carry out?

1. Turn the client onto the side facing the nurse.
2. Notify the physician.
3. Aspirate the fluid with the syringe.
4. Instill another 30 mL of fluid and then check for drainage.

29. When conducting a physical exam and assessing the apical pulse in an adult client, where should the nurse place the stethoscope?

1. Second left intercostal space at the midclavicular line
2. Fourth left intercostal space at the sternal margin
3. Fourth left intercostal space at the midclavicular line
4. Fifth left intercostal space at the midclavicular line

30. Which of thc following findings place a client at a high risk for suicide? *Select all that apply*.

1. Older age
2. A previous violent suicide attempt (using a knife or gun)
3. A previous suicide attempt at an isolated site
4. A history of depression 10 years previously
5. A current history of mental illness and disordered thinking

31. Under which delivery care model would the nurse expect to be responsible for the least number of clients?

1. Functional
2. Total patient care
3. Team nursing
4. Modified primary care

32. Following a stroke, a client has impaired swallowing and is unable to feed himself. What is the best position to place the client in when preparing to assist him with meals?

1. Semi-Fowler's position with head in midline and chin tilted upward
2. Supine position with head in midline and chin tilted downward
3. Upright position with head in midline and chin tilted downward
4. Upright position with head in midline and chin tilted upward

33. The nurse is caring for a dying client. Which of the following symptoms indicate that death will occur within a few days? *Select all that apply*.

1. The client is increasingly lethargic and disoriented.
2. The client has increasing dysphagia.
3. The client is extremely weak, gaunt, and pale.
4. The client is drinking only four or five ounces of water at a time.
5. The client is incontinent of a small amount of concentrated urine.
6. The client has a decreased cardiac rate.

34. Which of the following drugs is the appropriate antidote for an overdose of acetaminophen?

1. Protamine sulfate
2. Folic acid
3. Naloxone
4. *N*-acetylcysteine

35. Which of the following positions may result in blood pooling in the extremities, decreased blood pressure (BP) and cardiac output, increased respiratory effort, decreased lung compliance, and decreased cerebral circulation?

1. Trendelenburg
2. Right side-lying
3. Supine
4. Prone

36. A client with severe diarrhea, nausea, and vomiting has become increasingly lethargic and weak with tingling in the hands and feet, muscle cramps and tetany, hypotension, and dysrhythmias with ECG abnormalities that include PVCs and flattened T waves. Based on these signs and symptoms, which of the following electrolyte imbalances should the nurse suspect?

1. Hypokalemia
2. Hyperkalemia
3. Hyponatremia
4. Hypernatremia

37. Which of the following are HIPAA violations? *Select all that apply.*

1. The nurse shares information about the client with the client's sister.
2. The nurse allows another nurse to "shoulder surf" the client's HER.
3. The nurse accesses the history and physical of a client assigned to the nurse.
4. The nurse discusses the client's concerns about treatment with the physician.
5. The nurse tells the client's physician that the client expressed suicidal ideation.

38. The team leader has asked the nurse to change the tracheostomy tube on a client, but the nurse has never done this procedure before. Which of the following is the correct action for the nurse to take?

1. Ask another nurse on the team to assist with the procedure.
2. Look up the procedure in the procedure manual before attempting it.
3. Ask the registered nurse for assistance with the procedure.
4. Use a smartphone to access a YouTube video showing how to do the procedure.

39. In the normal electrocardiogram (ECG) complex, the QRS complex represents which of the following?

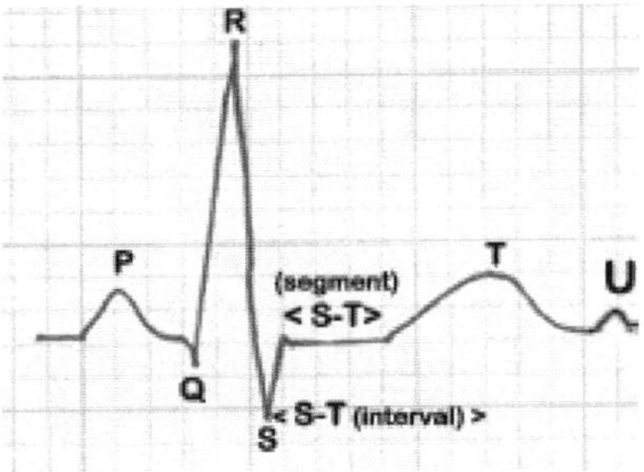

1. Ventricular repolarization
2. AV mode depolarization
3. Atrial depolarization
4. Ventricular depolarization

40. A client has been exploring different types of complementary therapies. Which of the following statements by the client indicate a need for education? *Select all that apply.*

1. "I don't need to worry about taking herbs because they're natural."
2. "Acupuncture may help to relieve back pain."
3. "Homeopathic medicine is better for infections than antibiotics."
4. "Relaxation exercises can help to reduce anxiety."
5. "I should check with the doctor before taking herbal preparations."
6. "I've heard that there is an herbal cure for cancer in Mexico."

41. The nurse is monitoring a woman in labor. During which stage of labor does the nurse expect that the woman will become fully dilated (10 cm)?

1. First stage
2. Second stage
3. Third stage
4. Fourth stage

42. The nurse is instructing a client with Addison's disease (adrenocortical insufficiency) about the signs and symptoms of Addisonian crisis. Which of the following should the nurse include? *Select all that apply.*

1. Hypertension
2. Pallor
3. Bradycardia
4. Nausea and abdominal pain
5. Tachycardia
6. Confusion and restlessness

43. A client is to have continuous measuring of his oxygen saturation with a pulse oximeter. However, he has a constant tremor in both of his hands and tends to pick at the covers. Which of the following is the best solution?

1. Apply the oximeter to the little finger because the tremors will not interfere.
2. Apply the oximeter to the little finger, and tape it in place.
3. Advise the physician that pulse oximetry is not possible.
4. Apply an earlobe oximeter.

44. When doing nasotracheal suctioning, during which of the following should the catheter be inserted?

1. Inhalation
2. Exhalation
3. Swallowing
4. Coughing

45. A client with pancreatic cancer is prescribed fentanyl patches to control pain. Which statement by the client indicates the need for more education?

1. "The patch will give better pain control if I apply heat over it."
2. "I should rotate the sites of administration."
3. "I can dispose of the patch by rolling it up and flushing it down the toilet."
4. "I should cover the patch with plastic when showering."

46. A client involved in a motorcycle accident has a complete spinal cord injury at level C8. Which of the following functional abilities would the nurse expect to observe?

1. The client requires an electric wheelchair with breath or head controls and assistance with all activities of daily living (ADLs).
2. The client is able to use a manual wheelchair on level surfaces only, and she can shave, brush her hair, and feed herself with adaptive equipment.
3. The client is able to use a manual wheelchair on most surfaces, and she is independent in transferring and personal care.
4. The client requires an electric wheelchair with hand controls, and she is able to feed herself with adaptive equipment.

47. When inserting a nasogastric feeding tube, the nurse pauses after inserting about 25 cm of tubing, listens at the distal end of the tubing, and hears air exchange. Which of the following is the most appropriate response?

1. Continue to insert tube but withdraw if coughing becomes excessive.
2. Continue to slowly insert tube while the patient swallows sips of water.
3. Pull the tube back approximately 10 cm and then reinsert.
4. Remove the tube and start the procedure again.

48. The nurse has inserted a nasogastric tube and aspirated gastric contents to check the pH with color-coded pH paper. The aspirate is dark brown, and the pH measures slightly less than 5 according to the color chart. What does this pH usually indicate?

1. Gastric aspirate
2. Intestinal aspirate
3. Respiratory aspirate
4. Inconclusive results

Questions 49–54 are a set that will test your clinical judgment skills. Read through the information you are given before answering the questions that follow. As you progress through the set, you will be given additional information that you will need to consider before answering subsequent questions.

SETTING

The nurse is caring for a 58-year-old male on the cardiac unit.

NURSES' NOTES

Day 1, 0800: The client arrived on the unit after an episode of syncope at home that lasted 2 minutes. The client is now alert and oriented to person, place, time, and situation. Lung sounds are clear, and pulses are strong in all extremities. Bowel sounds are hypoactive in all four quadrants. Skin is pale and dry. He denies any dizziness, light-headedness, or pain. The client has a history of hypercholesteremia, hypertension, gout, and a non-ST-elevation myocardial infarction (MI) 2 years ago. The client is a smoker with a 30 pack-year history. A telemetry monitor is applied that indicates normal sinus rhythm.

Day 1, 1215: The client called the nurse to the room and reported epigastric pain that radiates to his shoulder, with nausea and difficulty breathing. The client was restless and unable to lie still in bed. His heart rhythm is regular, but the rate is elevated. Radial and pedal pulses are weak, graded 1+. Lung sounds are clear.

VITAL SIGNS

	0800	1215
Temp	98.5 °F axillary	98.3 °F axillary
HR	89	120
BP	132/88	80/49
RR	18	30
Pulse oximetry	92%	87%

49. The nurse reviews the assessment data and vital signs. From the following list, select the assessment findings that require immediate follow-up. (Select all that apply)

1. Heart rate, 120
2. Blood pressure, 80/49
3. Lung sounds
4. Bowel sounds
5. Respirations, 30
6. Diaphoresis
7. Epigastric pain

50. For the list of client findings below, specify for each whether it is consistent with the disease processes of myocardial infarction (MI), systemic inflammatory response syndrome (SIRS), or cardiogenic shock. Select all supported disease processes for each finding.

Client Findings	MI	SIRS	Cardiogenic Shock
Epigastric pain	☐	☐	☐
Diaphoresis	☐	☐	☐
Restlessness	☐	☐	☐
Nausea	☐	☐	☐
Heart rate, 120	☐	☐	☐

NURSES' NOTES

Day 1, 1225: The primary physician was notified of the client's condition and arrived at the client's bedside. Electrocardiogram completed and showed tachycardia with ST segment elevation. The client was diagnosed with an acute MI per the physician. A plan was made for a stat cardiac catheterization.

51. The nurse should recognize that the client is at the most <u>immediate</u> risk of developing __________.

1. a pneumothorax
2. cardiac arrest
3. congestive heart failure

NURSES' NOTES

Day 1, 1230: The client is no longer responding to questions or physical touch. The pulse is not palpable to the femoral or carotid arteries. The telemetry monitor shows the following:

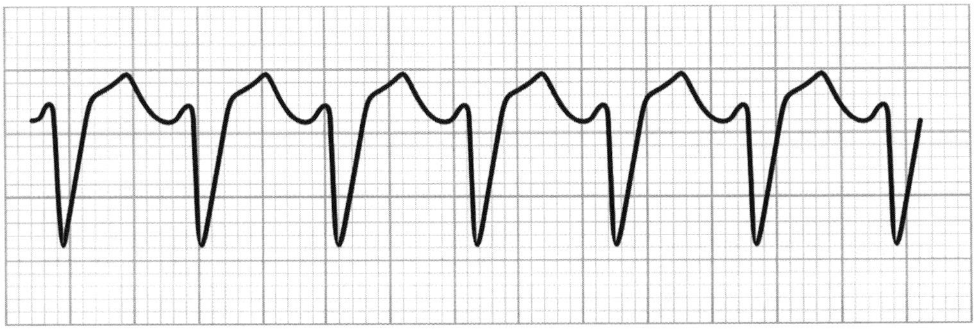

52. For the following list of potential interventions, specify whether each is indicated or not indicated.

Potential Nursing Interventions	Indicated	Not Indicated
Apply automatic external defibrillator pads, one to the upper right side of the chest and one to the lower left lateral side of the chest.	○	○
Administer a sublingual nitroglycerin 0.3 mg tablet per the facility's cardiac arrest protocol.	○	○
Apply a nonrebreather oxygen mask at 10 L/min.	○	○
Activate a code blue.	○	○
Begin chest compressions at 120 beats per minute.	○	○
Place the client in the semi-Fowler's position.	○	○

NURSES' NOTES

Day 1, 1235 (summary of code event): A code blue was activated, and the code team arrived. Chest compressions and rescue breaths were delivered via bag valve mask. Automatic external defibrillator pads were applied. A shock of 200 joules was delivered to the client. The cardiac monitor now shows the following rhythm. No femoral or carotid pulse is palpable.

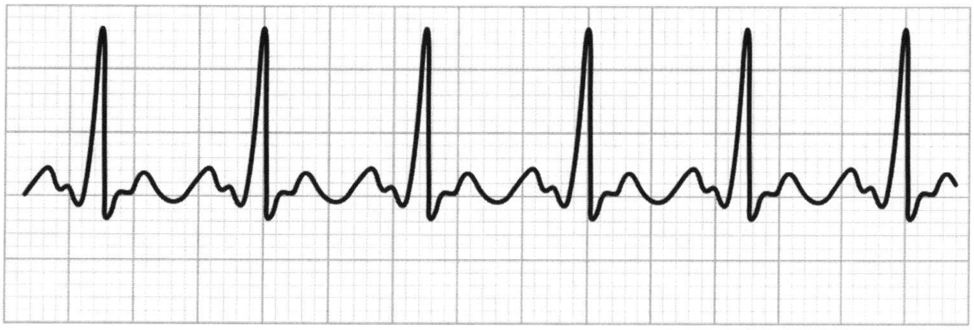

53. Highlight the orders from the following list that the nurse should anticipate based on the client's current status.

- Administer another shock of 200 joules to the client.
- Continue chest compressions at a rate of 120 times per minute.
- Stop the code because the heartbeat has returned to normal.
- Prepare a syringe of 1 mg IV epinephrine.
- Draw blood for laboratory tests: complete blood count, complete metabolic panel, arterial blood gas.

NURSES' NOTES

Day 3, 0800: The client is day 4 status post-MI and subsequent cardiac arrest. Pulse was reestablished following a code blue, and stat cardiac catheterization was performed with stent placement to the left anterior descending artery. The client has transferred back to the cardiac unit from the intensive care unit. Ongoing education has been provided to him in preparation for his eventual discharge.

54. Which of the following statements from the client indicates that he understands the education provided by the nurse? (Select all that apply)

1. "I will take clopidogrel daily for the next year."
2. "I will refrain from exercise for the next 2 months."
3. "I will stop taking atorvastatin."
4. "I will wait 6 months before returning to smoking again."
5. "I will follow up with the dietitian as soon as possible."

Questions 55–60 are a set that will test your clinical judgment skills. Read through the information you are given before answering the questions that follow. As you progress through the set, you will be given additional information that you will need to consider before answering subsequent questions.

Setting

A 65-year-old female arrives to the emergency department via ambulance.

Nurses' Notes

1600: A 65-year-old female client is brought into the emergency department via ambulance. The client reports that she called 911 after she had trouble getting out of bed that morning. She also states that she has been nauseous, complaining of generalized abdominal pain and chest pain since that morning. The client has a history of renal failure, hypertension, and diabetes mellites type 2. The client reports that she is on dialysis and that she had missed her appointment the day before. Emergency medical services (EMS) ran a 12-lead electrocardiogram (EKG) that revealed peaked T-waves. EMS also administered 324 mg aspirin to the client prior to her arrival at the hospital. The client is changed into a gown and placed on the cardiac monitor, an IV is started, labs are drawn, and vital sign measurements are taken.

Vital Signs

	1600
Temp	97.5°F temporal
HR	68
BP	185/95
RR	16
Pulse oximetry	96% on room air

Physical Assessment

Body System	**1600**
Neurological	The client is alert and oriented ×4. She is complaining of generalized weakness and an inability to get out of bed.
Pulmonary	The client's breath sounds are clear. Her breathing pattern is regular.
Cardiovascular	The client is complaining of chest pain. Her EKG shows peaked T-waves within what is otherwise a sinus rhythm. Also, +1 edema is noted to the bilateral lower extremities.
Integumentary	A fistula is noted on the left forearm. Her skin is otherwise normal in appearance.
Gastrointestinal	The client is complaining of nausea. Her abdomen is cramping throughout, but it is nontender.

Laboratory Results

Laboratory Test and Reference Range	**1600**
Red blood cell (RBC) count Adult female: 4.5–5.0 $\times 10^6$/mm^3	4.7
White blood cell (WBC) count Adult/child >2 years: 5,000–10,000/mm^3	9,000
Glucose Adult: 70–110 mg/dL	235
Troponin Adult: <0.4 ng/mL	0.00
Potassium Adult: 3.5–5.0 mmol/L	7.0
Creatinine 0.7–1.3 mg/dL	8.5

55. From the following list, select the assessment findings that require <u>immediate</u> follow-up. (Select all that apply)

1. Missed dialysis appointment
2. Serum glucose
3. Serum creatinine
4. Serum potassium
5. Blood pressure
6. Troponin

56. If left untreated, the client is <u>most</u> at risk of developing ________.

1. myocardial infarction
2. diabetic ketoacidosis
3. congestive heart failure
4. cardiac arrhythmia

57. The nurse receives the following orders. Highlight all orders from the following list that the nurse should consider a <u>priority</u>.

- Obtain a computed tomography (CT) scan of the abdomen with contrast.
- Administer IV dextrose and insulin.
- Administer IV calcium.
- Administer IV ondansetron.
- Obtain a chest x-ray.

NURSES' NOTES

1630: The nurse administers IV dextrose and insulin. The nurse then starts the IV calcium drip. A chest x-ray is obtained and shows no signs of pulmonary edema or cardiomegaly.

58. For the following list of potential nursing interventions, specify whether each is indicated or not indicated.

Potential Nursing Interventions	Indicated	Not Indicated
Request an order for a fluid bolus.	○	○
Request an order for a repeat basic metabolic panel.	○	○
Recheck at the bedside the serum glucose.	○	○
Start a second IV in the left arm.	○	○
Provide continuous cardiac monitoring.	○	○

NURSES' NOTES

1730: The client requests to walk to the bathroom. The client is steady on her feet without staff assistance. The client also states that her nausea has decreased and she would like to eat whenever able.

	1600	**1730**
Temp	97.5°F temporal	98.5°F temporal
HR	68	70
BP	185/95	175/80
RR	16	18
Pulse oximetry	96% on room air	97% on room air

LABORATORY RESULTS

Laboratory Test and Reference Range	1600	1730
Glucose Adult: 70–110 mg/dL	235	75
Troponin Adult: <0.4 ng/mL	0.00	0.01
Potassium Adult: 3.5–5.0 mmol/L	7.0	5.2
Creatinine 0.7–1.3 mg/dL	8.5	8.4

59. For the following list of assessment findings, specify whether each one indicates that the client's condition has improved, is unchanged, or has worsened.

Assessment Findings	Improved	Unchanged	Worsened
Glucose, 75	○	○	○
Troponin, 0.01	○	○	○
Potassium, 5.2	○	○	○
Client's neurological assessment	○	○	○
Client's gastrointestinal assessment	○	○	○

60. The client is being admitted to the floor. The nurse anticipates that the plan of care will include __________, __________, and __________. (Select three answers)

1. dialysis
2. telemetry monitoring
3. a continuous insulin drip
4. IV furosemide
5. repeat serum potassium labs

Answer Key and Explanations for Test #1

1. 75: In order to complete the calculation, the time needs to be converted to minutes. Three hours and 20 minutes equals 200 minutes. Then, the flow rate (mL per minute) is calculated by dividing the total volume by the minutes:

$$(1{,}000 \text{ mL})/(200 \text{ min}) = 5 \text{ mL/min}$$

Then, the drip rate (drops per minute) is calculated by multiplying the drop factor by the flow rate:

$$(15 \text{ drops/mL}) \times (5 \text{ mL/min}) = 75 \text{ drops/min}$$

2. 1: Loop diuretics, such as furosemide, block chloride and sodium resorption in the ascending limb of the loop of Henle, bringing about rapid diuresis but with major electrolyte disturbance, especially hypokalemia and hyponatremia and to a lesser degree hypocalcemia. Hypokalemia is of most importance because it can result in dysrhythmias with ECG abnormalities, hypotension, lethargy, weakness, nausea and vomiting, paresthesias, muscle cramping, and tetany. Normal values are 3.5–5.5 mEq/L. Potassium supplementation is often given routinely with loop diuretics.

3. 4: A client with a severe cough and fever requires both standard precautions and droplet precautions. The best action is to provide the client with a face mask and seat the client in a separate area as far away from other clients as possible to reduce the chance of the infection spreading. A client who is ill should not be sent away or asked to wait outside. The nurse should thoroughly wash his or her hands after contact with the client.

4. 4: These symptoms are consistent with mild pacemaker syndrome and occur when the atrial and ventricular contractions are not synchronized properly. This causes decreased cardiac output because the atria do not adequately fill the ventricles. Peripheral vascular resistance increases to compensate initially. Moderate pacemaker syndrome is characterized by increasing dyspnea and orthopnea, dizziness, vertigo, confusion, and sensation of choking. Severe pacemaker syndrome includes pulmonary edema with rales and marked dyspnea, syncope, and heart failure.

5. 2: The AED kit contains cutting shears so that the nurse can quickly expose the chest. The nurse should use the shears to cut away bras with metal wires because the wires may cause arcing during defibrillation. Likewise, any metal piercings on the chest, such as nipple rings, should be removed. The defibrillator electrodes are placed on the right upper chest (negative) and below and lateral to the heart on the left side (positive). AEDs provide spoken messages and diagrams to guide people through the process.

6. 1: "What aspects of the dying process are you most concerned about?" is the best response because it encourages the client to express her concerns and allows the nurse to assess what can be done to alleviate those concerns. For example, many people facing death are afraid of dying in pain, and the nurse can assure the client that adequate control of pain is almost always possible. This also provides a good opportunity to discuss hospice care. Some clients may express concern about family or financial obligations. These clients may benefit from the assistance of a social worker.

7. 1: The initial intervention when a client reports disturbed sleeping is to complete an assessment of sleep patterns. This should involve questions regarding hours of sleep, quality of sleep, arousals, as well as the number and duration of naps during the day. The client may be asked to keep a sleep diary around the clock, recording sleeping and awakening times, for a few days. Some other initial conservative interventions may include limiting naps and increasing daytime activity, limiting caffeine, maintaining room heat at 70–75 °F, and playing soft soothing music at bedtime.

8. 1: Careful observation can detect hearing deficits at an early age. By 3 months, an infant should exhibit a positive Moro reflex (startle) to sound and may awaken with noise and react to sound by opening or blinking the eyes. Between 3 and 6 months, an infant should begin to coo, try to emulate sounds, look in the direction of sounds such as a ringing telephone, and respond to his or her name. By 12 to 15 months, babies usually begin to say their first words, imitate sounds, and follow vocal directions.

9. 2: The referral that may be most effective for this client is an occupational therapist. Occupational therapists can assess clients' needs and assist them with improving fine motor skills or compensating for the loss of those skills. The occupational therapist can provide guidance regarding assistive devices and the performance of activities of daily living.

10. 15: In this case, the calculation involves multiplying the weight in kilograms by the number of milligrams per kilogram: 60 kg × 0.5 mg/kg per 24 hours. Since the drug is to be given in two equal doses (30/2), each dose is 15 mg.

11. 1: First-time mothers, especially, often have little experience with children and are unsure of what to expect. If the mother is concerned that her child cannot crawl at 6 months, then she needs factual information about when to expect the child to crawl, making "Most infants can crawl by 9 months" the best response. The nurse should also assure the mother that infants may vary in their development. A 6-month-old child should be able to sit in tripod position and roll in both directions. Crawling generally follows this, and the child's gross motor skills should improve over the next 3 months.

12. 2, 3, 4: This is a sigmoid colostomy, so many of the reabsorptive properties of the colon remain. Because of this, the stool may range from soft to solid. Many clients only expel stool every 2 to 3 days, so the client needs to find what is normal for him. Clients with sigmoid colostomies can often use irrigations to control bowel movements, and some are even able to trigger movements with certain foods or expel stool on a predictable schedule. Clients should be advised of all of the options for appliances and stoma covers.

13. 1: The nurse should always remember the five rights of delegation: right task, right circumstances, right person, right direction or communication, and right supervision. The nurse should never delegate tasks for which assistive personnel have not been trained, and this includes administration of medications and blood therapy. Assistive personnel can monitor vital signs during blood therapy and should be taught to recognize and report signs of adverse effects, but the responsibility for primary monitoring lies with the nurse.

14. 3: Piggyback units should be hung at least 6 inches higher than the primary intravenous unit. Because of the force of gravity when the piggyback unit is infusing, the flow from the primary unit stops until the piggyback unit is empty and then it starts again, so clamping the primary unit tubing is not necessary. During infusion of the piggyback unit, a backcheck valve prevents the piggyback solution from flowing up into the primary unit.

15. 4: Heberden's nodes are characteristic of osteoarthritis. Other findings may include radial deviation of the distal phalanx (fingertip tilted toward the thumb) and Bouchard's nodes (nodules on the proximal interphalangeal joints). Osteoarthritis is usually caused by a previous injury to the joints, so it may occur on one side only, and it is associated with cartilage deterioration. It is slowly progressive with symptoms usually occurring after age 60.

16. 3: According to the American Medical Association, informed consent must include the following:

- Explanation of diagnosis
- Nature and reason for treatment or procedure
- Risks and benefits
- Alternative options (regardless of cost or insurance coverage)
- Risks and benefits of alternative options
- Risks and benefits of not having a treatment or procedure

Providing informed consent is a requirement of all states. The client should be given full and clear information prior to signing the consent form and should be encouraged to ask questions to clarify any information that is not clear.

17. 1: Because the onset of symptoms is rapid, these findings are consistent with pulmonary embolism. Acute pulmonary embolism occurs when a thrombus from the venous system or the right side of the heart travels to the lungs and blocks a pulmonary artery or arteriole, resulting in increased alveolar dead space in which ventilation occurs but gas exchange is impaired because of ventilation/perfusion mismatching or intrapulmonary shunting. Common originating sites for thrombus formation are the deep veins in the legs, the pelvic veins, and the right atrium.

18. 2. An infiltration occurs when IV fluid leaks into the surrounding tissue, often causing swelling, discomfort (depending on the solution that has leaked), and cooling of the skin. The cooling of the skin results from the fluid being dispersed in the tissue and is what separates this complication from the others. Sometimes fluid can also be seen leaking from the injection site. In the case of an infiltration, the infusion should be stopped, the IV removed and dressed, the limb elevated, and the registered nurse notified. If the medication being infused is a known irritant, then medications may need to be administered to counteract any damage the solution could do to the tissue.

19. 1: The symptoms are consistent with diabetes mellitus type 1, so the laboratory assessment that is most indicated is blood glucose and HbA1c. The blood glucose level indicates the current level of glucose in the blood (normal value ≤100 mg/dL), but the level may fluctuate throughout the day and vary according to dietary intake. HbA1c provides a more accurate assessment because it shows the average glucose level over a 3-month period. The normal value for HbA1c is <6%.

20. 1: When implementing change, the best action to carry out first is to identify and gain support of key staff. In all organizations, there are staff members who are influential for various reasons, and they are usually easy to identify. Once these key staff members (key informants) are on board, they can often influence others to comply.

21. 3: A diet with very little protein will slow the healing process due to a lack of amino acids needed to repair tissue. Clients with wounds need extra protein to promote the healing process, so the client should be carefully assessed by a nutritionist to determine an adequate diet. Usual requirements for healing are 1.25–1.5 g/kg/day of protein.

22. 1, 3, 4: If the nurse is discussing the use of a condom, information that is important to share includes:

- Use a condom every time for every sexual encounter.
- Use latex rather than natural membrane condoms for better protection.
- Use only water-based lubricants.

- Use spermicide if trying to prevent pregnancy.
- Hold the condom in place when withdrawing the penis after ejaculation.
- Leave a 1-inch space at the end of the condom to contain ejaculate.

The nurse should also demonstrate how the condom is applied, using a model if one is available.

23. 2: The client's pressure injury is stage II. Wound staging is done according to the following:

- Stage I: Localized intact skin with nonblanchable redness
- Stage II: Partial thickness loss of dermis and red/pink wound surface without slough
- Stage III: Full thickness loss of dermis with subcutaneous tissue exposed. Slough, undermining, and tunneling may be present.
- Stage IV: Full thickness loss of dermis with muscle, tendons, or bones exposed. Slough or eschar may be present.

24. 2, 3: With peripheral arterial insufficiency, the foot exhibits rubor on dependency and pallor on elevation. The skin often feels cool and appears pale and shiny with loss of hair on the leg, foot, and toes. Because of impaired circulation, the toenails may appear thick and ridged. Pedal pulses are weak or absent. Ulcers tend to occur on the tips of toes, between toes, on heels, or on other pressure areas. Ulcers are usually deep, circular, and painful and may be necrotic. Because the venous system may be intact, peripheral edema is usually minimal.

25. 4: If a client with preeclampsia experiences a seizure (indicating eclampsia), the client should be placed in the most protective position for herself and the fetus, the left lateral position. This position decreases the risk that she will aspirate, and it relieves the pressure of the uterus against the vena cava, increasing blood flow to the fetus. The side rails should be raised if the client is in bed, but they should be padded with a blanket or pillows to prevent her from injuring herself.

26. 1: The most common route of entry of microbial agents into the lungs is aspiration. Most aspiration does not result in pneumonia, depending on the microbial load and the patient's condition, because a healthy lung is able to handle small amounts of aspirant. Inhalation is also a common route, either from people who are infected or from contaminated equipment. Vascular spread (bacteremia) is fairly rare but can occur, resulting in pneumonia. In some cases, bacteria and toxins may translocate from the GI system to the lungs per the mesenteric lymph nodes.

27. 4: The best solution to an influx of clients during an emergency situation is to carry out early discharge for low-risk, noncritical clients. Often, elective procedures, such as ambulatory surgeries and testing, are canceled and rescheduled. Clients may be sent home with home health care or transferred to other facilities, such as convalescent hospitals. Each facility should have a disaster plan in place that outlines the steps to take in an emergency.

28. 1: Because Foley catheters are usually maintained on continuous drainage, the bladder may be essentially empty when it is irrigated, so the small amount of irrigant may pool away from the end of the catheter. Therefore, the best solution if no fluid returns is to turn the client onto the side facing the nurse, being careful to maintain the sterile field. If the irrigant still does not return, then the nurse should gently aspirate using the syringe.

29. 4: The apical pulse is assessed at the fifth left intercostal space at the midclavicular line, which is the point of maximal impulse. The nurse first locates the sternal notch, and from there the second intercostal space. Then, moving fingers lightly down the side of the sternum to the fifth intercostal space and over to the midclavicular line, the nurse should be able to auscultate the S1 and S2 normal heart sounds.

30. 2, 3, 4: Clients who have previously attempted violent suicide, such as with a gun or knife; who attempted suicide at an isolated site with little chance of rescue; or who have a current history of mental illness and disordered thinking are at a high risk for suicide. Other risk factors include current severe depression and lack of an adequate social support system. Clients with these risk factors should be monitored carefully. Anyone who has previously attempted suicide in any manner has an increased risk of making another attempt.

31. 2: Total patient care is when a nurse is assigned to do all of the care for only one or two clients. Modified primary care is when a nurse is responsible for the same group of clients every day, usually with assistive personnel. Team nursing involves a team leader overseeing a group that comprises unlicensed assistive personnel, licensed vocational/practical nurses, and other registered nurses (RNs) to care for a fairly large group of clients, often ranging from 10 to 20 clients. Functional nursing is when tasks are divided between nurses; for example, one nurse may give medications to all clients, and another nurse might do all the dressing changes.

32. 3: The best position for a client with impaired swallowing is upright with the head midline and the chin down (flexed about 75% of the way toward the chest) because this position provides better protection of the airway and decreases the risk of choking and aspirating. The patient may be positioned with the arms on the overbed table with positioning aids used, if necessary, to maintain body alignment. The client should continue to remain in the upright position for at least 30 minutes after the feeding is completed.

33. 1, 2, 3, 5: Typical indications that death will occur within a few days include lethargy, disorientation, and increasing dysphagia. Clients are usually unable to take foods or swallow medications. The client appears very weak, gaunt, and pale and is able to take only sips of fluid. Clients usually have decreased urinary output and may be incontinent of concentrated urine. The cardiac rate and respiratory rate both increase, but the strength of cardiac contractions weakens, and the pulse may become irregular.

34. 4: *N*-acetylcysteine is the antidote for an acetaminophen overdose. Acetaminophen toxicity occurs with a single dose greater than 140 mg/kg of body weight or with greater than 7.5 g in 24 hours. The antidote is given for serum levels greater than 150. It is most effective if given with 8 hours of ingestion. *N*-acetylcysteine is given at the rate of 140 mg/kg initially and repeated with 70 mg/kg every 4 hours for 17 additional doses, either by mouth or intravenously.

35. 4: The prone position may cause blood to pool in the extremities, and pressure on the abdomen may result in a decrease in blood pressure (BP), preload, and cardiac output. Respiratory effort increases, and lung compliance decreases. The head positioned sharply to one side may interfere with cerebral circulation. If the head is turned laterally, the dependent eye must be observed carefully for external compression. Bilateral bolsters or other supports should be used to support the thorax (clavicle to iliac crest) to relieve abdominal compression, which may impede respirations and venous return.

36. 1: These signs and symptoms indicate hypokalemia. Potassium influences the activity of both skeletal and cardiac muscles. Normal values range from 3.5–5.5 mEq/L. Hypokalemia occurs with levels of less than 3.4 mEq/L and critical values of less than 2.5 mEq/L.

37. 1, 2: HIPAA privacy and security rules protect personal health information about a client, so it is a HIPAA violation to share information about the client with family and friends other than parents of a minor child or a spouse without specific permission to do so. It is a security violation to allow unauthorized access to the EHR, and this includes not only sharing passwords but also allowing others to "shoulder surf" in order to gain information.

38. 3: Because the team leader is ultimately responsible for care that has been delegated to other staff members, the nurse should tell the team leader that she has never changed a tracheostomy tube before and ask for assistance. The team leader should make the decision as to whether to assist her or assign the task of assisting to another nurse on the team. The nurse should never attempt a procedure for which she is not prepared or knowledgeable.

39. 4: In the normal electrocardiogram (ECG) complex, the QRS complex represents ventricular depolarization:

- P wave: Start of electrical impulse in the sinus node and spreading through the atria, muscle depolarization
- QRS complex: Ventricular muscle depolarization and atrial repolarization. The width of the complex represents intraventricular conduction time.
- T wave: Ventricular muscle repolarization (resting state) as cells regain negative charge
- U wave: Repolarization of the Purkinje fibers

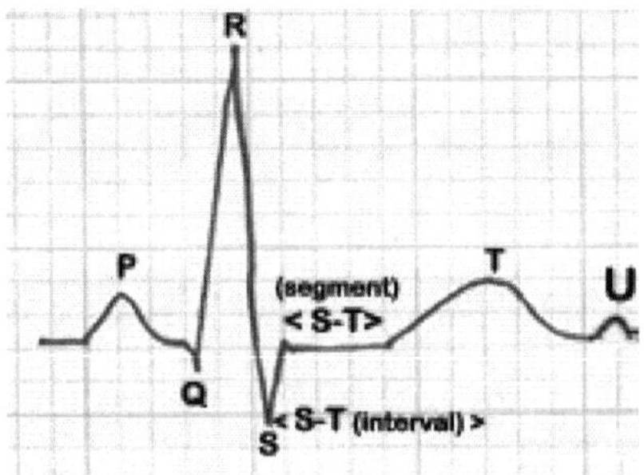

40. 1, 3, 6: If a client has been exploring different types of complementary therapies and states, "I don't need to worry about taking herbs because they're natural," the client needs to be aware that many prescription medications are derived from herbs, and herbs may interact with medications and increase or decrease their actions. Additionally, "Homeopathic medicine is better for infections than antibiotics," is not supported by any research and may pose a risk to the client if an infection goes untreated. "I've heard that there is an herbal cure for cancer in Mexico" suggests the client is relying on unsubstantiated claims.

41. 1: There are four stages of labor:

Stage 1: The period between the onset of labor and full dilation (10 cm). Comprises two phases: latent (cervical effacement and beginning dilation) and active (continued dilation from 4 to 10 cm).
Stage 2: The period from full dilation through the delivery of the infant.
Stage 3: The period after delivery of the infant through delivery of the placenta.
Stage 4: The postpartum period lasting two hours after delivery.

42. 2, 4, 5, 6: Addisonian crisis is an acute episode of adrenal insufficiency that is life threatening and precipitated by a stressor, such as gastrointestinal infection, fever, or surgery. Addisonian crisis may be misdiagnosed as an acute abdomen because clients may present with nausea and severe abdominal pain. Shock, with hypotension and pallor, is common, and clients may exhibit tachycardia, confusion, and restlessness. Because temperature regulation is impaired, clients may exhibit hypothermia or hyperthermia. Suspected Addisonian crisis must be treated immediately because clients may die while awaiting test results.

43. 4: The nurse should apply an earlobe oximeter. A digit pulse oximeter should be avoided if the client has tremors or if he is likely to move his hand frequently. The skin should be clean and dry when the oximeter is applied. If using a digit oximeter, a client should not have artificial nails or wear colored nail polish because these may interfere with readings. If a client is severely obese, the clip on the oximeter may not stay in place, so a disposable (single-use) sensor pad may be necessary.

44. 1: When doing nasotracheal suctioning, the catheter should be inserted only during inhalation because this is when the epiglottis is open. However, suction should not be applied during insertion. During suctioning, a normal reaction is for the client to cough, but if the client begins to gag or becomes nauseated, the catheter may be in the esophagus. Tracheal suctioning should be completed before pharyngeal because the pharynx contains more bacteria than the trachea.

45. 1: Clients must avoid placing direct sources of heat, such as a heating pad, over a fentanyl patch because this action increases the rate of absorption and may cause the client to have an overdose. Clients are allowed to bathe or shower while wearing the patch, but this may cause the patch to loosen. To prevent this, clients may cover the patch with plastic wrap taped in place. A patch should be disposed of by rolling it and flushing it down the toilet because some medication will remain in the patch.

46. 2: A client with a complete spinal cord injury at level C8 is a quadriplegic and should be able to use a manual wheelchair independently on most surfaces but may require adaptive devices for activities of daily living (ADLs). The client should have full extension and flexion of her elbows and wrists and some movement in the fingers and thumbs. She should be able to transfer independently and drive a car with hand controls. The client may need some assistance with ADLs, such as lower body dressing.

47. 4: If, when inserting a nasogastric feeding tube, the nurse pauses after inserting the tube 25 cm, this is at the level of the carina. If the nurse listens at the distal end of the tube and hears air exchange, this is an indication that the tube is in the respiratory tract and not the esophagus. The tube should be immediately completely withdrawn, allowing the client time to relax and stop coughing, before insertion is attempted again. Note, even if there is no sound of air exchange, this cannot be used as confirmation of correct placement.

48. 2: The pH in this situation usually indicates intestinal aspirate rather than gastric aspirate. Gastric aspirate may vary in color from cloudy to green to tan to brown with a pH less than 4, while intestinal aspirate may be yellow or brown but the pH is usually greater than 4. Respiratory secretions may look like saliva and have a pH greater than 5.5.

49. 1, 2, 5, 6, and 7: The nurse should follow up on symptoms of a potential cardiac problem (epigastric pain and diaphoresis) and signs of altered perfusion (elevated heart rate, decreased blood pressure, and tachypnea) due to the risk of serious injury or even death to the client. Although the client is hypoxic and tachypneic, his lung sounds are normal and do not require follow-up at this time. Although his bowel sounds should be monitored going forward, they would not be a priority for follow-up with the existence of more urgent symptoms.

50.

Client Findings	MI	SIRS	Cardiogenic Shock
Epigastric pain	■	□	□
Diaphoresis	■	□	□
Restlessness	■	■	■
Nausea	■	□	□
Heart rate, 120	□	■	■

The client is presenting with several symptoms of an MI, including radiating chest pain (sometimes described by clients as epigastric pain), diaphoresis, restlessness, and nausea. Although not always present, clients will also commonly experience tachycardia when having an MI due to anxiety, pain, or the strain placed on the heart. In order to be diagnosed with SIRS, a client must have at least two of the following four symptoms: tachycardia, tachypnea, alteration in normal temperature (either fever or hypothermia), and alteration in white blood cell count (either >12,000/mm^3 or <4,000/mm^3). Restlessness can also be present due to the systemic effects of SIRS. Cardiogenic shock is a result of such severe damage to the heart that it can no longer adequately supply the body with blood and oxygen, resulting in symptoms such as tachycardia, hypotension, tachypnea, and restlessness. Although cardiogenic shock can be due to a heart attack, it can also be caused by chronic conditions such as congestive heart failure, and it is not always associated with acute cardiac symptoms such as chest pain.

51. 2: The client is demonstrating the signs of cardiogenic shock, which can rapidly progress to cardiac arrest due to lack of perfusion to the heart. Although a client may develop heart failure if the heart suffers permanent damage from an MI, this would be a long-term problem and would not be the most immediate risk to the client. A pneumothorax develops when air enters the pleural space and places pressure on the lung, causing it to collapse. This is most often caused by trauma or surgery that allows air to enter the pleural space and is not the most immediate risk to the client.

52.

Potential Nursing Interventions	Indicated	Not Indicated
Apply automatic external defibrillator pads, one to the upper right side of the chest and one to the lower left lateral side of the chest.	●	○
Administer a sublingual nitroglycerin 0.3 mg tablet per the facility's cardiac arrest protocol.	○	●
Apply a nonrebreather oxygen mask at 10 L/min.	○	●
Activate a code blue.	●	○
Begin chest compressions at 120 beats per minute.	●	○
Place the client in the semi-Fowler's position.	○	●

The client is experiencing cardiac arrest; it is essential that the nurse begin compressions and activate a code blue as soon as possible. The nurse or one of her team members should apply automatic external defibrillator pads in the appropriate positions (the upper right side of the chest and the lower left side of the chest), especially because pulseless ventricular tachycardia is a shockable rhythm. Although nitroglycerin would typically be administered during an MI, it would not be indicated during cardiac arrest. A nonrebreather mask would also not be indicated for a client without a pulse because the client requires bag-valve-mask ventilation per the advanced cardiac life support protocol. The client should be placed in the supine position with a backboard beneath his torso in order for the code team to provide optimal compressions.

53.

- Administer another shock of 200 joules to the client.
- Continue chest compressions at a rate of 120 times per minute.
- Stop the code because the heartbeat has returned to normal.
- Prepare a syringe of 1 mg IV epinephrine.
- Draw blood for laboratory tests: complete blood count, complete metabolic panel, arterial blood gas.

Although the cardiac monitor shows a sinus rhythm, the client still has no pulse, so he is experiencing pulseless electrical activity, which is not a shockable rhythm. The nurse and the code team should continue the code and continue chest compressions at 100–120 beats per minute. During cardiac arrest, epinephrine 1 mg should be administered every 3–5 minutes IV while the client remains pulseless. A member of the code team should also prepare to draw blood for laboratory tests while the code is underway in order to help the team determine the underlying cause of the client's arrest.

54. 1 and 5: Following stent placement, it is essential that the client take an antiplatelet medication, such as clopidogrel, daily for up to 1 year to prevent occlusion of the stent and subsequent MI. The client should also meet with a dietitian, if possible, to learn about the impact of diet on cardiovascular disease. The client should continue to take atorvastatin to lower his cholesterol levels and to prevent further occlusion of the coronary arteries. It is important after an MI to return to exercise as soon as possible—albeit gradually and slowly—to help regain strength, and many clients benefit from specific cardiac rehabilitation programs. The client should be counseled to give up smoking altogether because it increases the likelihood for further cardiac events as well as other diseases.

55. 1, 4, and 5: Any client who has missed a dialysis appointment is at increased risk of fluid overload and electrolyte imbalances. It is important that all dialysis clients understand the danger of missing appointments. The client's serum potassium is critically high and should be the nurse's top concern in this case because it could lead to deadly outcomes. The client's elevated blood pressure (along with the swelling in her limbs) is also concerning, as it shows a sign of possible fluid overload caused by missing her dialysis appointment the day before. The nurse should continue to monitor the patient for further increases in blood pressure because severely high blood pressures can lead to hypertensive emergencies and stroke. Although the client's serum glucose is elevated, this is not a level that is considered critical in most diabetic clients. The client's serum creatinine is also elevated, but this is expected in a renal failure client (especially in those due for dialysis). The client's troponin level is currently within normal limits and is not concerning.

56. 4: Because of the client's missed dialysis appointment and critically high potassium level, the client is currently at highest risk of developing a cardiac arrhythmia such as ventricular tachycardia, ventricular fibrillation, or even asystole. It is critical that this risk is addressed first to prevent cardiac arrest. Although the client is having chest pain and has an abnormal EKG, her troponin is normal, revealing that the peaked T-waves are more likely caused by elevated potassium than a blockage in the heart. Therefore, myocardial infarction is unlikely. Diabetic ketoacidosis is also unlikely given that the client's blood sugar is not critically high for an adult with diabetes and her other assessment findings (normal mentation and breathing) do not suggest this. Additional labs, such as blood gases, would be indicated to further rule out diabetic ketoacidosis. Finally, congestive heart failure may eventually occur in the client that is fluid overloaded, but this is a lower risk because it is generally a chronic condition and treatment is not as emergent for this potential complication.

57.

- Obtain a computed tomography (CT) scan of the abdomen with contrast.
- Administer IV dextrose and insulin.
- Administer IV calcium.
- Administer IV ondansetron.
- Obtain a chest x-ray.

Emergent treatment of the client's elevated potassium is indicated at this time. This is done by administering IV insulin, which can allow the excess serum potassium to pass through the cell membrane. IV dextrose is necessary to prevent the likely hypoglycemia that IV insulin administration can cause. IV calcium is also given in these cases to decrease the risk of cardiac arrhythmia. Although the physician may want a CT scan of the client's abdomen to diagnose a possible cause of her abdominal pain, this diagnosis is not as emergent as preventing potential cardiac arrhythmias from the hyperkalemia. Additionally, the nurse may want to question this order because CT contrast can be nephrotoxic and may cause further damage to the client's already injured kidneys. IV ondansetron may be indicated to help the client feel more comfortable with less nausea, but it is not emergently needed at this time. A chest x-ray may also be indicated to rule out pulmonary edema due to fluid overload. However, the client is not currently presenting with signs of respiratory distress, so this intervention can be delayed.

58.

Potential Nursing Interventions	Indicated	Not Indicated
Request an order for a fluid bolus.	○	●
Request an order for a repeat basic metabolic panel.	●	○
Recheck at the bedside the serum glucose.	●	○
Start a second IV in the left arm.	○	●
Provide continuous cardiac monitoring.	●	○

The client's basic metabolic panel (which includes serum potassium) and serum glucose should be monitored periodically after the administration of IV insulin. This is to ensure that the treatment was effective and to ensure that the client does not become hypoglycemic. Continuous cardiac monitoring is also indicated to monitor for signs that the client's rhythm is worsening or improving. Although the nurse may believe that an IV fluid bolus could help the decrease the client's serum potassium, this is not indicated for a client who is already fluid overloaded. Nurses should always be cautious in administering too much fluid to clients with conditions such as renal failure or congestive heart failure because this can lead to pulmonary edema. Starting a second IV may be a good idea for this client so that more than one medication can be administered at a time in case of emergency. However, it is contraindicated to start an IV in an arm that has a fistula and the nurse should look elsewhere for additional IV access. The nurse should also document the limb restriction in the client's chart and place her on limb restriction precautions, such as placing a "restricted limb" bracelet on the limb, to prevent other healthcare professionals from manipulating that side unknowingly.

59.

Assessment Findings	Improved	Unchanged	Worsened
Glucose, 75	○	○	●
Troponin, 0.01	○	●	○
Potassium, 5.2	●	○	○
Client's neurological assessment	●	○	○
Client's gastrointestinal assessment	●	○	○

Although the client's serum glucose is now considered within normal limits for the average adult, it has dropped significantly since the IV insulin was administered. To prevent further dropping and hypoglycemia, the nurse should encourage glucose intake. If possible, the client should be given food and a sugary beverage. If the physician states that this is contraindicated or it is not safe for the client to take things by mouth, the nurse should advocate for further IV dextrose administration. The client's troponin is slightly higher than the initial reading, but it is still considered normal and is thus considered unchanged. The client's potassium is still elevated and requires intervention, but it is much closer to the normal range and has improved. The client is now no longer too weak to get up; thus, her neurological assessment has improved. Finally, the client is requesting food, which is a likely indication that her nausea and abdominal pain (gastrointestinal assessment) have improved.

60. 1, 2, and 5: While the client's potassium level has improved with the insulin administration, it is still important to monitor for signs of arrhythmias and to continue to check her potassium levels. Insulin is a temporary fix, and potassium levels can rebound if the cause of hyperkalemia is not treated. Therefore, the client should have dialysis soon. An insulin drip is not indicated for this client. In fact, given the drop in her glucose after one dose of IV insulin, an insulin drip would likely be contraindicated. This treatment is meant more for clients with critically high glucose levels. Finally, although IV furosemide may help decrease the client's potassium and fluid overload through her urine, this medication is unlikely to be ordered for a renal client with such a high creatinine level. Furosemide can be nephrotoxic and should be used with caution in this case.

Fundamentals of Nursing Practice Test #2

1. A client with extensive burns of the lower extremities is treated with topical agents, and the burns are wrapped with several layers of dressings. On examination, the nurse finds that the peripheral pulses are diminished. Which is the best initial action for the nurse?

1. Elevate the extremities to reduce edema.
2. Remove the dressings.
3. Loosen the dressings.
4. Reevaluate the peripheral pulses after 15 minutes.

2. A 48-year-old female client complains of episodes of severe right upper quadrant abdominal pain lasting two to six hours, indigestion, nausea and vomiting, and clay-colored stools. The nurse suspects the client may have which of the following diagnoses?

1. Colitis
2. Pancreatitis
3. Cholecystitis
4. Diverticulitis

3. To facilitate the client's right of autonomy, which of the following assessments by the nurse is the most important?

1. The client's cognitive ability
2. Legal obligations
3. The physician's wishes
4. The client's physical ability

4. A client who has been taking digoxin presents in the emergency department with an irregular pulse, bradycardia of 22–28 bpm, nausea, vomiting, diarrhea, headache, and halo vision. Which of the following interventions should the nurse anticipate? *Select all that apply.*

1. Administer an increased dose of digoxin.
2. Administer digoxin immune fab.
3. Administer atropine.
4. Provide supportive treatment.
5. Conduct laboratory tests for digoxin and electrolyte levels.
6. Carry out continuous cardiac monitoring.

5. A client has terminal cancer. For months, the client's spouse has been teary and obviously grieving about the impending death, but now that death is imminent, the spouse seems detached and relatively unemotional. Which of the following is the most likely reason for the spouse's reaction?

1. Lack of feelings for the spouse
2. State of emotional shock
3. Dulling of responses because of substance abuse
4. Premature completion of anticipatory grief

6. A client is recovering from placement of an implantable cardioverter-defibrillator (ICD) and suddenly exhibits hypotension with narrowing pulse pressure, pulsus paradoxus, distant heart sounds, restlessness, bulging neck veins, and increasing cyanosis. Which of the following is the most likely cause of these signs and symptoms?

1. A perforation of the ventricle with cardiac tamponade
2. Incorrect positioning of the leads
3. A myocardial infarction
4. Heart failure

7. A client receiving chemotherapy for breast cancer (stage 2) tells the nurse that she is considering complementary therapy to relieve her almost constant nausea and asks the nurse for advice. Which of the following complementary therapies is most likely to be safe and effective?

1. Acupuncture
2. Therapeutic touch
3. Magnetic therapy
4. Herbal therapies

8. When changing a colostomy appliance, with which of the following should the skin about the stoma be cleansed after the pouch is removed?

1. Soap and water
2. Alcohol swabs
3. Tap water
4. Baby wipes

9. The hospital receives news that a train has crashed half a mile away and that a cloud of nonlethal hazardous material has blanketed the area. Which of the following emergency responses should the nurse anticipate?

1. Evacuation
2. Shelter in place
3. Relocation of staff and clients to the interior of building
4. Partial evacuation—children and critically ill only

10. A client has developed signs of tardive dyskinesia with repetitive behavior, including lip smacking and tongue protrusion with choreiform movements of the trunk and extremities. Which of the following medications is most likely the cause of these symptoms?

1. Donepezil HCl (Aricept)
2. Fluoxetine HCl (Prozac)
3. Celecoxib (Celebrex)
4. Haloperidol (Haldol)

11. A client brought to the emergency department has been exposed to cold temperatures, and his core body temperature is 34 °C. Which of the following rewarming techniques is most indicated?

1. Cardiopulmonary bypass
2. Warm IV fluid administration
3. Warm peritoneal lavage
4. Forced-air warming blankets

12. Which of the following are examples of personal protective equipment (PPE)? *Select all that apply.*

1. Back belts
2. Goggles
3. Personal radiation dosimeters
4. Respirators
5. Gloves

13. Which of the following are true regarding premature ventricular contractions? *Select all that apply.*

1. PVCs can be harmless abnormalities.
2. Frequent PVCs signify a myocardial infarction.
3. PVCs can occur in conjunction with underlying dysrhythmias.
4. PVCs can be caused by caffeine, nicotine, or alcohol.

14. A client newly diagnosed with schizophrenia has been exhibiting both negative and positive symptoms. Which of the following symptoms would be categorized as negative?

1. Inappropriate affect
2. Visual hallucinations
3. Delusions of grandeur
4. Disheveled appearance

15. A client with diabetes mellitus type 2 is being discharged, and the nurse is instructing the client about safe disposal of syringes and needles at home. Which of the following information should the nurse provide when educating the client? *Select all that apply.*

1. "Place needles and syringes in a sharps disposal container immediately after use."
2. "Keep the container in a safe place out of reach of children and pets."
3. "Dispose of the sharps container in the regular trash can."
4. "Dispose of the sharps container in accordance with community guidelines."
5. "Dispose of the sharps container when it is three-quarters full."
6. "Needles can be flushed down the toilet."

16. Which of the following is the primary purpose in the nurse administering the Apgar (appearance, pulse, grimace, activity, respiration) test to a neonate?

1. To determine the infant's biophysical profile
2. To determine if the infant needs emergency medical care
3. To determine if the infant has congenital defects
4. To determine if the infant is preterm, full term, or post-term

17. The physician has ordered that a client with diabetes insipidus receive 50 mcg of desmopressin acetate by oral tabs twice daily. The tablets are labeled 0.2 mg per tablet. How many tablets will the nurse administer for each dose? *Record your answer as a decimal.*

18. A client with 2+ peripheral edema and increasing complaints of lethargy has the following laboratory results:

Test	Result
BUN	172 mg/dL
Serum creatinine	16.4 mg/dL
Glucose	98 mg/dL

Which further testing should the nurse expect based on these findings?

1. Testing for diabetes
2. Testing for liver disease
3. Testing for heart disease
4. Testing for kidney disease

19. The nurse has inserted a Foley catheter into a male client who is bedridden. Which of the following is the best position in which to secure the catheter?

1. The penis is positioned down with the Foley catheter taped to the front of the inner thigh, and then the tubing is looped to allow for turning and it is taped to the edge of the bed.
2. The penis is positioned up with the Foley catheter taped to the right or left lower abdomen, and then the tubing is looped to allow for turning and it is taped to the edge of the bed.
3. The penis is left unpositioned with the catheter curved over one leg, and the tubing is looped and secured only to the edge of the bed.
4. The penis is positioned downward with the catheter secured to the posterior thigh, and the tubing is looped and secured to the edge of the bed.

20. If the nurse is to give a client two oral medications (capsules) per the enteral feeding tube, which of the following is the correct procedure?

1. Open the capsules directly into the feeding formula and instill.
2. Open the capsules together and dilute with water before instilling.
3. Open the capsules separately and dilute each with water before instilling.
4. Oral medications cannot be given per the enteral feeding tube.

21. The nurse is administering an intermittent tube feeding to a client per an NG tube. The nurse has checked the placement of the tube, checked for gastric residual, and aspirated 150 mL of gastric contents. Which of the following next actions is most appropriate?

1. Hold feeding and notify MD of gastric residual.
2. Proceed with tube feeding.
3. Return the aspirated gastric contents to the stomach and flush the tubing with 30 mL water.
4. Return 100 mL of aspirated gastric contents to the stomach followed by the tube feeding.

22. Which of the following ensures minimal proper identification prior to administering medication?

1. The nurse recognizes client.
2. The nurse asks the client's name and checks their hospital ID bracelet.
3. The nurse reads the client's name on the intake and output record at the foot of the client's bed.
4. The nurse asks for the client's name.

23. An adult client has instilled drops into the ear to soften cerumen, and the nurse is to irrigate the ear to remove the cerumen. Which of the following statements are correct about ear irrigations? *Select all that apply.*

1. 50 mL of irrigant should be instilled rapidly to dislodge the cerumen.
2. The tip of the syringe should be used to occlude the ear canal.
3. The pinna should be pulled up and back.
4. Allow fluid to drain out during the procedure.
5. Position client in sitting or lying position.
6. Ask client to turn the head away from the affected ear.

24. The nurse must administer 5 mL of acetaminophen solution through the nasogastric (NG) tube of a client, but the NG tube is attached to suction. How long (in minutes) should the nurse discontinue the suction after administering the medication? *Record your answer as a whole number.*

________ minutes

25. The nurse must give an intramuscular injection to an adult. What length of needle is most appropriate?

1. 0.5 in
2. 0.625 in
3. 1 in
4. 1.5 in

26. A client is receiving warfarin for venous thrombosis, and the client's INR is 4.0 with no evidence of bleeding. What action does the nurse anticipate?

1. Administer warfarin as prescribed.
2. Administer increased dosage of warfarin until INR increases.
3. Hold or administer reduced dosage until INR decreases.
4. Hold warfarin and administer vitamin K orally.

27. Which metabolic effect is most common if a client is taking a loop diuretic?

1. Hypouricemia
2. Hyperglycemia
3. Hyperkalemia
4. Hypokalemia

28. A new mother is concerned that her neonate is having periods of apnea. What duration of apnea is of concern in the neonate?

1. All periods of apnea
2. 2–3 seconds
3. 6–8 seconds
4. >15–20 seconds

29. A physician has ordered the HbA1c test for a client who complains of increased thirst and urination. Which of the following results (on two separate testings) is the lowest value considered diagnostic for diabetes mellitus?

1. 3.5–4.5%
2. 4.5–6.0%
3. 5.7–6.4%
4. ≥6.5%

30. A client is receiving enteral feedings through a nasogastric tube, and the nurse is administering the client's medications. Which of the following can be administered through the NG tube? *Select all that apply.*

1. Hard extended-release capsules (opened, crushed, and dissolved)
2. Pills (crushed and dissolved)
3. Enteric-coated tablets (crushed and dissolved)
4. Liquid suspension
5. Soft-gel capsules (dissolved)
6. Sublingual wafer (dissolved)

31. The nurse must collect a urine sample for a routine urinalysis from a client who has had an indwelling Foley catheter with a sampling port for three days. After initially clamping the catheter tubing for 20 minutes, which of the following is the correct procedure?

1. The nurse collects a urine sample by inserting a needleless syringe into the sampling port and withdrawing 1 mL of urine.
2. The nurse wipes the sampling port with alcohol and then withdraws the urine using a 10-mL needleless syringe.
3. The nurse disconnects the Foley catheter from the drainage tube and allows urine to drip from the catheter into a sterile urine specimen container.
4. The nurse wipes the sampling port with alcohol, then uses a 3-ml syringe with a 1-inch 21-gauge needle to withdraw urine from the port.

32. When reviewing dietary restrictions with an immunocompromised client following kidney transplantation, the client should be advised to avoid which of the following food products?

1. Raw bean sprouts
2. Strawberries
3. All citrus fruits
4. Milk products

33. A client has suffered an ischemic stroke in the right hemisphere. Which of the following should the nurse anticipate?

1. Left-sided paralysis and visual field defects
2. Expressive, receptive, and/or global aphasia
3. Uncharacteristic positive attitude and outlook
4. Difficulty with mathematics, reading, and writing

34. A client's medication order is for 300 mg of a liquid medication that is available at 75 mg per mL. How many mL should the nurse administer to the client? *Record your answer as a whole number.*

_______ mL

35. A client has had a central catheter inserted for administration of parenteral nutrition. An X-ray was taken to ensure correct positioning prior to commencing infusions. The X-ray report indicates that the catheter tip is in the right atrium. Which of the following actions by the nurse is correct?

1. Hold the infusion and notify the MD.
2. Gently withdraw the catheter 2–3 inches.
3. Begin the infusion as the catheter is placed correctly.
4. Gently insert the catheter 2–3 inches further.

36. A client has accidentally splashed a toxic (although not caustic) substance in his right eye, and the nurse must flush the eye. Which of the following steps are correct? *Select all that apply.*

1. Position the client's head down until level and on the left side.
2. Irrigate with a bulb syringe tip about a half-inch above the eye.
3. Flush for about 5 minutes.
4. Hold the eyelid open with thumb and index finger while flushing.
5. Hold an emesis basin against the left side of the client's face to contain the irrigant.

37. During which stage of injury repair does the wound show evidence of erythema and edema and phagocytosis begin?

1. Proliferation
2. Inflammation
3. Hemostasis
4. Maturation

38. A client has been admitted through the emergency department after an acute episode of GI hemorrhage. The client's hemoglobin is 6.1 and hematocrit is 18.3. The client is a Jehovah's Witness and has refused transfusions even though his hemoglobin and hematocrit are still falling; the physician has advised him that he might die without transfusions. Which of the following is the most appropriate response for the nurse?

1. Provide supportive care and respect the client's right to refuse treatment.
2. Urge the client to consider his family and reconsider his decision.
3. Tell the client that his decision is unreasonable.
4. Ask the client's family members to reason with the client.

39. A client with a head injury is being admitted into the intensive care unit with a score on the Glasgow Coma Scale of 6. Based on this score, what is the severity of the client's head injury?

1. Mild head injury
2. Severe head injury
3. Coma
4. Moderate head injury

40. A client has recurrent episodes of constipation and fecal impaction. The nurse is assisting the client with a bowel-training regimen. Which of the following interventions should be included? *Select all that apply.*

1. Scheduled toileting
2. Stool softeners
3. High-fiber diet
4. Daily laxatives
5. Periodic enemas
6. Routine exercise

41. A client is to be discharged with a tracheostomy. Which of the following should the nurse most stress when educating the client about home management? *Select all that apply.*

1. Bowel care
2. Pulmonary hygiene
3. Dietary supplements
4. Tracheostomy care
5. Exercise program

42. If a long-time user of opioids is administered naloxone (Narcan) for an opioid overdose, which of the following may occur as a result of the reversal agent?

1. Parkinsonian-like tremors
2. Confusion and disorientation
3. Hyperthermia
4. Acute withdrawal symptoms

43. The nurse is opening a sterile dressing pack to change the dressing on a client's abdominal wound. Which of the following actions will contaminate the contents of the pack?

1. The nurse holds the sterile dressing below waist level when transferring it to the sterile drape.
2. The nurse holds the package in his nondominant hand while peeling the wrapper over the nondominant hand with his other hand.
3. The nurse positions the bottom half of the sterile drape over the top half of the work surface before placing the top half of the drape over the bottom half of the work surface.
4. The nurse opens the outermost flap of the sterile kit away from his body.

44. A client with heart failure has a left ventricular ejection fraction of 38%. When educating the client about managing the condition, which of the following advice should the nurse include? *Select all that apply.*

1. The client should take frequent rest periods.
2. The client should avoid strenuous activities.
3. The client should stop all exercises.
4. The client should stop smoking.
5. The client should limit alcohol intake to 2–3 drinks daily.

45. A client with a brain tumor has exhibited changes in mood and personality and has developed weakness on her right side. Based on these symptoms, the nurse suspects the tumor is located in which part of the brain?

1. Occipital lobe
2. Frontal lobe
3. Temporal lobe
4. Cerebellum

46. The nurse is to administer 250 mL of normal saline intravenously with a flow rate of 15 drops per minute and a drop factor of 15 drops/mL. How many minutes will it take to complete the infusion? *Record your answer as a whole number.*

_______ minutes

47. When assessing a client's skin, the nurse notes a scattered red rash on the trunk. The individual lesions are about 0.5 cm in diameter and are flat, nonpalpable, and circumscribed. How would this type of lesion be classified?

1. Papule
2. Nodule
3. Macule
4. Patch

48. The nurse is assessing a client's cardiac monitoring and notes the following electrocardiogram (ECG) recording:

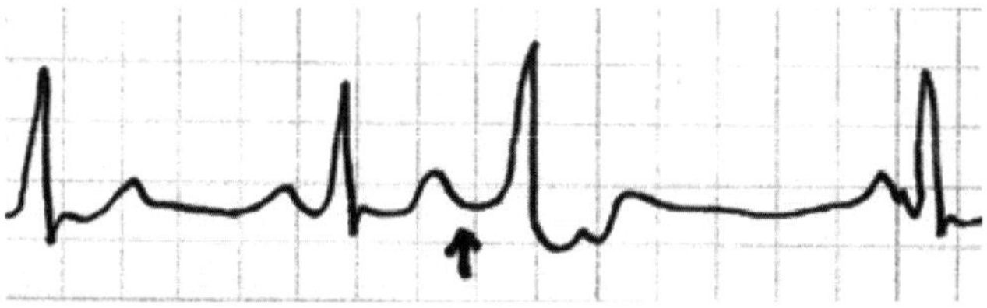

How would the nurse classify this cardiac abnormality?

1. Atrial flutter
2. Premature junctional contraction
3. Ventricular tachycardia
4. Premature ventricular contraction

Questions 49–54 are a set that will test your clinical judgment skills. Read through the information you are given before answering the questions that follow. As you progress through the set, you will be given additional information that you will need to consider before answering subsequent questions.

SETTING

The nurse in the emergency department is caring for a 69-year-old male client.

NURSES' NOTES

1115: The client presents to the emergency department reporting shortness of breath (dyspnea), wheezing, and a cough for the past week. He has a barrel-shaped chest on inspection and reports coughing "more often than normal" with increased thick sputum. The client states that he has been using his albuterol inhaler every 3 hours and typically only needs it after moderate exertion. His daughter reports that he has smoked a half a pack of cigarettes per day for the past 46 years and that he usually has dyspnea with moderate exertion but it has progressed to dyspnea at rest within the past week. The client has a history of prostate cancer, hypertension, chronic obstructive pulmonary disease (COPD), and type 2 diabetes mellitus. The client reports that his fasting blood glucose at 0800 today was 104 mg/dL. On assessment, the client is experiencing dyspnea when answering questions and is only able to speak a few words at a time. The client's daughter states that he has appeared to be increasingly anxious over the past 3 days. His skin is warm and dry, and inspiratory and expiratory wheezing is auscultated bilaterally.

VITAL SIGNS

	1115
Temp	98.4 °F axillary
HR	102, irregular
BP	184/74
RR	23
Pulse oximetry	86% on room air

49. From the following list, select the assessment findings that require immediate follow-up. (Select all that apply)

1. Fasting blood glucose
2. Dyspnea and cough
3. Pulse oximetry reading
4. Anxiety
5. Barrel-shaped chest
6. Pulse, respirations, and blood pressure
7. Warm, dry skin
8. Medical history

50. Based on the client's current clinical picture, he is at the highest risk for developing __________.

1. respiratory alkalosis
2. respiratory acidosis
3. diabetic ketoacidosis
4. metabolic acidosis

Nurses' Notes

1130: The client is sitting in a tripod position with increased work of breathing. His pulse oximetry reading is 83% on room air. The client states "I can't catch my breath," pausing to take a breath between each word. The client is less responsive to questions and appears tired. The primary physician was notified, and new orders are being placed.

Vital Signs

	1115	1130
Temp	98.4 °F axillary	98.4 °F axillary
HR	102, irregular	104, irregular
BP	184/74	180/74
RR	23	27
Pulse oximetry	86% on room air	83% on room air

51. The nurse receives the following orders. Highlight all orders from the following list that the nurse should consider a priority.

- Administer oxygen, 4 L/min via nasal cannula.
- Chest x-ray.
- Administer albuterol nebulization treatment.
- Collect samples for laboratory tests: sputum culture, complete blood count (CBC), and arterial blood gas (ABG).

Nurses' Notes

1200: The client's ABGs are taken at the bedside by the respiratory therapist, and the physician is notified of the results.

Laboratory Results

Laboratory Test and Reference Range	Result
pH Adult: 7.35–7.45	7.32
PaO_2 Adult: >90 mmHg	58
$PaCO_2$ Adult: 35–45 mmHg	48
HCO^3 Adult: 18–24 mEq/L	25

52. Based on the results of the arterial blood gases collected bedside, the nurse anticipates interventions to address the client's __________ using __________.

Blank 1:

1. compensated respiratory alkalosis
2. uncompensated respiratory alkalosis
3. compensated respiratory acidosis
4. uncompensated respiratory acidosis

Blank 2:

1. mechanical ventilation
2. BiPAP
3. increased oxygen via nasal cannula
4. extracorporeal membrane oxygenation

53. For the following list of potential nursing interventions, specify whether each one is indicated or not indicated.

Potential Nursing Interventions	Indicated	Not Indicated
Anticipate an order for a Foley catheter.	○	○
Assist the client into a supine position.	○	○
Apply a bordered foam dressing to protect the client's skin.	○	○
Educate the patient and family on the reason for using BiPAP.	○	○
Monitor the patient for abdominal distension.	○	○

NURSES' NOTES

1300: The client is resting in his room, interacting appropriately with his daughter. Repeat ABGs are taken at the bedside by a respiratory therapist. The client is able to answer assessment questions in short sentences and denies anxiety, pain, and discomfort at this time.

VITAL SIGNS

	1115	**1130**	**1300**
Temp	98.4 °F axillary	98.4 °F axillary	98.5 °F axillary
HR	102, irregular	104, irregular	121, irregular
BP	184/74	180/74	172/80
RR	23	27	19
Pulse oximetry	86% on room air	83% on room air	92% on BiPAP

LABORATORY RESULTS

Laboratory Test and Reference Range	Result
pH Adult: 7.35–7.45	7.37
PaO_2 Adult: >90 mmHg	82
$PaCO_2$ Adult: 35–45 mmHg	43
HCO^3 Adult: 18–24 mEq/L	23

54. The client has been reevaluated to determine his response to the initial interventions provided. Of the following list of assessment findings, specify whether each one indicates that the client's condition has improved, is unchanged, or has worsened.

Assessment Findings	Improved	Unchanged	Worsened
Dyspnea while talking	O	O	O
Respirations, 19	O	O	O
Temperature, 98.5 °F axillary	O	O	O
Pulse oximetry reading, 92%	O	O	O
Heart rate, 121 and irregular	O	O	O
pH, 7.37	O	O	O
$PaCO_2$, 43	O	O	O

Questions 55–60 are a set that will test your clinical judgment skills. Read through the information you are given before answering the questions that follow. As you progress through the set, you will be given additional information that you will need to consider before answering subsequent questions.

SETTING

A 68-year-old female client is brought into the emergency department via ambulance.

NURSES' NOTES

2100: A 68-year-old female arrives to the emergency department via ambulance. Emergency medical services (EMS) reports that at 2030 the client was getting ready for bed when her spouse noticed that her face was drooping and her words were no longer making sense. The client presents with a right-sided facial droop, her gaze is deviated to the left, and she does not respond when asked questions. When asked to make a fist with her right hand, the client makes a fist with her left. The client is able to blink her eyes when instructed. The client responds to touch on the left, but not on the right, and she is unable to move her right side. EMS reports that the client has a history of hypertension, type 2 diabetes, and atrial fibrillation. The client has been on lisinopril and apixaban, but she reportedly ran out last week and has been unable to get the prescriptions refilled. The client is placed on the cardiac monitor, an 18-gauge IV is placed in her left antecubital fossa, and her vital sign measurements are obtained. A bedside blood sugar level is obtained and found to be 125 mg/dL.

VITAL SIGNS

	2100
Temp	97.5 °F temporal
HR	86
BP	195/90
RR	20
Pulse oximetry	92% on room air

PHYSICAL ASSESSMENT

Body System	2100
Neurological	The client is unable to speak. She has right-sided facial droop, left gaze deviation, and no sensation or movement on the right side of her body.
Pulmonary	Lung sounds are clear; respirations are regular and unlabored.

Body System	2100
Cardiovascular	The client is in atrial fibrillation at an irregular rate of 85–90 bpm. Heart sounds are strong; pulses are regular. No signs of chest pain. No edema noted to the extremities.

55. From the following list, select the assessment findings that require immediate follow-up. (Select all that apply.)

1. Temperature
2. Cardiovascular assessment findings
3. Neurological assessment findings
4. Blood pressure
5. Blood sugar
6. Medical history

56. For the list of client findings below, specify for each whether it is consistent with the disease processes of seizures, strokes, or hypoglycemia. Select all supported disease processes for each finding.

Client Findings	Seizure	Stroke	Hypoglycemia
Aphasia	□	□	□
Gaze deviation	□	□	□
Unilateral loss of sensation	□	□	□
Inability to follow commands	□	□	□
Facial droop	□	□	□

57. Based on the clinical picture, the client is most likely experiencing a(n) _________.

1. ischemic stroke secondary to an embolism
2. ischemic stroke secondary to diabetes
3. hemorrhagic stroke secondary to a missed dose of apixaban
4. hemorrhagic stroke secondary to a fall

58. The nurse receives the following orders. Highlight all orders from the following list that the nurse should consider a priority. (Select all that apply.)

- Obtain serum blood sugar.
- Collect blood for a complete blood count (CBC), basic metabolic panel (BMP), and troponin level.
- Obtain an EKG.
- Provide education on medication compliance.
- Obtain a CT scan of the head.
- Administer IV labetalol.

NURSES' NOTES

2110: IV labetalol is administered on the way to the CT scan per the physician's orders. The client is taken to CT with the nurse and the on-call neurologist present.

2130: Upon viewing the CT scan, the neurologist confirms that there is no head bleed present, suspects that an ischemic stroke is the cause of the client's symptoms, and orders administration of a thrombolytic. Because the client is currently unable to speak, the neurologist obtains consent over the phone with the client's family. The neurologist calculates the client's initial National Institutes of Health Stroke Scale (NIHSS) score to be 24.

2135: The nurse administers the ordered thrombolytic.

VITAL SIGNS

	2100	2130
Temp	97.5 °F temporal	98.5 °F temporal
HR	86	90
BP	195/90	165/90
RR	20	18
Pulse oximetry	92% on room air	94% on room air

59. For the following list of potential nursing interventions, specify whether each is indicated or not indicated.

Potential Nursing Interventions	Indicated	Not Indicated
Regularly reassess the client's neurological symptoms.	O	O
Request an order for oral lisinopril.	O	O
Regularly recheck the client's vital signs.	O	O
Monitor for signs of facial swelling.	O	O
Request an order for physical therapy.	O	O

NURSES' NOTES

2230: The client is now able to answer orientation questions, but her speech is slurred. She still has a facial droop. The client is also now able to feel on her right side, but she states that the sensation is weaker than her left side. She is still unable to move her right side. Her gaze is still to the left, but she is now able to look to the right when directed. The nurse calculates the client's new NIHSS score to be 14.

VITAL SIGNS

	2100	2130	2230
Temp	97.5 °F temporal	98.5 °F temporal	97.4 °F temporal
HR	86	90	75
BP	195/90	165/76	190/85
RR	20	18	22
Pulse oximetry	92% on room air	93% on room air	92% on room air

60. For the following list of assessment findings, specify whether each one indicates that the client's condition has improved, is unchanged, or has worsened.

Assessment Findings	Improved	Unchanged	Worsened
Blood pressure, 190/85	O	O	O
Pulse oximetry reading, 92%	O	O	O
NIHSS score, 14	O	O	O
Facial droop	O	O	O
Gaze deviation	O	O	O

Answer Key and Explanations for Test #2

1. 3: Edema is a common problem related to burns, so the nurse must check peripheral pulses frequently (at least every two hours) and keep the extremities elevated on two pillows. If the pulses become diminished, the first step is to loosen the dressings and recheck the pulses to determine if the dressings are restricting blood flow. Burns are often treated with topical agents and several layers of dressings, which should be applied on the lower extremities distally to proximally.

2. 3: Cholecystitis may result in severe episodes of pain in the right upper quadrant of the abdomen, often lasting two to six hours, and sometimes radiating to the back. Clients may also experience indigestion, nausea and vomiting, and clay-colored stools if the bile duct is blocked. In severe cases, jaundice may be evident. Cholecystitis may result from calculi or pancreatitis and is most common in overweight females ages 20–40, but it also may occur in women who are pregnant.

3. 1: The ethical principle of autonomy recognizes that clients have the right to make their own informed decisions about their care. The most important assessment is of the client's cognitive ability because the client needs to be able to understand and consider information that is given by healthcare providers. Children may be able to make informed decisions, but the law does not allow them to do so unless they are emancipated, so the right of autonomy passes to the parents or guardians. Likewise, clients who have cognitive impairment may not be able to make informed decisions.

4. 2, 4, 5, 6: These signs and symptoms are consistent with severe digoxin toxicity. The nurse should anticipate administering digoxin immune fab to counteract the digoxin. The client should have laboratory tests for digoxin and electrolyte levels (hypokalemia is common) and continuous cardiac monitoring. Supportive treatment should be provided for GI symptoms.

5. 4: The most likely reason for the spouse's reaction is premature completion of anticipatory grief. The spouse began the grieving process early, anticipating the loss and the emotions, and may be quite spent and emotionally withdrawn when this process completes. A different type of grieving will occur when the client actually dies.

6. 1: These symptoms are indications of cardiac tamponade resulting from perforation of the ventricle and bleeding into the pericardial sac. This is a medical emergency, and the nurse must immediately notify the physician and prepare the client for surgery. Although nonhemorrhagic tamponade will usually respond well to pericardiocentesis, hemorrhagic tamponade requires a thoracotomy because the bleeding will continue until its cause is corrected.

7. 1: Acupuncture has been demonstrated to relieve chemotherapy-induced nausea and vomiting in a number of studies. Some studies also seem to indicate that ginger (usually in tea form) can reduce the intensity of nausea but not vomiting. The nurse may recommend both of these therapies. However, there is no evidence to suggest that therapeutic touch or magnetic therapy are effective in relieving nausea, and herbal therapies must be evaluated individually as some may interact negatively with the client's medications.

8. 3: When changing a colostomy appliance, the skin about the stoma should be cleansed with warm tap water. Alcohol may be irritating to the tissue, and soap or baby wipes may leave residue on the tissue that interferes with adhesion. If any soap is used, it should be mild and without oils or perfume and should be rinsed off thoroughly with warm water. If skin paste is present, it should be removed before wetting the skin.

9. 2: Because attempting to evacuate clients from the facility is likely to increase exposure to the hazardous material, the most likely emergency response is to shelter in place. This applies to both staff and clients. Guidelines may vary according to the type of waste but can include locking doors, sealing doors and windows, and shutting off air-conditioning and forced-air systems. Many facilities have windows that do not open, but if not, windows should be closed immediately. Staff should monitor news reports because emergency personnel may not be readily available to provide information.

10. 4: Tardive dyskinesia (TD) is a chronic adverse effect associated with haloperidol and other neuroleptic drugs as well as anticholinergics and substances of abuse. Elderly clients and those with schizophrenia and other neuropsychiatric diseases have an increased risk of developing TD, so these drugs should be used with care or avoided. Once symptoms develop, up to 50% of clients remain afflicted, even if the medication is discontinued. No established treatment is available, although different approaches can be tried, including herbal medicines.

11. 4: If a client is experiencing hypothermia, treatment depends on the core body temperature. For a core body temperature of 28–32.2°C, active internal rewarming procedures are carried out. These include cardiopulmonary bypass, warm IV fluid administration, and warm peritoneal lavage. However, for a core body temperature of 32.2–35°C, passive or active external rewarming procedures are used. These include over-the-bed heaters and forced-air warming blankets. Patients with hypothermia have reduced sensation, so they must be carefully monitored to prevent burns.

12. 2, 3, 4, 5: The purpose of personal protective equipment (PPE) is to protect the wearer against hazards in the workplace, so the equipment may vary from one workplace to another. Goggles, respirators, masks, gloves, and gowns are commonly used PPE in nursing, but personal radiation dosimeters may also be considered as PPE if the nurse is exposed to radiation in the workplace and needs to monitor the exposure. Back belts have not been shown in studies to reduce the risk of back injuries, are not considered PPE, and are not recommended for use.

13. 1, 3, 4: The following ECG tracing represents premature ventricular contraction. If occurring without other abnormalities in clients who are otherwise healthy, PVCs are usually of no particular concern and are not generally treated. PVCs may result from intake of caffeine, nicotine, or alcohol. Frequent PVCs do not signify a myocardial infarction (MI), though they can signify ventricular tachycardia if there is a run of more than 3 PVCs in a row. The presence of frequent PVCs following an MI does increase the mortality risk and must be carefully monitored. PVCs may occur in conjunction with underlying supraventricular dysrhythmias.

14. 1: Inappropriate affect is a negative symptom. Schizophrenia is characterized by both negative and positive symptoms:

Positive	Negative
Hallucinations (auditory, visual, olfactory, gustatory, tactile)	Affective flattening (poor eye contact, diminished expression, inappropriate affect)
Delusions (persecution, grandeur, reference, control, somatic)	Alogia [poverty of speech] (decreased fluency and content)
Disorganized thinking and speech (echolalia, word salad, incoherence, loose association)	Avolition/Apathy (inability to initiate goal-directed activities, lack of interest in work, grooming, hygiene)
Disorganized behavior (disheveled appearance, restlessness, agitation, inappropriate sexual behavior)	Anhedonia (lack of pleasure in social activities and diminished interest in intimacy)
	Social isolation

15. 1, 2, 4, 5: The client should dispose of syringes and needles in a sharps disposal container (or glass jar) immediately after use, being sure to maintain the container out of reach of children and pets. The container should be disposed of when it is about three-quarters full because if the container is too full, the risk of accidental puncture increases. While the container may be disposed of in the regular trash in some areas, other areas are more restrictive, so the client must check with the local community garbage disposal company for guidelines. Needles should never be flushed down the toilet.

16. 2: The Apgar test is given at one minute and five minutes after birth to determine if emergency care is needed. A total score of 7 or above is a sign of good health.

Sign	0	1	2
Appearance (skin color)	Cyanosis or pallor over entire body	Normal, except for extremities	Entire body is normal
Pulse (heart rate)	Absent	<100 bpm	>100 bpm
Grimace (reflex irritability)	Unresponsive	Grimace	Infant sneezes, coughs, and recoils
Activity (muscle tone)	Absent	Flexed extremities	Infant moves freely
Respiration (breathing rate and effort)	Absent	Bradypnea, dyspnea	Good breathing and crying

17. 0.25: To complete the calculation, first convert micrograms (mcg) to milligrams (mg), and then dived the desired dose by the available dose:

$$(50 \text{ mcg})\left(\frac{1 \text{ mg}}{1{,}000 \text{ mcg}}\right) = 0.05 \text{ mg}$$

$$\frac{0.05 \text{ mg}}{0.2 \text{ mg/tablet}} = 0.25 \text{ tablets}$$

18. 4: The glucose is high normal, but both kidney function tests, the BUN and serum creatinine, are markedly elevated. This indicates a probable kidney failure, so further testing for kidney disease is indicated.

Test	Result	Normal value
BUN	172 mg/dL	7-17 mg/dL
Serum creatinine	16.4 mg/dL	8.4-10.2 mg/dL
Glucose	98 mg/dL	70-99 mg/dL

19. 2: After insertion of a Foley catheter into a male client, his penis should be positioned upward so that the catheter does not catch on his legs. It should be secured by tape to the right or left lower abdomen, with the tubing looped so the client has slack to turn from side to side. Then, the tube is taped to the edge of the bed. The tubing should hang vertically down from the mattress to the collection bag so the urine drains properly.

20. 3: If a client is to receive two oral medications (capsules) per the enteral feeding tube, the nurse should open the capsules separately and dilute each with water. They should be drawn up in separate syringes for instilling. If the client has continuous feeding, the feeding should be stopped and the tube flushed with about 15 mL of water before instilling the first drug and then flushed again with the same volume after instillation to empty the tube of the medication before the second drug instillation. Then, the tube is flushed again before restarting the feeding.

21. 1: While protocols regarding tube feedings may vary somewhat, generally if gastric residual is less than 100 mL, it is returned to the stomach and the tubing flushed with 30 mL of water. If it is more than 100mL (in this case 150 mL), it may indicate that an obstruction has occurred, and the nurse should hold the feeding and notify the MD before proceeding. The amount of residual gastric contents should be aspirated and measured at least every 8 hours.

22. 2: Two forms of identifiers should always be used prior to administering medication to any client, even if the nurse recognizes the client and is relatively sure of the client's identity. Asking the client's name and checking the hospital ID bracelet meet minimal requirements. In some cases, clients may be identified by asking their names and birthdates. The nurse should always double check the name on the medication as well. An ID bracelet that is not on the client but elsewhere, such as on a bedside stand, should not be used for identification.

23. 3, 4, 5: The irrigating syringe should be filled with about 50 mL of irrigant, but it should be instilled slowly, using care not to occlude the ear canal with the syringe tip, as this may result in increased pressure and rupture of the eardrum. The client should be positioned lying flat or sitting with the head turned toward the affected ear to facilitate drainage and help secure the drainage basin. On those over 3 years old, the pinna is pulled up and back. The solution should drain out freely during the irrigation.

24. 30: Administration of medications through an NG tube under suction should be avoided if possible because some of the medication may be suctioned out; however, if medication is ordered, the nurse must disconnect the suction prior to administration, ensure the NG tube is properly placed (injecting air and listening for gurgling, aspirating, and checking the pH), flush the NG tube with 30 mL water, administer the medication, flush the tubing with another 30 mL water, and leave it disconnected from the suction for 30 minutes to allow time for the medication to be absorbed.

25. 4: Intramuscular (IM) injections are almost always given to adults with a needle that is 1.5 inches in length. A shorter length (1 inch) should be reserved for children or for very thin adults. The needle gauge usually varies from 21–25, although very thick preparations may require a gauge of 18 or 19. IM injections are usually given with a 3-mL syringe, although the maximum amount of medication in each injection should not exceed 2 mL. If larger volumes are ordered, then the dose should be divided and administered in two injections.

26. 3: The nurse should anticipate that the dosage of warfarin will be held or reduced until the INR decreases. The INR level should be maintained at 2.0–3.0 for venous thrombosis, pulmonary embolism, and valvular heart disease, and at 2.5–3.5 for clients with mechanical heart valves or recurrent systemic emboli. Vitamin K is generally not indicated as a reversal agent with an INR below 5.0, especially with no evidence of bleeding.

27. 4: The metabolic effect that is most common if a client is taking a loop diuretic is hypokalemia. Therefore, clients are often prescribed supplementary potassium to take with the loop diuretic and have regular monitoring of electrolytes. Other metabolic effects that may occur are hyperglycemia and hyperuricemia. Some people may develop gastrointestinal problems, such as nausea, vomiting, and diarrhea. Other adverse effects include thrombocytopenia, neutropenia, agranulocytosis, headache, tinnitus, dizziness, and blurred vision.

28. 4: If a mother is concerned that her neonate is having periods of apnea, the nurse should reassure her that slight pauses in breathing, referred to as periodic breathing, are normal in the neonate. Usually the pause is only 2–3 seconds, but it may be longer in some cases. However, if the periods persist for more than 15–20 seconds or increase in frequency, the mother should notify the physician, especially if the episodes are accompanied by other changes, such as pallor, cyanosis, bradycardia, or hypotonia.

29. 4: While there is not total agreement about the results of HbA1c tests, generally levels at or above 6.5% are considered diagnostic of diabetes mellitus. Values of 5.7–6.4% are considered pre-diabetic by most authorities. Lower values are within normal limits. Because hemoglobin retains excess blood glucose and red blood cells live about 120 days, the HbA1c test shows the average blood glucose levels over a 3-month period. HbA1c is used to diagnose diabetes and monitor long-term diabetic therapy.

30. 2, 4, 5: Pills may be crushed and diluted in 10–15 mL of water to be added to the NG tube feedings. Liquid forms of medications are easiest to add. Soft-gel capsules can be opened at one end and drained, but some dosage is usually lost, so dissolving the capsule in warm water first (and removing the remains of the gel capsule) is a better solution. Extended-release capsules should be opened but NOT crushed before adding to the tube. Enteric-coated tablets should not be crushed or administered per NG tube, and sublingual wafers are not absorbed through the GI tract.

31. 2: The integrity of the closed system of drainage should be maintained. The correct procedure for collecting a urine specimen from a Foley catheter with a sample port is to first wipe the port with alcohol and allow the alcohol to dry. Next, insert a 10-mL needleless syringe into the port and withdraw the sample.

32. 1: When reviewing dietary restriction with an immunocompromised client following kidney transplantation, the client should be advised to avoid raw bean sprouts because of the chance they may harbor pathogenic organisms. Clients should also be advised to avoid grapefruit and grapefruit juice, which may interfere with some medications, as well as raw or undercooked meats and uncooked dough that contains raw eggs, such as cookie dough. Clients should also be advised to limit or avoid foods from buffets or salad bars, as they may not be properly prepared or may sit for prolonged periods, encouraging the growth of bacteria.

33. 1: If a client has suffered an ischemic stroke in the right hemisphere, the nurse should anticipate that the client has left paralysis and left visual field defect. Language skills usually remain intact, although the client may have some short-term memory loss and difficulty following directions. Clients may also act impulsively and have poor judgement. The client's fine motor skills may be impaired, resulting in difficulty dressing and carrying out tasks that involve the use of tools.

34. 4: If a client's medication order is for 300 mg of a liquid medication that is available at 75 mg per mL, the nurse should administer 4 mL of medication.

$$\frac{(300 \text{ mg})}{75 \text{ mg/mL}} = 4 \text{ mL}$$

35. 1: The nurse should hold the infusion and notify the MD that the catheter tip is incorrectly placed, as it should be in the superior vena cava rather than the right atrium. Infusing the solutions directly into the right atrium may result in tissue damage. While the catheter needs to be withdrawn a few inches and another X-ray taken to ensure correct placement, this procedure should only be done by a physician or a specially trained nurse.

36. 2, 4: If a client has accidentally splashed a toxic (although not caustic) substance in the right eye, the steps to flushing the eye include:

- Place the client on their right side and elevate their head to 20 degrees.
- Hold the emesis basin against the right side of their face.
- Fill bulb syringe with NS irrigant.
- Hold the right eyelid open with the thumb and index finger.
- Hold the tip of the syringe about a half-inch above the eye and direct the flow of the irrigant toward the lower conjunctival sac, from inner to outer canthus.
- Flush for about 1 minute.

37. 2: The wound shows evidence of erythema and edema, and phagocytosis begins during the inflammation stage of injury repair. Stages:

1. Hemostasis: During first few minutes. Platelets seal off the vessels and secrete substances that cause vasoconstriction. Thrombin stimulates the clotting mechanism, forming a fibrin mesh.
2. Inflammation: Over days 1–4. Inflammatory response and phagocytosis occur.
3. Proliferation: Over days 5–20. Fibroblasts produce collagen and granulation tissue starts to form. Epithelialization contracts wound.
4. Maturation: After day 21 to 2 years. Collagen tightens to reduce scarring. The tissue gains tensile strength.

38. 1: In this situation, the best response is to provide supportive care as indicated and respect the client's right to refuse treatment. While it is appropriate to tell the client that he can change his mind at any time, pressuring the client or his family is not appropriate.

39. 2: A Glasgow Coma Scale (GCS) score of 6 indicates a severe head injury. GCS is based on scores assigned for three parameters: eye-opening response, verbal response, and motor response. Scores range from 3 (worst possible) to 15 (best possible). Head injuries are classified according to the following scores:

- Severe head injury: GCS score of 8 or less
- Moderate head injury: GCS score of 9–12
- Mild head injury: GCS score of 13–15

40. 1, 2, 3, 6: If a client has recurrent episodes of constipation and fecal impaction, interventions that should be part of bowel training include scheduled toileting, such as attempting to defecate at the same time each day. The client should be advised to increase fluid intake and eat high-fiber foods. Stool softeners may be taken but not daily laxatives, which may in time make constipation worse. Stimulants, such as a suppository or a hot cup of coffee, may help to promote defecation. Routine exercise may help to stimulate intestinal contractions.

41. 1, 2, 4: Clients with a tracheostomy are at increased risk of fecal impaction because they cannot perform the Valsalva maneuver to bear down, so they need to be educated about bowel care and advised to use stool softeners routinely and laxatives and suppositories as needed. Additionally, they need to understand the importance of pulmonary hygiene to prevent atelectasis and infection and should be confident in all aspects of tracheostomy care, including information about what to do if the tracheostomy tube falls out.

42. 4: Because naloxone (Narcan) reverses the action of opioids, if administered to a long-time opioid user, it may trigger an acute withdrawal reaction. The dosage of naloxone should be titrated carefully and the client should be monitored throughout treatment. Withdrawal symptoms may occur within minutes of administration of the drug, depending on the dosage of medication and the degree of opioid dependence.

43. 1: The sterile field extends from the waist to the shoulders, and sterile gowns are considered sterile only between these points. Any sterile item that is held out of the line of sight or below the waist is considered contaminated. The sterile field should be placed on a table that is waist high. The drape is considered sterile except for one inch around the perimeter of the drape, so no contents should come in contact with that area. Sterile items should be dropped toward the center of the drape.

44. 1, 2, 4: If a client with heart failure has a left ventricular fraction of 38%, this is classified as heart failure (<40% EF). Normal EF is 50–70%. Risk of dysrhythmias occurs if the EF falls to below 35%. While the client should avoid strenuous exercise and should take frequent rest periods, maintaining a routine of regular exercise, such as walking, is important to maintain adequate cardiac output. The client should stop smoking and limit alcohol intake to one to two drinks daily.

45. 2: Brain tumors or traumatic brain injuries to different parts of the brain can result in specific types of symptoms:

- Frontal lobe: Changes in mood and personality, as well as hemiparesis
- Occipital lobe: Visual disturbances and visual hallucinations
- Temporal lobe: Loss of memory, speech abnormalities, and lack of coordination
- Parietal lobe: Loss of sensation; difficulty with fine motor skills, such as writing; and loss of half-body awareness
- Cerebellum: Lack of balance and coordination
- Brain stem: Dysphagia, facial pain, weakness, and cranial nerve dysfunction

46. 250: Calculation:

$$\left(\frac{15 \text{ drops}}{1 \text{ min}}\right) \times \left(\frac{1 \text{ ml}}{15 \text{ drops}}\right) = 1 \text{ ml/min}$$

$$(250 \text{ ml}) \times (1 \text{ ml/min}) = 250 \text{ min}$$

47. 3: This type of lesion would be classified as a macule. Macular lesions include those associated with petechiae, measles, and scarlet fever. Freckles are benign macules. A patch is similar to a macule but larger than 1 cm. Papules are solid, elevated, and less than 1 cm in diameter. Nodules are similar to papules but larger than 1 cm.

48. 4:

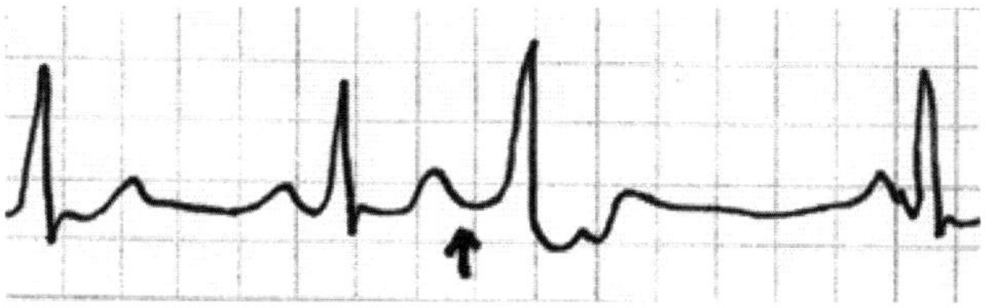

This ECG recording represents premature ventricular contraction (PVC). PVCs are ectopic beats that can occur early in otherwise healthy individuals, although they are of concern in those with preexisting heart disease because they may indicate a risk for more severe ventricular arrhythmias, such as ventricular tachycardia. The impulse for the ectopic beat originates within the ventricles prior to the sinus impulse. PVCs may occur singly, in pairs, or in a recurring pattern and are often followed by a compensatory pause.

49. 2, 3, 6, and 8: The client's dyspnea with cough, low pulse oximetry reading, and pulse/respirations/blood pressure all require immediate follow-up because they are indicative of respiratory distress, which can quickly escalate to respiratory failure if left without intervention. These factors, in conjunction with the client's history of COPD, support the client's risk for rapid respiratory decline. Although clients with COPD generally have lower oxygen saturation, 86% is low even in this context and must be addressed. A barrel-shaped appearance to the chest is normal in clients with chronic COPD due to the hyperinflation of the lungs secondary to air trapping in the alveoli, and it does not represent an emergent condition. The client's fasting blood glucose was within normal parameters. The client's warm, dry skin is also a normal finding. Although the client's anxiety and productive cough should be addressed and treated, they are not of immediate concern.

50. 2: The client is demonstrating the signs and symptoms of respiratory distress, which could lead to respiratory failure if left untreated. These include dyspnea at rest, decreased oxygen saturation, tachypnea, and wheezing. COPD disrupts the body's ability to properly ventilate due to the air trapping that occurs in the lungs. This can result in a buildup of carbon dioxide (CO_2) because it is not being released. An increase in CO_2 secondary to insufficient ventilation results in respiratory acidosis, which is a complication of COPD exacerbations.

51.

- Administer oxygen, 4 L/min via nasal cannula.
- Chest x-ray.
- Administer albuterol nebulization treatment.
- Collect samples for laboratory tests: sputum culture, complete blood count (CBC), and arterial blood gas (ABG).

The client's oxygen saturation level has decreased, and his overall respiratory status has declined (evidenced by the tripod position and the client only being able to speak one word at a time). The highest priority intervention is to administer oxygen in order to increase his oxygen saturation level and support his respiratory efforts. The nebulization treatment is a priority because it will help open up the client's airway and treat his dyspnea. The sputum culture and CBC will reveal if the client has an infection, and the ABG will demonstrate the severity of the client's respiratory status. The x-ray is not a priority intervention because it will not have an immediate effect on the client's respiratory status and can be performed once the client has been stabilized.

52. 4 and 2: The client's COPD exacerbation has resulted in respiratory acidosis demonstrated by his elevated $PaCO_2$ and decreased pH readings. The kidneys are attempting to compensate for the acidosis by retaining HCO^3 (demonstrated by a slightly elevated HCO^3 level), but they are unable to do so because the pH level remains below normal. This leaves the client with uncompensated respiratory acidosis. The most effective treatment of respiratory acidosis is bilevel positive airway pressure (BiPAP), which assists in opening the alveoli and releasing the trapped air. This would be done prior to invasive mechanical ventilation. Increasing oxygen via nasal cannula would be insufficient, and extracorporeal membrane oxygenation is not indicated unless the patient continues to decline with a pH of less than 7.2.

53.

Potential Nursing Interventions	Indicated	Not Indicated
Anticipate an order for a Foley catheter.	○	●
Assist the client into a supine position.	○	●
Apply a bordered foam dressing to protect the client's skin.	●	○
Educate the client and family on the reasoning for using BiPAP.	●	○
Monitor the patient for abdominal distension.	●	○

There is no indication for a Foley catheter at this time: A bedpan or urinal could be used to avoid introducing infection risks. Moving the client into a supine position will put more pressure on his lungs, and it may worsen his current respiratory status. The client is at risk for skin breakdown related to the pressure caused by the BiPAP mask. Applying a bordered foam dressing to the client's skin will help protect it. It is important to explain the use of BiPAP to the client and family in order to lessen anxiety and ensure understanding of the purpose of the device. The client and family should be informed of the importance of removing excess CO_2 and increasing oxygenation. The client should be monitored for abdominal distension—a potential complication from BiPAP that may cause discomfort.

54.

Assessment Findings	Improved	Unchanged	Worsened
Dyspnea while talking	●	○	○
Respirations, 19	●	○	○
Temperature, 98.5 °F axillary	○	●	○
Pulse oximetry reading, 92%	●	○	○
Heart rate, 121 and irregular	○	○	●
pH, 7.37	●	○	○
$PaCO_2$, 43	●	○	○

During the 1130 assessment, the client was only able to speak one word at a time; however, he is now able to speak in short sentences, which demonstrates improvement of his dyspnea. The client's respiratory rate has decreased from 23 to 19, showing improvement because he is no longer tachypneic. The client remains afebrile; therefore, this component is unchanged. The client's pulse oximetry reading increased from 83% to 92%, which represents an improvement to an acceptable oximetry reading for an individual with COPD. The client's heart rate has increased from 102 to 121, which represents worsening tachycardia. The client's pH and $PaCO_2$ are now within the normal range, which indicates that the client's respiratory acidosis has resolved.

55. 3, 4, and 6: The client's temperature, cardiovascular assessment, and blood sugar are all expected findings given her medical history. The client's neurological assessment and elevated blood pressure are abnormal findings that require further testing emergently. The client's medical history shows that she has an increased risk of poor health outcomes. For example, being older than age 65 and having a history of hypertension, type 2 diabetes, and atrial fibrillation all increase the client's risk of cardiovascular and neurological diseases. Additionally, the client missing her lisinopril and apixaban medications for the past week increases her risk of elevated blood pressure and of developing clots.

56.

Client Findings	Seizure	Stroke	Hypoglycemia
Aphasia	■	■	■
Gaze deviation	■	■	□
Unilateral loss of sensation	□	■	□
Inability to follow commands	■	■	■
Facial droop	□	■	□

Seizures and strokes are both neurological in origin and therefore have overlapping signs and symptoms, including aphasia, gaze deviation, and the inability to follow commands. A stroke is differentiated from a seizure in that the infarct in the brain often results in unilateral deficits, including a unilateral loss of sensation or a facial droop. Hypoglycemia can cause mental status changes, such as the inability to follow commands and even aphasia, but it does not cause unilateral deficits or gaze deviation.

57. 1: The client is most likely experiencing an ischemic stroke based on her symptoms and her recent medical history. Clients with a history of atrial fibrillation who are off of their blood thinning medication are at a higher risk of developing an embolism that could travel to the brain and cause ischemia. The client's symptoms also indicate that she is vision, aphasia, neglect (VAN) positive. This screening assessment is conducted by a trained healthcare provider (generally a paramedic, ED/ICU/stroke nurse, advanced practice provider, or physician) to determine if the client is likely having a large vessel occlusion. Although diabetes puts the client at a greater risk for strokes, it is unlikely to be considered a direct cause of the stroke. A hemorrhagic stroke is also possible and should be ruled out as soon as possible. However, a hemorrhagic stroke is less likely in this case because the client has not complained of a severe headache and has not had any reported head trauma (such as a fall). Also, missing a dose of a blood thinner such as apixaban is unlikely to cause hemorrhage and more likely to lead to an embolism.

58.

- Obtain serum blood sugar.
- Collect blood for a CBC, BMP, and troponin level.
- Obtain an EKG.
- Provide education on medication compliance.
- Obtain a CT scan of the head.
- Administer IV labetalol.

When dealing with a suspected stroke, it is important to remember that the longer that care is delayed, the more likely the client is to have worse outcomes. Treating a stroke quickly increases the odds that the client will either recover, or at the very least not have worsening symptoms from lack of brain perfusion. Generally, thrombolytics must be administered within 4.5 hours of the onset of stroke symptoms, and endovascular thrombectomy for large vessel occlusions must be done within 24 hours of the onset of symptoms. A computed tomography (CT) scan of the client should be obtained within 25 minutes of arrival to the emergency department to rule out a hemorrhagic stroke. If indicated, as soon as a hemorrhagic stroke is ruled out (and an ischemic stroke is diagnosed), thrombolytic medication may be administered. Additionally, the client's elevated blood pressure must be treated because a systolic blood pressure above 185 is considered a contraindication for thrombolytics. While it is important to obtain a bedside blood sugar early because hypo-/hyperglycemia can present similarly to a stroke, this was already taken via fingerstick and did not have a concerning finding. Secondary testing such as an electrocardiogram (EKG) and lab work may be done, but this is not a priority and should not delay the initial CT scan or the administration of thrombolytics. Providing patient education about the importance of medication compliance may be important later in the client's care, but it would not be appropriate for the current emergency situation.

59.

Potential Nursing Interventions	Indicated	Not Indicated
Regularly reassess the client's neurological symptoms.	●	○
Request an order for oral lisinopril.	○	●
Regularly recheck the client's vital signs.	●	○
Monitor for signs of facial swelling.	●	○
Request an order for physical therapy.	○	●

When administering thrombolytics, it is important to monitor the client's vital signs and neurological status closely and routinely. Although it is important to note any improvements that the medication may cause, it is also important to quickly recognize and treat any worsening symptoms. Thrombolytics increase the client's risk of hemorrhage, including intracranial hemorrhage. Having an elevated blood pressure can also increase this risk. Additionally, thrombolytics can cause angioedema, which causes facial swelling, that should be recognized and treated early. Although blood pressure medications may be indicated for this client, the client should remain on a strict nothing-by-mouth status until a swallow screening has been completed and shows that she is not at risk of aspiration. Physical therapy will likely be indicated following the client's hospital admission for rehabilitation because she is currently unable to move the right side of her body and would be at a high risk of falling during a physical therapy assessment at this time.

60.

Assessment Findings	Improved	Unchanged	Worsened
Blood pressure, 190/85	○	○	●
Pulse oximetry reading, 92%	○	●	○
NIHSS score, 14	●	○	○
Facial droop	○	●	○
Gaze deviation	●	○	○

The client's overall respiratory assessment has remained unchanged throughout her stay, with the pulse oximetry reading hovering between 92 and 93%. These minor changes remain at suboptimal levels, as a normal pulse oximetry reading is >95% (except for those with conditions such as COPD which is not indicated here). The physician should be notified, as oxygen delivery via nasal cannula may be initiated to increase her oxygenation status to normal range. Her tachypnea (demonstrated by a respiratory rate of >20 breaths per minute) may also improve with oxygen support. The client's overall neurological assessment has improved. The client still seems to have gaze deviation and possible neglect on one side, but she is now able to look to the other side when prompted. Her NIHSS score went from 22 to 14, which is also an improvement (the closer the score is to 0, the better). Her facial droop and most of her vital signs (including her pulse oximetry reading) remain unchanged. However, her blood pressure has worsened. The physician should be notified of this finding immediately. Although the thrombolytic medication was administered nearly 1 hour prior to this, the client is still at risk of intracranial hemorrhage, and her blood pressure needs to be controlled to help prevent that outcome.

How to Overcome Test Anxiety

Just the thought of taking a test is enough to make most people a little nervous. A test is an important event that can have a long-term impact on your future, so it's important to take it seriously and it's natural to feel anxious about performing well. But just because anxiety is normal, that doesn't mean that it's helpful in test taking, or that you should simply accept it as part of your life. Anxiety can have a variety of effects. These effects can be mild, like making you feel slightly nervous, or severe, like blocking your ability to focus or remember even a simple detail.

If you experience test anxiety—whether severe or mild—it's important to know how to beat it. To discover this, first you need to understand what causes test anxiety.

Causes of Test Anxiety

While we often think of anxiety as an uncontrollable emotional state, it can actually be caused by simple, practical things. One of the most common causes of test anxiety is that a person does not feel adequately prepared for their test. This feeling can be the result of many different issues such as poor study habits or lack of organization, but the most common culprit is time management. Starting to study too late, failing to organize your study time to cover all of the material, or being distracted while you study will mean that you're not well prepared for the test. This may lead to cramming the night before, which will cause you to be physically and mentally exhausted for the test. Poor time management also contributes to feelings of stress, fear, and hopelessness as you realize you are not well prepared but don't know what to do about it.

Other times, test anxiety is not related to your preparation for the test but comes from unresolved fear. This may be a past failure on a test, or poor performance on tests in general. It may come from comparing yourself to others who seem to be performing better or from the stress of living up to expectations. Anxiety may be driven by fears of the future—how failure on this test would affect your educational and career goals. These fears are often completely irrational, but they can still negatively impact your test performance.

Elements of Test Anxiety

As mentioned earlier, test anxiety is considered to be an emotional state, but it has physical and mental components as well. Sometimes you may not even realize that you are suffering from test anxiety until you notice the physical symptoms. These can include trembling hands, rapid heartbeat, sweating, nausea, and tense muscles. Extreme anxiety may lead to fainting or vomiting. Obviously, any of these symptoms can have a negative impact on testing. It is important to recognize them as soon as they begin to occur so that you can address the problem before it damages your performance.

The mental components of test anxiety include trouble focusing and inability to remember learned information. During a test, your mind is on high alert, which can help you recall information and stay focused for an extended period of time. However, anxiety interferes with your mind's natural processes, causing you to blank out, even on the questions you know well. The strain of testing during anxiety makes it difficult to stay focused, especially on a test that may take several hours. Extreme anxiety can take a huge mental toll, making it difficult not only to recall test information but even to understand the test questions or pull your thoughts together.

Effects of Test Anxiety

Test anxiety is like a disease—if left untreated, it will get progressively worse. Anxiety leads to poor performance, and this reinforces the feelings of fear and failure, which in turn lead to poor performances on subsequent tests. It can grow from a mild nervousness to a crippling condition. If allowed to progress, test anxiety can have a big impact on your schooling, and consequently on your future.

Test anxiety can spread to other parts of your life. Anxiety on tests can become anxiety in any stressful situation, and blanking on a test can turn into panicking in a job situation. But fortunately, you don't have to let anxiety rule your testing and determine your grades. There are a number of relatively simple steps you can take to move past anxiety and function normally on a test and in the rest of life.

Physical Steps for Beating Test Anxiety

While test anxiety is a serious problem, the good news is that it can be overcome. It doesn't have to control your ability to think and remember information. While it may take time, you can begin taking steps today to beat anxiety.

Just as your first hint that you may be struggling with anxiety comes from the physical symptoms, the first step to treating it is also physical. Rest is crucial for having a clear, strong mind. If you are tired, it is much easier to give in to anxiety. But if you establish good sleep habits, your body and mind will be ready to perform optimally, without the strain of exhaustion. Additionally, sleeping well helps you to retain information better, so you're more likely to recall the answers when you see the test questions.

Getting good sleep means more than going to bed on time. It's important to allow your brain time to relax. Take study breaks from time to time so it doesn't get overworked, and don't study right before bed. Take time to rest your mind before trying to rest your body, or you may find it difficult to fall asleep.

Along with sleep, other aspects of physical health are important in preparing for a test. Good nutrition is vital for good brain function. Sugary foods and drinks may give a burst of energy but this burst is followed by a crash, both physically and emotionally. Instead, fuel your body with protein and vitamin-rich foods.

Also, drink plenty of water. Dehydration can lead to headaches and exhaustion, especially if your brain is already under stress from the rigors of the test. Particularly if your test is a long one, drink water during the breaks. And if possible, take an energy-boosting snack to eat between sections.

Along with sleep and diet, a third important part of physical health is exercise. Maintaining a steady workout schedule is helpful, but even taking 5-minute study breaks to walk can help get your blood pumping faster and clear your head. Exercise also releases endorphins, which contribute to a positive feeling and can help combat test anxiety.

When you nurture your physical health, you are also contributing to your mental health. If your body is healthy, your mind is much more likely to be healthy as well. So take time to rest, nourish your body with healthy food and water, and get moving as much as possible. Taking these physical steps will make you stronger and more able to take the mental steps necessary to overcome test anxiety.

Mental Steps for Beating Test Anxiety

Working on the mental side of test anxiety can be more challenging, but as with the physical side, there are clear steps you can take to overcome it. As mentioned earlier, test anxiety often stems from lack of preparation, so the obvious solution is to prepare for the test. Effective studying may be the most important weapon you have for beating test anxiety, but you can and should employ several other mental tools to combat fear.

First, boost your confidence by reminding yourself of past success—tests or projects that you aced. If you're putting as much effort into preparing for this test as you did for those, there's no reason you should expect to fail here. Work hard to prepare; then trust your preparation.

Second, surround yourself with encouraging people. It can be helpful to find a study group, but be sure that the people you're around will encourage a positive attitude. If you spend time with others who are anxious or cynical, this will only contribute to your own anxiety. Look for others who are motivated to study hard from a desire to succeed, not from a fear of failure.

Third, reward yourself. A test is physically and mentally tiring, even without anxiety, and it can be helpful to have something to look forward to. Plan an activity following the test, regardless of the outcome, such as going to a movie or getting ice cream.

When you are taking the test, if you find yourself beginning to feel anxious, remind yourself that you know the material. Visualize successfully completing the test. Then take a few deep, relaxing breaths and return to it. Work through the questions carefully but with confidence, knowing that you are capable of succeeding.

Developing a healthy mental approach to test taking will also aid in other areas of life. Test anxiety affects more than just the actual test—it can be damaging to your mental health and even contribute to depression. It's important to beat test anxiety before it becomes a problem for more than testing.

Study Strategy

Being prepared for the test is necessary to combat anxiety, but what does being prepared look like? You may study for hours on end and still not feel prepared. What you need is a strategy for test prep. The next few pages outline our recommended steps to help you plan out and conquer the challenge of preparation.

Step 1: Scope Out the Test

Learn everything you can about the format (multiple choice, essay, etc.) and what will be on the test. Gather any study materials, course outlines, or sample exams that may be available. Not only will this help you to prepare, but knowing what to expect can help to alleviate test anxiety.

Step 2: Map Out the Material

Look through the textbook or study guide and make note of how many chapters or sections it has. Then divide these over the time you have. For example, if a book has 15 chapters and you have five days to study, you need to cover three chapters each day. Even better, if you have the time, leave an extra day at the end for overall review after you have gone through the material in depth.

If time is limited, you may need to prioritize the material. Look through it and make note of which sections you think you already have a good grasp on, and which need review. While you are studying, skim quickly through the familiar sections and take more time on the challenging parts.

Write out your plan so you don't get lost as you go. Having a written plan also helps you feel more in control of the study, so anxiety is less likely to arise from feeling overwhelmed at the amount to cover.

Step 3: Gather Your Tools

Decide what study method works best for you. Do you prefer to highlight in the book as you study and then go back over the highlighted portions? Or do you type out notes of the important information? Or is it helpful to make flashcards that you can carry with you? Assemble the pens, index cards, highlighters, post-it notes, and any other materials you may need so you won't be distracted by getting up to find things while you study.

If you're having a hard time retaining the information or organizing your notes, experiment with different methods. For example, try color-coding by subject with colored pens, highlighters, or post-it notes. If you learn better by hearing, try recording yourself reading your notes so you can listen while in the car, working out, or simply sitting at your desk. Ask a friend to quiz you from your flashcards, or try teaching someone the material to solidify it in your mind.

Step 4: Create Your Environment

It's important to avoid distractions while you study. This includes both the obvious distractions like visitors and the subtle distractions like an uncomfortable chair (or a too-comfortable couch that makes you want to fall asleep). Set up the best study environment possible: good lighting and a comfortable work area. If background music helps you focus, you may want to turn it on, but otherwise keep the room quiet. If you are using a computer to take notes, be sure you don't have any other windows open, especially applications like social media, games, or anything else that could distract you. Silence your phone and turn off notifications. Be sure to keep water close by so you stay hydrated while you study (but avoid unhealthy drinks and snacks).

Also, take into account the best time of day to study. Are you freshest first thing in the morning? Try to set aside some time then to work through the material. Is your mind clearer in the afternoon or evening? Schedule your study session then. Another method is to study at the same time of day that you will take the test, so that your brain gets used to working on the material at that time and will be ready to focus at test time.

Step 5: Study!

Once you have done all the study preparation, it's time to settle into the actual studying. Sit down, take a few moments to settle your mind so you can focus, and begin to follow your study plan. Don't give in to distractions or let yourself procrastinate. This is your time to prepare so you'll be ready to fearlessly approach the test. Make the most of the time and stay focused.

Of course, you don't want to burn out. If you study too long you may find that you're not retaining the information very well. Take regular study breaks. For example, taking five minutes out of every hour to walk briskly, breathing deeply and swinging your arms, can help your mind stay fresh.

As you get to the end of each chapter or section, it's a good idea to do a quick review. Remind yourself of what you learned and work on any difficult parts. When you feel that you've mastered the material, move on to the next part. At the end of your study session, briefly skim through your notes again.

But while review is helpful, cramming last minute is NOT. If at all possible, work ahead so that you won't need to fit all your study into the last day. Cramming overloads your brain with more information than it can process and retain, and your tired mind may struggle to recall even previously learned information when it is overwhelmed with last-minute study. Also, the urgent nature of cramming and the stress placed on your brain contribute to anxiety. You'll be more likely to go to the test feeling unprepared and having trouble thinking clearly.

So don't cram, and don't stay up late before the test, even just to review your notes at a leisurely pace. Your brain needs rest more than it needs to go over the information again. In fact, plan to finish your studies by noon or early afternoon the day before the test. Give your brain the rest of the day to relax or focus on other things, and get a good night's sleep. Then you will be fresh for the test and better able to recall what you've studied.

Step 6: Take a Practice Test

Many courses offer sample tests, either online or in the study materials. This is an excellent resource to check whether you have mastered the material, as well as to prepare for the test format and environment.

Check the test format ahead of time: the number of questions, the type (multiple choice, free response, etc.), and the time limit. Then create a plan for working through them. For example, if you have 30 minutes to take a 60-question test, your limit is 30 seconds per question. Spend less time on the questions you know well so that you can take more time on the difficult ones.

If you have time to take several practice tests, take the first one open book, with no time limit. Work through the questions at your own pace and make sure you fully understand them. Gradually work up to taking a test under test conditions: sit at a desk with all study materials put away and set a timer. Pace yourself to make sure you finish the test with time to spare and go back to check your answers if you have time.

After each test, check your answers. On the questions you missed, be sure you understand why you missed them. Did you misread the question (tests can use tricky wording)? Did you forget the information? Or was it something you hadn't learned? Go back and study any shaky areas that the practice tests reveal.

Taking these tests not only helps with your grade, but also aids in combating test anxiety. If you're already used to the test conditions, you're less likely to worry about it, and working through tests until you're scoring well gives you a confidence boost. Go through the practice tests until you feel comfortable, and then you can go into the test knowing that you're ready for it.

Test Tips

On test day, you should be confident, knowing that you've prepared well and are ready to answer the questions. But aside from preparation, there are several test day strategies you can employ to maximize your performance.

First, as stated before, get a good night's sleep the night before the test (and for several nights before that, if possible). Go into the test with a fresh, alert mind rather than staying up late to study.

Try not to change too much about your normal routine on the day of the test. It's important to eat a nutritious breakfast, but if you normally don't eat breakfast at all, consider eating just a protein bar. If you're a coffee drinker, go ahead and have your normal coffee. Just make sure you time it so that the caffeine doesn't wear off right in the middle of your test. Avoid sugary beverages, and drink enough water to stay hydrated but not so much that you need a restroom break 10 minutes into the test. If your test isn't first thing in the morning, consider going for a walk or doing a light workout before the test to get your blood flowing.

Allow yourself enough time to get ready, and leave for the test with plenty of time to spare so you won't have the anxiety of scrambling to arrive in time. Another reason to be early is to select a good seat. It's helpful to sit away from doors and windows, which can be distracting. Find a good seat, get out your supplies, and settle your mind before the test begins.

When the test begins, start by going over the instructions carefully, even if you already know what to expect. Make sure you avoid any careless mistakes by following the directions.

Then begin working through the questions, pacing yourself as you've practiced. If you're not sure on an answer, don't spend too much time on it, and don't let it shake your confidence. Either skip it and come back later, or eliminate as many wrong answers as possible and guess among the remaining ones. Don't dwell on these questions as you continue—put them out of your mind and focus on what lies ahead.

Be sure to read all of the answer choices, even if you're sure the first one is the right answer. Sometimes you'll find a better one if you keep reading. But don't second-guess yourself if you do immediately know the answer. Your gut instinct is usually right. Don't let test anxiety rob you of the information you know.

If you have time at the end of the test (and if the test format allows), go back and review your answers. Be cautious about changing any, since your first instinct tends to be correct, but make sure you didn't misread any of the questions or accidentally mark the wrong answer choice. Look over any you skipped and make an educated guess.

At the end, leave the test feeling confident. You've done your best, so don't waste time worrying about your performance or wishing you could change anything. Instead, celebrate the successful completion of this test. And finally, use this test to learn how to deal with anxiety even better next time.

Review Video: Test Anxiety
Visit mometrix.com/academy and enter code: 100340

Important Qualification

Not all anxiety is created equal. If your test anxiety is causing major issues in your life beyond the classroom or testing center, or if you are experiencing troubling physical symptoms related to your anxiety, it may be a sign of a serious physiological or psychological condition. If this sounds like your situation, we strongly encourage you to seek professional help.

Online Resources

Due to our efforts to try to keep this book to a manageable length, we've created a link that will give you access to all of your online resources:

mometrix.com/resources719/fundnursing

It's Your Moment, Let's Celebrate It!

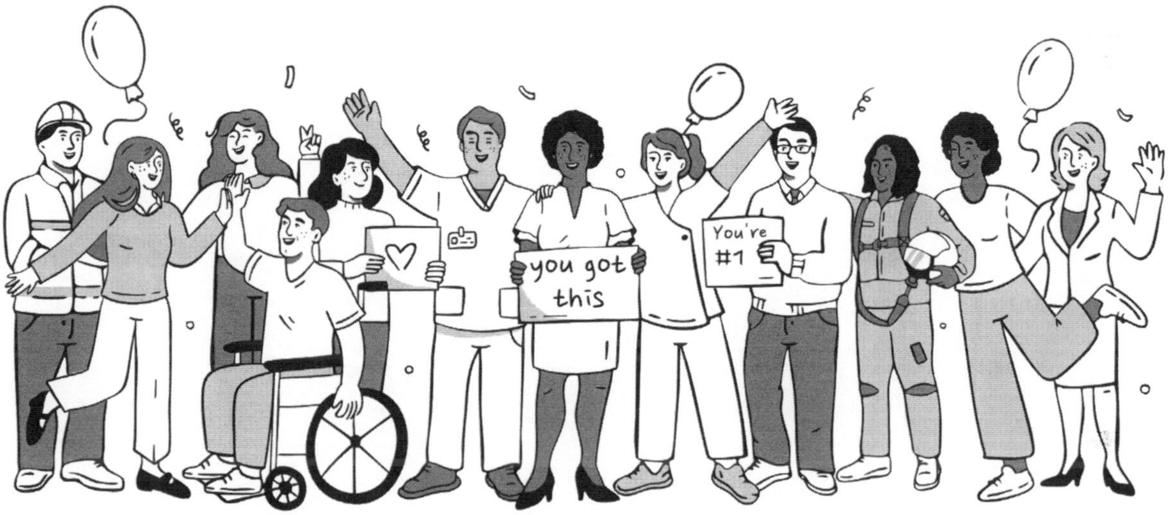

Share your story @mometrixtestpreparation

Mometrix
TEST PREPARATION

Fundamentals of Nursing Secrets Study Guide Part 1 of 2

DEAR FUTURE EXAM SUCCESS STORY

First of all, **THANK YOU** for purchasing Mometrix study materials!

Second, congratulations! You are one of the few determined test-takers who are committed to doing whatever it takes to excel on your exam. **You have come to the right place.** We developed these study materials with one goal in mind: to deliver you the information you need in a format that's concise and easy to use.

In addition to optimizing your guide for the content of the test, we've outlined our recommended steps for breaking down the preparation process into small, attainable goals so you can make sure you stay on track.

We've also analyzed the entire test-taking process, identifying the most common pitfalls and showing how you can overcome them and be ready for any curveball the test throws you.

Standardized testing is one of the biggest obstacles on your road to success, which only increases the importance of doing well in the high-pressure, high-stakes environment of test day. Your results on this test could have a significant impact on your future, and this guide provides the information and practical advice to help you achieve your full potential on test day.

Your success is our success

We would love to hear from you! If you would like to share the story of your exam success or if you have any questions or comments in regard to our products, please contact us at **800-673-8175** or **support@mometrix.com**.

Thanks again for your business and we wish you continued success!

Sincerely,
The Mometrix Test Preparation Team

Table of Contents

Introduction

Thank you for purchasing this resource! You have made the choice to prepare yourself for a test that could have a huge impact on your future, and this guide is designed to help you be fully ready for test day. Obviously, it's important to have a solid understanding of the test material, but you also need to be prepared for the unique environment and stressors of the test, so that you can perform to the best of your abilities.

For this purpose, the first section that appears in this guide is the **Secret Keys**. We've devoted countless hours to meticulously researching what works and what doesn't, and we've boiled down our findings to the five most impactful steps you can take to improve your performance on the test. We start at the beginning with study planning and move through the preparation process, all the way to the testing strategies that will help you get the most out of what you know when you're finally sitting in front of the test.

We recommend that you start preparing for your test as far in advance as possible. However, if you've bought this guide as a last-minute study resource and only have a few days before your test, we recommend that you skip over the first two Secret Keys since they address a long-term study plan.

If you struggle with **test anxiety**, we strongly encourage you to check out our recommendations for how you can overcome it. Test anxiety is a formidable foe, but it can be beaten, and we want to make sure you have the tools you need to defeat it.

Secret Key #1 – Plan Big, Study Small

There's a lot riding on your performance. If you want to ace this test, you're going to need to keep your skills sharp and the material fresh in your mind. You need a plan that lets you review everything you need to know while still fitting in your schedule. We'll break this strategy down into three categories.

Information Organization

Start with the information you already have: the official test outline. From this, you can make a complete list of all the concepts you need to cover before the test. Organize these concepts into groups that can be studied together, and create a list of any related vocabulary you need to learn so you can brush up on any difficult terms. You'll want to keep this vocabulary list handy once you actually start studying since you may need to add to it along the way.

Time Management

Once you have your set of study concepts, decide how to spread them out over the time you have left before the test. Break your study plan into small, clear goals so you have a manageable task for each day and know exactly what you're doing. Then just focus on one small step at a time. When you manage your time this way, you don't need to spend hours at a time studying. Studying a small block of content for a short period each day helps you retain information better and avoid stressing over how much you have left to do. You can relax knowing that you have a plan to cover everything in time. In order for this strategy to be effective though, you have to start studying early and stick to your schedule. Avoid the exhaustion and futility that comes from last-minute cramming!

Study Environment

The environment you study in has a big impact on your learning. Studying in a coffee shop, while probably more enjoyable, is not likely to be as fruitful as studying in a quiet room. It's important to keep distractions to a minimum. You're only planning to study for a short block of time, so make the most of it. Don't pause to check your phone or get up to find a snack. It's also important to **avoid multitasking**. Research has consistently shown that multitasking will make your studying dramatically less effective. Your study area should also be comfortable and well-lit so you don't have the distraction of straining your eyes or sitting on an uncomfortable chair.

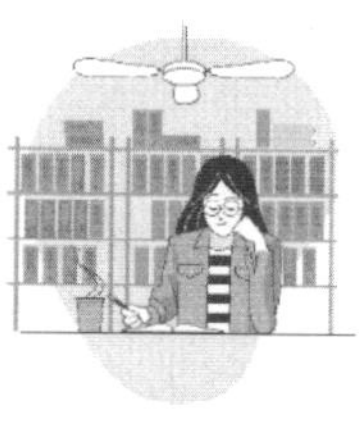

The time of day you study is also important. You want to be rested and alert. Don't wait until just before bedtime. Study when you'll be most likely to comprehend and remember. Even better, if you know what time of day your test will be, set that time aside for study. That way your brain will be used to working on that subject at that specific time and you'll have a better chance of recalling information.

Finally, it can be helpful to team up with others who are studying for the same test. Your actual studying should be done in as isolated an environment as possible, but the work of organizing the information and setting up the study plan can be divided up. In between study sessions, you can discuss with your teammates the concepts that you're all studying and quiz each other on the details. Just be sure that your teammates are as serious about the test as you are. If you find that your study time is being replaced with social time, you might need to find a new team.

Secret Key #2 – Make Your Studying Count

You're devoting a lot of time and effort to preparing for this test, so you want to be absolutely certain it will pay off. This means doing more than just reading the content and hoping you can remember it on test day. It's important to make every minute of study count. There are two main areas you can focus on to make your studying count.

Retention

It doesn't matter how much time you study if you can't remember the material. You need to make sure you are retaining the concepts. To check your retention of the information you're learning, try recalling it at later times with minimal prompting. Try carrying around flashcards and glance at one or two from time to time or ask a friend who's also studying for the test to quiz you.

To enhance your retention, look for ways to put the information into practice so that you can apply it rather than simply recalling it. If you're using the information in practical ways, it will be much easier to remember. Similarly, it helps to solidify a concept in your mind if you're not only reading it to yourself but also explaining it to someone else. Ask a friend to let you teach them about a concept you're a little shaky on (or speak aloud to an imaginary audience if necessary). As you try to summarize, define, give examples, and answer your friend's questions, you'll understand the concepts better and they will stay with you longer. Finally, step back for a big picture view and ask yourself how each piece of information fits with the whole subject. When you link the different concepts together and see them working together as a whole, it's easier to remember the individual components.

Finally, practice showing your work on any multi-step problems, even if you're just studying. Writing out each step you take to solve a problem will help solidify the process in your mind, and you'll be more likely to remember it during the test.

Modality

Modality simply refers to the means or method by which you study. Choosing a study modality that fits your own individual learning style is crucial. No two people learn best in exactly the same way, so it's important to know your strengths and use them to your advantage.

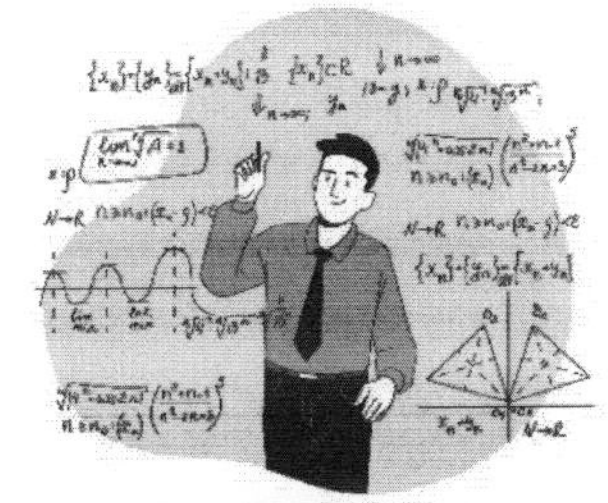

For example, if you learn best by visualization, focus on visualizing a concept in your mind and draw an image or a diagram. Try color-coding your notes, illustrating them, or creating symbols that will trigger your mind to recall a learned concept. If you learn best by hearing or discussing information, find a study partner who learns the same way or read aloud to yourself. Think about how to put the information in your own words. Imagine that you are giving a lecture on the topic and record yourself so you can listen to it later.

For any learning style, flashcards can be helpful. Organize the information so you can take advantage of spare moments to review. Underline key words or phrases. Use different colors for different categories. Mnemonic devices (such as creating a short list in which every item starts with the same letter) can also help with retention. Find what works best for you and use it to store the information in your mind most effectively and easily.

Secret Key #3 – Practice the Right Way

Your success on test day depends not only on how many hours you put into preparing, but also on whether you prepared the right way. It's good to check along the way to see if your studying is paying off. One of the most effective ways to do this is by taking practice tests to evaluate your progress. Practice tests are useful because they show exactly where you need to improve. Every time you take a practice test, pay special attention to these three groups of questions:

- The questions you got wrong
- The questions you had to guess on, even if you guessed right
- The questions you found difficult or slow to work through

This will show you exactly what your weak areas are, and where you need to devote more study time. Ask yourself why each of these questions gave you trouble. Was it because you didn't understand the material? Was it because you didn't remember the vocabulary? Do you need more repetitions on this type of question to build speed and confidence? Dig into those questions and figure out how you can strengthen your weak areas as you go back to review the material.

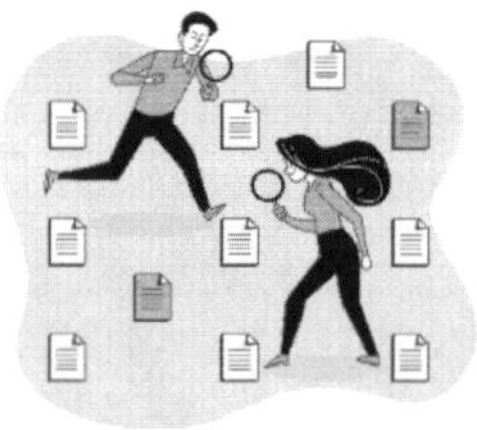

Additionally, many practice tests have a section explaining the answer choices. It can be tempting to read the explanation and think that you now have a good understanding of the concept. However, an explanation likely only covers part of the question's broader context. Even if the explanation makes perfect sense, **go back and investigate** every concept related to the question until you're positive you have a thorough understanding.

As you go along, keep in mind that the practice test is just that: practice. Memorizing these questions and answers will not be very helpful on the actual test because it is unlikely to have any of the same exact questions. If you only know the right answers to the sample questions, you won't be prepared for the real thing. **Study the concepts** until you understand them fully, and then you'll be able to answer any question that shows up on the test.

It's important to wait on the practice tests until you're ready. If you take a test on your first day of study, you may be overwhelmed by the amount of material covered and how much you need to learn. Work up to it gradually.

On test day, you'll need to be prepared for answering questions, managing your time, and using the test-taking strategies you've learned. It's a lot to balance, like a mental marathon that will have a big impact on your future. Like training for a marathon, you'll need to start slowly and work your way up. When test day arrives, you'll be ready.

Start with the strategies you've read in the first two Secret Keys—plan your course and study in the way that works best for you. If you have time, consider using multiple study resources to get different approaches to the same concepts. It can be helpful to see difficult concepts from more than one angle. Then find a good source for practice tests. Many times, the test website will suggest potential study resources or provide sample tests.

Practice Test Strategy

If you're able to find at least three practice tests, we recommend this strategy:

Untimed and Open-Book Practice

Take the first test with no time constraints and with your notes and study guide handy. Take your time and focus on applying the strategies you've learned.

Timed and Open-Book Practice

Take the second practice test open-book as well, but set a timer and practice pacing yourself to finish in time.

Timed and Closed-Book Practice

Take any other practice tests as if it were test day. Set a timer and put away your study materials. Sit at a table or desk in a quiet room, imagine yourself at the testing center, and answer questions as quickly and accurately as possible.

Keep repeating timed and closed-book tests on a regular basis until you run out of practice tests or it's time for the actual test. Your mind will be ready for the schedule and stress of test day, and you'll be able to focus on recalling the material you've learned.

Secret Key #4 – Pace Yourself

Once you're fully prepared for the material on the test, your biggest challenge on test day will be managing your time. Just knowing that the clock is ticking can make you panic even if you have plenty of time left. Work on pacing yourself so you can build confidence against the time constraints of the exam. Pacing is a difficult skill to master, especially in a high-pressure environment, so **practice is vital**.

Set time expectations for your pace based on how much time is available. For example, if a section has 60 questions and the time limit is 30 minutes, you know you have to average 30 seconds or less per question in order to answer them all. Although 30 seconds is the hard limit, set 25 seconds per question as your goal, so you reserve extra time to spend on harder questions. When you budget extra time for the harder questions, you no longer have any reason to stress when those questions take longer to answer.

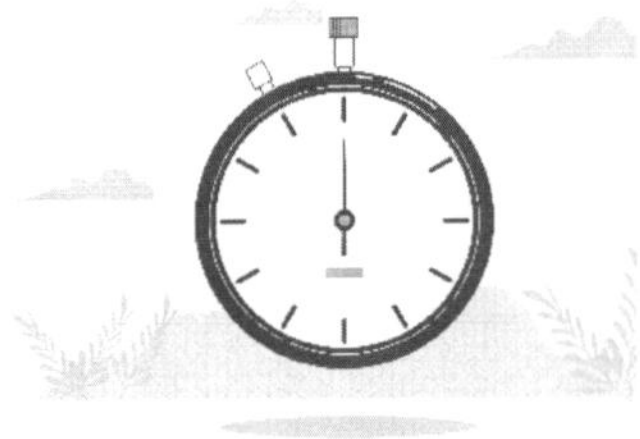

Don't let this time expectation distract you from working through the test at a calm, steady pace, but keep it in mind so you don't spend too much time on any one question. Recognize that taking extra time on one question you don't understand may keep you from answering two that you do understand later in the test. If your time limit for a question is up and you're still not sure of the answer, mark it and move on, and come back to it later if the time and the test format allow. If the testing format doesn't allow you to return to earlier questions, just make an educated guess; then put it out of your mind and move on.

On the easier questions, be careful not to rush. It may seem wise to hurry through them so you have more time for the challenging ones, but it's not worth missing one if you know the concept and just didn't take the time to read the question fully. Work efficiently but make sure you understand the question and have looked at all of the answer choices, since more than one may seem right at first.

Even if you're paying attention to the time, you may find yourself a little behind at some point. You should speed up to get back on track, but do so wisely. Don't panic; just take a few seconds less on each question until you're caught up. Don't guess without thinking, but do look through the answer choices and eliminate any you know are wrong. If you can get down to two choices, it is often worthwhile to guess from those. Once you've chosen an answer, move on and don't dwell on any that you skipped or had to hurry through. If a question was taking too long, chances are it was one of the harder ones, so you weren't as likely to get it right anyway.

On the other hand, if you find yourself getting ahead of schedule, it may be beneficial to slow down a little. The more quickly you work, the more likely you are to make a careless mistake that will affect your score. You've budgeted time for each question, so don't be afraid to spend that time. Practice an efficient but careful pace to get the most out of the time you have.

Secret Key #5 – Have a Plan for Guessing

When you're taking the test, you may find yourself stuck on a question. Some of the answer choices seem better than others, but you don't see the one answer choice that is obviously correct. What do you do?

The scenario described above is very common, yet most test takers have not effectively prepared for it. Developing and practicing a plan for guessing may be one of the single most effective uses of your time as you get ready for the exam.

In developing your plan for guessing, there are three questions to address:

- When should you start the guessing process?
- How should you narrow down the choices?
- Which answer should you choose?

When to Start the Guessing Process

Unless your plan for guessing is to select C every time (which, despite its merits, is not what we recommend), you need to leave yourself enough time to apply your answer elimination strategies. Since you have a limited amount of time for each question, that means that if you're going to give yourself the best shot at guessing correctly, you have to decide quickly whether or not you will guess.

Of course, the best-case scenario is that you don't have to guess at all, so first, see if you can answer the question based on your knowledge of the subject and basic reasoning skills. Focus on the key words in the question and try to jog your memory of related topics. Give yourself a chance to bring the knowledge to mind, but once you realize that you don't have (or you can't access) the knowledge you need to answer the question, it's time to start the guessing process.

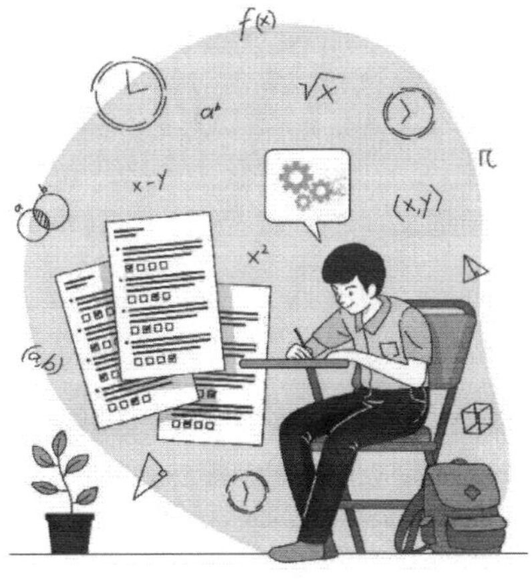

It's almost always better to start the guessing process too early than too late. It only takes a few seconds to remember something and answer the question from knowledge. Carefully eliminating wrong answer choices takes longer. Plus, going through the process of eliminating answer choices can actually help jog your memory.

Summary: Start the guessing process as soon as you decide that you can't answer the question based on your knowledge.

How to Narrow Down the Choices

The next chapter in this book (**Test-Taking Strategies**) includes a wide range of strategies for how to approach questions and how to look for answer choices to eliminate. You will definitely want to read those carefully, practice them, and figure out which ones work best for you. Here though, we're going to address a mindset rather than a particular strategy.

Your odds of guessing an answer correctly depend on how many options you are choosing from.

Number of options left	5	4	3	2	1
Odds of guessing correctly	20%	25%	33%	50%	100%

You can see from this chart just how valuable it is to be able to eliminate incorrect answers and make an educated guess, but there are two things that many test takers do that cause them to miss out on the benefits of guessing:

- Accidentally eliminating the correct answer
- Selecting an answer based on an impression

We'll look at the first one here, and the second one in the next section.

To avoid accidentally eliminating the correct answer, we recommend a thought exercise called **the $5 challenge**. In this challenge, you only eliminate an answer choice from contention if you are willing to bet $5 on it being wrong. Why $5? Five dollars is a small but not insignificant amount of money. It's an amount you could afford to lose but wouldn't want to throw away. And while losing $5 once might not hurt too much, doing it twenty times will set you back $100. In the same way, each small decision you make—eliminating a choice here, guessing on a question there—won't by itself impact your score very much, but when you put them all together, they can make a big difference. By holding each answer choice elimination decision to a higher standard, you can reduce the risk of accidentally eliminating the correct answer.

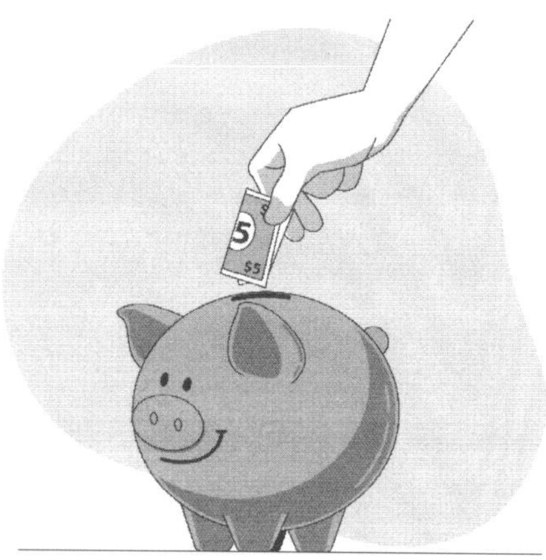

The $5 challenge can also be applied in a positive sense: If you are willing to bet $5 that an answer choice *is* correct, go ahead and mark it as correct.

Summary: Only eliminate an answer choice if you are willing to bet $5 that it is wrong.

Which Answer to Choose

You're taking the test. You've run into a hard question and decided you'll have to guess. You've eliminated all the answer choices you're willing to bet $5 on. Now you have to pick an answer. Why do we even need to talk about this? Why can't you just pick whichever one you feel like when the time comes?

The answer to these questions is that if you don't come into the test with a plan, you'll rely on your impression to select an answer choice, and if you do that, you risk falling into a trap. The test writers know that everyone who takes their test will be guessing on some of the questions, so they intentionally write wrong answer choices to seem plausible. You still have to pick an answer though, and if the wrong answer choices are designed to look right, how can you ever be sure that you're not falling for their trap? The best solution we've found to this dilemma is to take the decision out of your hands entirely. Here is the process we recommend:

Once you've eliminated any choices that you are confident (willing to bet $5) are wrong, select the first remaining choice as your answer.

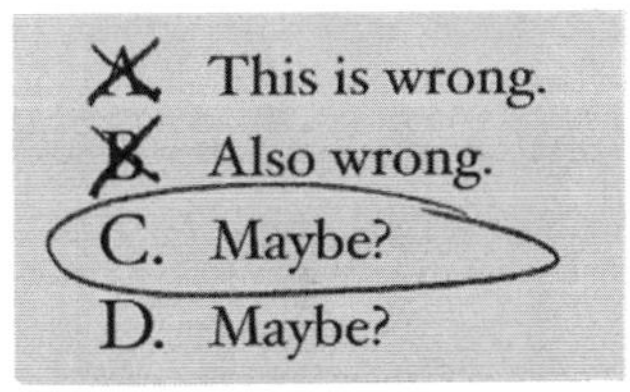

Whether you choose to select the first remaining choice, the second, or the last, the important thing is that you use some preselected standard. Using this approach guarantees that you will not be enticed into selecting an answer choice that looks right, because you are not basing your decision on how the answer choices look.

This is not meant to make you question your knowledge. Instead, it is to help you recognize the difference between your knowledge and your impressions. There's a huge difference between thinking an answer is right because of what you know, and thinking an answer is right because it looks or sounds like it should be right.

Summary: To ensure that your selection is appropriately random, make a predetermined selection from among all answer choices you have not eliminated.

Test-Taking Strategies

This section contains a list of test-taking strategies that you may find helpful as you work through the test. By taking what you know and applying logical thought, you can maximize your chances of answering any question correctly!

It is very important to realize that every question is different and every person is different: no single strategy will work on every question, and no single strategy will work for every person. That's why we've included all of them here, so you can try them out and determine which ones work best for different types of questions and which ones work best for you.

Question Strategies

✓ Read Carefully

Read the question and the answer choices carefully. Don't miss the question because you misread the terms. You have plenty of time to read each question thoroughly and make sure you understand what is being asked. Yet a happy medium must be attained, so don't waste too much time. You must read carefully and efficiently.

✓ Contextual Clues

Look for contextual clues. If the question includes a word you are not familiar with, look at the immediate context for some indication of what the word might mean. Contextual clues can often give you all the information you need to decipher the meaning of an unfamiliar word. Even if you can't determine the meaning, you may be able to narrow down the possibilities enough to make a solid guess at the answer to the question.

✓ Prefixes

If you're having trouble with a word in the question or answer choices, try dissecting it. Take advantage of every clue that the word might include. Prefixes can be a huge help. Usually, they allow you to determine a basic meaning. *Pre-* means before, *post-* means after, *pro-* is positive, *de-* is negative. From prefixes, you can get an idea of the general meaning of the word and try to put it into context.

✓ Hedge Words

Watch out for critical hedge words, such as *likely, may, can, often, almost, mostly, usually, generally, rarely,* and *sometimes*. Question writers insert these hedge phrases to cover every possibility. Often an answer choice will be wrong simply because it leaves no room for exception. Be on guard for answer choices that have definitive words such as *exactly* and *always*.

✓ Switchback Words

Stay alert for *switchbacks*. These are the words and phrases frequently used to alert you to shifts in thought. The most common switchback words are *but, although,* and *however*. Others include *nevertheless, on the other hand, even though, while, in spite of, despite,* and *regardless of*. Switchback words are important to catch because they can change the direction of the question or an answer choice.

✓ Face Value

When in doubt, use common sense. Accept the situation in the problem at face value. Don't read too much into it. These problems will not require you to make wild assumptions. If you have to go beyond creativity and warp time or space in order to have an answer choice fit the question, then you should move on and consider the other answer choices. These are normal problems rooted in reality. The applicable relationship or explanation may not be readily apparent, but it is there for you to figure out. Use your common sense to interpret anything that isn't clear.

Answer Choice Strategies

⊘ Answer Selection

The most thorough way to pick an answer choice is to identify and eliminate wrong answers until only one is left, then confirm it is the correct answer. Sometimes an answer choice may immediately seem right, but be careful. The test writers will usually put more than one reasonable answer choice on each question, so take a second to read all of them and make sure that the other choices are not equally obvious. As long as you have time left, it is better to read every answer choice than to pick the first one that looks right without checking the others.

⊘ Answer Choice Families

An answer choice family consists of two (in rare cases, three) answer choices that are very similar in construction and cannot all be true at the same time. If you see two answer choices that are direct opposites or parallels, one of them is usually the correct answer. For instance, if one answer choice says that quantity *x* increases and another either says that quantity *x* decreases (opposite) or says that quantity *y* increases (parallel), then those answer choices would fall into the same family. An answer choice that doesn't match the construction of the answer choice family is more likely to be incorrect. Most questions will not have answer choice families, but when they do appear, you should be prepared to recognize them.

⊘ Eliminate Answers

Eliminate answer choices as soon as you realize they are wrong, but make sure you consider all possibilities. If you are eliminating answer choices and realize that the last one you are left with is also wrong, don't panic. Start over and consider each choice again. There may be something you missed the first time that you will realize on the second pass.

⊘ Avoid Fact Traps

Don't be distracted by an answer choice that is factually true but doesn't answer the question. You are looking for the choice that answers the question. Stay focused on what the question is asking for so you don't accidentally pick an answer that is true but incorrect. Always go back to the question and make sure the answer choice you've selected actually answers the question and is not merely a true statement.

⊘ Extreme Statements

In general, you should avoid answers that put forth extreme actions as standard practice or proclaim controversial ideas as established fact. An answer choice that states the "process should be used in certain situations, if..." is much more likely to be correct than one that states the "process should be discontinued completely." The first is a calm rational statement and doesn't even make a definitive, uncompromising stance, using a hedge word *if* to provide wiggle room, whereas the second choice is far more extreme.

⊘ Benchmark

As you read through the answer choices and you come across one that seems to answer the question well, mentally select that answer choice. This is not your final answer, but it's the one that will help you evaluate the other answer choices. The one that you selected is your benchmark or standard for judging each of the other answer choices. Every other answer choice must be compared to your benchmark. That choice is correct until proven otherwise by another answer choice beating it. If you find a better answer, then that one becomes your new benchmark. Once you've decided that no other choice answers the question as well as your benchmark, you have your final answer.

⊘ PREDICT THE ANSWER

Before you even start looking at the answer choices, it is often best to try to predict the answer. When you come up with the answer on your own, it is easier to avoid distractions and traps because you will know exactly what to look for. The right answer choice is unlikely to be word-for-word what you came up with, but it should be a close match. Even if you are confident that you have the right answer, you should still take the time to read each option before moving on.

General Strategies

⊘ TOUGH QUESTIONS

If you are stumped on a problem or it appears too hard or too difficult, don't waste time. Move on! Remember though, if you can quickly check for obviously incorrect answer choices, your chances of guessing correctly are greatly improved. Before you completely give up, at least try to knock out a couple of possible answers. Eliminate what you can and then guess at the remaining answer choices before moving on.

⊘ CHECK YOUR WORK

Since you will probably not know every term listed and the answer to every question, it is important that you get credit for the ones that you do know. Don't miss any questions through careless mistakes. If at all possible, try to take a second to look back over your answer selection and make sure you've selected the correct answer choice and haven't made a costly careless mistake (such as marking an answer choice that you didn't mean to mark). This quick double check should more than pay for itself in caught mistakes for the time it costs.

⊘ PACE YOURSELF

It's easy to be overwhelmed when you're looking at a page full of questions; your mind is confused and full of random thoughts, and the clock is ticking down faster than you would like. Calm down and maintain the pace that you have set for yourself. Especially as you get down to the last few minutes of the test, don't let the small numbers on the clock make you panic. As long as you are on track by monitoring your pace, you are guaranteed to have time for each question.

⊘ DON'T RUSH

It is very easy to make errors when you are in a hurry. Maintaining a fast pace in answering questions is pointless if it makes you miss questions that you would have gotten right otherwise. Test writers like to include distracting information and wrong answers that seem right. Taking a little extra time to avoid careless mistakes can make all the difference in your test score. Find a pace that allows you to be confident in the answers that you select.

⊘ KEEP MOVING

Panicking will not help you pass the test, so do your best to stay calm and keep moving. Taking deep breaths and going through the answer elimination steps you practiced can help to break through a stress barrier and keep your pace.

Final Notes

The combination of a solid foundation of content knowledge and the confidence that comes from practicing your plan for applying that knowledge is the key to maximizing your performance on test day. As your foundation of content knowledge is built up and strengthened, you'll find that the strategies included in this chapter become more and more effective in helping you quickly sift through the distractions and traps of the test to isolate the correct answer.

Now that you're preparing to move forward into the test content chapters of this book, be sure to keep your goal in mind. As you read, think about how you will be able to apply this information on the test. If you've already seen sample questions for the test and you have an idea of the question format and style, try to come up with questions of your own that you can answer based on what you're reading. This will give you valuable practice applying your knowledge in the same ways you can expect to on test day.

Good luck and good studying!

Safe, Effective Care Environment: Management of Care

Health Care Delivery Systems

HEALTH CARE DELIVERY SYSTEMS

In the United States, healthcare delivery systems are traditionally fragmented, unique, and quite complex in nature. In contrast to the United States, most other countries in developed nations have national health insurance systems, which are commonly referred to as **universal access systems**. Such universal access systems are managed by the government and are funded by taxes. Healthcare delivery systems in the United States consist of subcategories such as managed care, military, vulnerable populations, and integrated service delivery. **Managed care healthcare delivery systems** are the predominant systems for the delivery of health care in the United States.

MANAGED CARE HEALTHCARE DELIVERY SYSTEM

The managed care healthcare delivery system promotes efficiency by integrating all the basic functions of healthcare delivery and using management strategies to control healthcare service usage. Managed healthcare delivery systems also determine the **prices** of services and provider reimbursement. The government and employers primarily provide the financing for managed care systems. Managed care delivery systems act like insurance companies in that they use a contract health plan that is an agreement between the managed care system and the subscriber. Subscribers under a managed care delivery system are usually required to use selected healthcare providers.

LEVELS OF HEALTH CARE

- **Acute care** is short-term medical treatment, usually in a hospital, for episodic illness or injury.
- **Long-term care** applies to major trauma patients or those with chronic and multiple medical, mental, and social problems who cannot take care of themselves.
- **Custodial care** is mainly for the purpose of assisting clients with their home personal care and does not necessarily require the provider to have specialized skills or training.
- **Intermediate care** applies to patients requiring more than custodial care and might require nursing supervision. Unless true skilled care is required, insurance companies group intermediate and custodial care under the same benefit guidelines.
- **Sub-acute care** is used for patients who are medically stable but still require active care from trained medical professionals. Treatments in this level include frequent or complex wound care, rehabilitation, complex intravenous therapy, and combination therapies. Patients are usually in an extended care facility (ECF), such as a nursing home or a **skilled nursing facility**.

TRANSITIONAL HOSPITALS

Transitional hospitals are acute care facilities for patients that are medically stable and whose rehabilitation plan is too complex for an **extended care facility (ECF)**. Transitional hospitals that specialize in medically complex care do so at a lower cost than a traditional hospital because of their specialization. Some transitional hospitals supply only basic patient care, also at a lower cost than a traditional hospital. Examples of transitional hospitals are: burn or extensive wound care, hemodialysis, hospice, infectious disease management, intravenous (IV) medication therapies, neurobehavioral rehabilitation, pain control therapies, rehabilitation, total parenteral nutrition, and ventilator care/weaning from ventilators.

Telehealth

Telehealth refers to the delivery of healthcare services to patients who are not physically present with the healthcare professional, usually due to remote location, disability, or pandemic (such as the recent outbreak of COVID-19). Telehealth can be delivered over a telephone, via email, or by video conference. The primary benefits of telehealth are that it allows for the extension of precious healthcare resources, lowers the overall cost of healthcare, and allows patients to receive healthcare who would not normally have access to it.

There are a number of **ways in which telehealth is useful** to healthcare professionals:

- Consultation with colleagues
- Patient interviews
- Monitor a patient's biometric values and assess their condition
- Evaluate diagnostic images which allows physicians to remotely view and evaluate these images even if they are located overseas (e.g., India)
- Evaluation of microscope slides and laboratory reports

Primary Nursing Model

The primary nursing model of care is an individualized and comprehensive model in which the same nurse gives care during the entire period of care. This method stresses care continuity and allows the nurse to provide direct patient care. The primary nurse has total 24-hour care responsibility for the patient. Such nursing care is oriented toward the goal of meeting the individualized needs of the patient. This model of primary nursing also utilizes the primary nurse to communicate with other members of the healthcare team regarding the patient's needs and total health care. Many institutions have rejected this care model as being cost prohibitive.

Case Management Model

The case management model of care originated in the 1990s. At that time, the model of nursing care was changed from a focus on the quality of care to a focus on the quality of care plus the cost of care. This model of care was used extensively in social work and in outpatient psychiatry. The core of the case management model of care is the case management team. The case management team is an interdisciplinary group that convenes on a regular schedule to discuss and monitor a patient's health care and progress. Many consider this model to be cost effective in the current healthcare system.

Public Health Nursing Model

The public health nursing model of care is based upon the idea that public health care is population based. This model of care primarily focuses on an entire population that has similar health issues. The public health model of care also focuses on the broad scope of the determinants of health. Public health care targets all levels of prevention, with its primary focus being that of primary prevention. Secondary prevention is an additional focus in the public healthcare model, and it tries to detect and treat healthcare problems in earlier stages. This model also focuses on tertiary prevention to hopefully prevent existing healthcare issues from worsening.

Family-Centered Model

The family-centered model of care gained prominence in the healthcare field at the end of the twentieth century. The family-centered model recognized that the family is usually the center of a patient's life and that the family often has the most insight about a patient's abilities and needs. This model enables the family to collaborate with the healthcare providers in helping the patient make informed decisions about healthcare services and supports. Strengths and weaknesses of all the family members are often also considered in this model of care. This model of care has resulted in increased patient satisfaction.

INTEGRATIVE MODEL

The integrative model of care is sometimes referred to as the **interdisciplinary model of care**. This model of care involves cooperation and communication between a team of healthcare professionals. Information sharing among such professionals allows for the development of a comprehensive treatment plan that encompasses the medical, psychological, and social needs of a patient. The integrative health team may include physicians, nurses, social workers, psychologists, and occupational/physical therapists. Such a coordinated model of care can improve quality of life, decrease healthcare costs, and provide a positive benefit to patients over their lifespan. This model of care may also include a focus on the holistic or "whole-person" aspects of a patient's care.

MEDICAL HOME MODEL

The medical home model is a healthcare approach to providing care (primary and comprehensive) to patients. This healthcare model serves to coordinate and improve relationships between patients, their families, and their personal physicians. In March 2007, the American Academy of Family Physicians, American Academy of Pediatrics, American College of Physicians, and American Osteopathic Association developed **joint principles** for the medical home model. The characteristics of these principles are a personal physician, physician-directed medical practice, focus on the whole person, coordinated care, focus on quality and safety of medical care, enhanced patient access, and payment.

CHRONIC CARE MODEL

According to the CDC about 133 million Americans are impacted by chronic disease, and approximately 40 million are limited in their usual activities due to chronic disease. The chronic care model was developed to manage patients with chronic medical conditions in a proactive manner as opposed to the traditional reactive manner. This model integrates the basic components for improving medical care in health systems at numerous levels. These levels of health systems are the **community**, the **organization**, the **provider practice**, and the **patient**. There are three basic themes in the chronic care model. The model is **evidence-based**, **population-based**, and **patient-centered**. The theme of evidence-based stresses the importance of evidence and excellence as opposed to autonomy.

COMMUNITY-BASED NURSING

Community-based nurses strive to promote health, screen for and prevent disease, contain infectious diseases, prevent trauma, manage chronic diseases, rehabilitate, and help maintain function. These nurses work in schools, workplaces, government agencies, county programs, public health agencies, ambulatory care clinics, mental and student health centers, physician offices, home health/hospice agencies, and religious parishes. They give direct care, act as managers and supervisors, do screening exams, and offer health programs. They teach people how to care for themselves and how to prevent injury and disease. They provide referrals to other community resources, working with those resources to provide a smooth transition that results in continuous care. Nurses work with others to write grants to obtain services for specific populations. **Community resources** used to meet healthcare needs include church programs such as food pantries, transportation programs, or visiting programs. Federal programs, mental health, domestic abuse services, senior citizen groups and services, and programs in workplaces and schools are other resources.

The Interprofessional Team

Facilitating Change

Performance improvement processes cannot occur without organizational change, and resistance to change is common for many people, so coordinating collaborative processes requires anticipating resistance and taking steps to achieve cooperation. Resistance often relates to concerns about job loss, increased responsibilities, and general denial or lack of understanding and frustration. Leaders can prepare others involved in the process of change by taking these steps:

- Be honest, informative, and tactful, giving people thorough information about anticipated changes and how the changes will affect them, including positives.
- Be patient in allowing people the time they need to contemplate changes and express anger or disagreement.
- Be empathetic in listening carefully to the concerns of others.
- Encourage participation, allowing staff to propose methods of implementing change, so they feel some sense of ownership.
- Establish a climate in which all staff members are encouraged to identify the need for change on an ongoing basis.
- Present further ideas for change to management.

Conflict Resolution

Conflict is an almost inevitable product of teamwork, and the leader must assume responsibility for conflict resolution. While conflicts can be disruptive, they can produce positive outcomes by opening dialogue and forcing team members to listen to different perspectives. The team should make a plan for dealing with conflict. The best time for conflict resolution is when differences emerge but before open conflict and hardening of positions occur. The leader must pay close attention to the people and problems involved, listen carefully, and reassure those involved that their points of view are understood. Steps to conflict resolution include:

- Allow both sides to present their side of conflict without bias, maintaining a focus on opinions rather than individuals.
- Encourage cooperation through negotiation and compromise.
- Maintain the focus, providing guidance to keep the discussions on track and avoid arguments.
- Evaluate the need for re-negotiation, formal resolution process, or third-party involvement.
- Utilize humor and empathy to diffuse escalating tensions.
- Summarize the issues, outlining key arguments.
- Avoid forcing resolution if possible.

Healthcare Team Members

Role of Nursing Care to Support Therapies Provided by Other Disciplines

Nursing care often involves providing support to therapies provided by other disciplines. The nurse works as a team member with physicians, occupational and physical therapists, respiratory therapists, social workers, and discharge planners. Floor nurses may work with nurses in other specializations, such as critical care or psychiatric nurses. As a primary coordinator of the care plan, the nurse ensures that the necessary therapies from all disciplines are administered as ordered, and maintains clear communication with all members of the patient's healthcare team. Nurses also support nutritional services by assuring that the patient receives the proper diet for the particular medical or surgical condition, and they communicate with housekeeping to ensure that the patient's environment is appropriate.

Occupational Therapy

The function of occupational therapy is to enable the patient to attain functional outcomes that enhance health, prevent further injury or impairment, and sustain or improve the highest attainable level of independence. The occupational therapist's role is to **facilitate interventions** that aid the patient in improving basic motor and cognitive skills and to **introduce strategies** for meeting challenges at work or at home. In cases of permanent disability or loss of mobility, the occupational therapist works with the patient on adaptive measures to improve function and the ability to perform daily living tasks. Occupational therapists may use physical exercises to improve muscle strength, balance, and dexterity, or cognitive exercises and strategies to improve problem-solving and memory. They help patients with disabilities or cognitive impairments adapt to particular environments, such as a private home or workplace, and teach patients how to use adaptive equipment like wheelchairs, orthotic devices, or computer programs.

Respiratory Therapy

The function of respiratory therapy is to provide care to patients with respiratory and cardiopulmonary disorders. The role of the respiratory therapist is to diagnose, evaluate, and treat patients with these disorders, and manage their therapeutic care. The respiratory therapist administers aerosolized medications and provides bronchopulmonary hygiene and postural drainage therapy. The role of the respiratory therapist is also to provide support for mechanically-ventilated patients and to maintain an artificial or natural airway. Many respiratory therapists perform pulmonary function testing as well as hemodynamic monitoring. Some respiratory therapists obtain arterial blood gases and other blood samples, as well as assemble and maintain respiratory equipment. They also teach patients how to self-administer aerosol medications and use life-support respiratory equipment in the home environment.

Case Manager

The case manager is an RN that works for a healthcare insurer as a **manager of the provision of healthcare services** to the people the company insures. One manager or a group of managers are given a caseload of patients with the same range of diagnoses. The case manager is an expert in the range of diagnoses and coordinates services to fulfill the healthcare needs of that particular group of patients. The patient is followed throughout the continuum of care to ensure quality and cost-effectiveness of treatments and care. Complications are prevented and the incidence of repeat hospitalization is decreased. The case manager utilizes evidence-based pathways, clinical pathways, or other plans to track the care and progress of the patient. They are the ones who precertify care, negotiate for payment, and authorize treatment. Patient progress reports from the hospital utilization review or other liaison to the case manager are required at periodic intervals during the hospital stay.

Ethical Responsibilities

Ethical Principles

Autonomy is the ethical principle that the individual has the right to make decisions about his or her own care. In the case of children or patients with dementia who cannot make autonomous decisions, parents or family members may serve as the legal decision maker. The nurse must keep the patient and/or family fully informed so that they can exercise their autonomy in informed decision-making.

Justice is the ethical principle that relates to the distribution of the limited resources of healthcare benefits to the members of society. These resources must be distributed fairly. This issue may arise if there is only one bed left and two sick patients. Justice comes into play in deciding which patient should stay and which should be transported or otherwise cared for. The decision should be made according to what is best or most just for the patients and not colored by personal bias.

Beneficence is an ethical principle that involves performing actions that are for the purpose of benefitting another person. In the care of a patient, any procedure or treatment should be done with the ultimate goal of benefitting the patient, and any actions that are not beneficial should be reconsidered. As conditions change, procedures need to be continually reevaluated to determine if they are still of benefit.

Nonmaleficence is an ethical principle that means healthcare workers should provide care in a manner that does not cause direct intentional harm to the patient:

- The actual act must be good or morally neutral.
- The intent must be only for a good effect.
- A bad effect cannot serve as the means to get to a good effect.
- A good effect must have more benefit than a bad effect has harm.

Nursing Code of Ethics

There is more interest in the **ethics** involved in healthcare due to technological advances that have made the prolongation of life, organ transplants, prenatal manipulation, and saving of premature infants possible, sometimes with poor outcomes. Couple these with healthcare's limited resources, and **ethical dilemmas** abound. Ethics is the study of **morality** as the value that controls actions. The American Nurses Association Code of Ethics contains nine statements defining **principles** the nurse can use when faced with moral and ethical problems. Nurses must be knowledgeable about the many ethical issues in healthcare and about the field of ethics in general. The nurse must help a patient to reveal their values and morals to the health care team so that the patient, family, and team can resolve moral issues pertaining to the patient's care. As part of the healthcare team, the nurse has a right to express personal values and moral concerns about medical issues.

Bioethics

Bioethics is a branch of ethics that involves making sure that the medical treatment given is the most morally correct choice given the different options that might be available and the differences inherent in the varied levels of treatment. In the health care unit, if the patients, family members, and the staff are in agreement when it comes to values and decision-making, then no ethical dilemma exists; however, when there is a difference in value beliefs between the patients/family members and the staff, there is a bioethical dilemma that must be resolved. Sometimes, discussion and explanation can resolve differences, but at times the institution's ethics committee must be brought in to resolve the conflict. The primary goal of bioethics is to determine the most morally correct action using the set of circumstances given.

Ethical Decision-Making Model

There are many ethical decision-making models. Some general guidelines to apply in using ethical decision-making models could be the following:

- Gather information about the identified problem
- State reasonable alternatives and solutions to the problem
- Utilize ethical resources (for example, clergy or ethics committees) to help determine the ethically important elements of each solution or alternative
- Suggest and attempt possible solutions
- Choose a solution to the problem

It is important to always consider the **ethical principles** of autonomy, beneficence, nonmaleficence, justice, and fidelity when attempting to facilitate ethical decision-making with family members, caregivers, and the healthcare team.

Professional Boundaries

Gifts

Over time, patients may develop a bond with nurses they trust and may feel grateful to the nurse for the care provided and want to express thanks, but the nurse must make sure to maintain professional boundaries. Patients often offer **gifts** to nurses to show their appreciation, but some adults, especially those who are weak and ill or have cognitive impairment, may be taken advantage of easily. Patients may offer valuables and may sometimes be easily manipulated into giving large sums of money. Small tokens of appreciation that can be shared with other staff, such as a box of chocolates, are usually acceptable (depending upon the policy of the institution), but almost any other gifts (jewelry, money, clothes) should be declined: "I'm sorry, that's so kind of you, but nurses are not allowed to accept gifts from patients." Declining may relieve the patient of the feeling of obligation.

Sexual Relations

When the boundary between the role of the professional nurse and the vulnerability of the patient is breached, a boundary violation occurs. Because the nurse is in the position of authority, the responsibility to maintain the boundary rests with the nurse; however, the line separating them is a continuum and sometimes not easily defined. It is inappropriate for nurses to engage in **sexual relations** with patients, and if the sexual behavior is coerced or the patient is cognitively impaired, it is **illegal**. However, more common violations with adults, particularly elderly patients, include exposing a patient unnecessarily, using sexually demeaning gestures or language (including off-color jokes), harassment, or inappropriate touching. Touching should be used with care, such as touching a hand or shoulder. Hugging may be misconstrued.

Attention

Nursing is a giving profession, but the nurse must temper giving with recognition of professional boundaries. Patients have many needs. As acts of kindness, nurses (especially those involved in home care) often give certain patients extra attention and may offer to do **favors**, such as cooking or shopping. They may become overly invested in the patients' lives. While this may benefit a patient in the short term, it can establish a relationship of increasing **dependency** and **obligation** that does not resolve the long-term needs of the patient. Making referrals to the appropriate agencies or collaborating with family to find ways to provide services is more effective. Becoming overly invested may be evident by the nurse showing favoritism or spending too much time with the patient while neglecting other duties. On the other end of the spectrum are nurses who are disinterested and fail to provide adequate attention to the patient's detriment. Lack of adequate attention may lead to outright neglect.

Coercion

Power issues are inherent in matters associated with professional boundaries. Physical abuse is both unprofessional and illegal, but behavior can easily border on abusive without the patient being physically injured. Nurses can easily **intimidate** older adults and sick patients into having procedures or treatments they do not want. Regardless of age, patients have the right to choose and the right to refuse treatment. Difficulties arise with cognitive impairment, and in that case, another responsible adult (often the patient's child or spouse) is designated to make decisions, but every effort should be made to gain patient cooperation. Forcing the patient to do something against his or her will borders on abuse and can sometimes degenerate into actual abuse if physical coercion is involved.

Personal Information

When pre-existing personal or business relationships exist, other nurses should be assigned care of the patient whenever possible, but this may be difficult in small communities. However, the nurse should strive to maintain a professional role separate from the personal role and respect professional boundaries. The nurse must respect and maintain the confidentiality of the patient and family members, but the nurse must also be very careful about **disclosing personal information** about him or herself because this establishes a social relationship that interferes with the professional role of the nurse and the boundary between the patient and the nurse. The nurse and patient should never share secrets. When the nurse divulges personal information, he or she may become vulnerable to the patient, a reversal of roles.

Ethical Assessment

While the terms *ethics* and *morals* are sometimes used interchangeably, ethics is a study of morals and encompasses concepts of right and wrong. When making **ethical assessments,** one must consider not only what people should do but also what they actually do, as these two things are sometimes at odds. Ethical issues can be difficult to assess because of personal bias, which is one of the reasons that sharing concerns with other internal sources and reaching consensus is so valuable. Issues of concern might include options for care, refusal of care, rights to privacy, adequate relief of suffering, and the right to self-determination. Internal sources might include the ethics committee, whose role is to make decisions regarding ethical issues. Risk management can provide guidance related to personal and institutional liability. External agencies might include government agencies, such as the public health department.

Ethical Analysis of a Situation

Assessment of the situation is done to reveal the ethical, legal, and professional **conflicts** that are present. Those who are involved are identified, including the patient, family, and healthcare personnel. The decision maker is determined if it is not the patient. Information about the situation is collected to determine medical facts about the disease and condition of the patient, options for treatment, and nursing diagnoses. Any pertinent legal information is included. The patient and family's cultural, religious, and moral values are determined. Possible courses of action are listed and compared in terms of outcomes for the patient using the utilitarian or deontological theory of ethics. Professional codes of ethics are also applied. A decision is made and evaluated as to whether it is the most morally correct action. Ethical arguments for and against the decision are given and responded to by the decision maker.

Patient Rights and Responsibilities

Empowering patients and families to act as their own advocates requires that they have a clear understanding of their **rights and responsibilities.** These should be given (in print form) and/or presented (audio/video) to patients and families on admission or as soon as possible:

- **Rights** include competent, non-discriminatory medical care that respects privacy and allows participation in decisions about care and the right to refuse care. They should have clear understandable explanations of treatments, options, and conditions, including outcomes. They should be apprised of transfers, changes in care plan, and advance directives. They should have access to medical records and billing information.
- **Responsibilities** include providing honest and thorough information about health issues and medical history. They should ask for clarification if they don't understand information that is provided to them, and they should follow the plan of care that is outlined or explain why that is not possible. They should treat staff and other patients with respect.

Review Video: Patient Advocacy
Visit mometrix.com/academy and enter code: 202160

Informed Consent

The patient or their legal guardian must provide informed consent for all treatment the patient receives. This includes a thorough explanation of all procedures and treatment and associated risks. Patients/guardians should be apprised of all options and allowed to have input on the decision-making process. They should be apprised of all reasonable risks and any complications that might be life threatening or increase morbidity. The American Medical Association has established **guidelines for obtaining informed consent:**

- Explanation of the diagnosis
- Nature and reason for the treatment or procedure
- Risks and benefits of the treatment or procedure
- Alternative options (regardless of cost or insurance coverage)
- Risks and benefits of alternative options, including no treatment

Obtaining informed consent is a requirement in all states; however, a patient may waive their right to informed consent. If this is the case, the nurse should document the patient's waiving of this right and proceed with the procedure. Informed consent is not necessary for procedures performed to save life or limb in which the patient or guardian is unable to consent.

Confidentiality

Confidentiality is the obligation that is present in a professional-patient relationship. Nurses are under an obligation to protect the information they possess concerning the patient and family. Care should be taken to safeguard that information and provide the privacy that the family deserves. This is accomplished through the use of required passwords when family calls for information about the patient and through the limitation of who is allowed to visit. There may be times when confidentiality must be broken to save the life of a patient, but those circumstances are rare. The nurse must make all efforts to safeguard patient records and identification. Computerized record keeping should be done in such a way that the screen is not visible to others, and paper records must be secured.

Legal Responsibilities

Regulation of Nursing by States' Nurse Practice Act

Each state's **nurse practice act** seeks to regulate nursing within the state. It specifies the amount and type of education required to become an RN or LPN/LVN. It defines the nurse's role and responsibilities in healthcare settings. It lists actions that the nurse may take and defines advanced practice education, experience, responsibilities, and limitations. It gives nurses the authorization to perform as required. It also regulates delegation and supervision responsibilities of the nurse. Nurse practice acts are administered by the state board of nursing, which is responsible for issuing and renewing nurse licenses as well as discipline and censure of nurses. Most state boards of nursing now have a website that provides state-specific information about licensure and nursing rights and responsibilities.

Nurse's Accountability for Nursing Care

Nurses are part of an interdisciplinary team responsible for patient outcomes. Nurses have the responsibility for the outcomes of nursing care as a professional group. This responsibility is outlined in each state's nurse practice act, the American Nurses Association (ANA) practice guidelines, and the nurse's job description. Tools, such as the nursing care plan that includes standardized nursing diagnoses, interventions, and expected outcomes, enable the nurse to fulfill this responsibility. Empowerment to act as the patient advocate allows the nurse to point out factors in the patient's individual situation that can be addressed to further improve outcome. Critical thinking during decision-making and detailed documentation are also important. The nurse is held accountable for delegation as well as supervising care by others and evaluation of the outcomes of that care as well. The nurse has personal **accountability** in terms of ethical and moral conduct. Since clinical knowledge is crucial to critical thinking, the nurse must strive to increase knowledge continuously through professional development throughout his or her career.

Advance Directives

In accordance to Federal and state laws, individuals have the right to self-determination in health care, including the right to make decisions about end of life care through **advance directives** such as living wills and the right to assign a surrogate person to make decisions through a durable power of attorney. Patients should routinely be questioned about an advanced directive as they may present at a healthcare provider without the document. Patients who have indicated that they desire a do-not-resuscitate (DNR) order should not receive resuscitative treatments for terminal illness or conditions in which meaningful recovery cannot occur. Patients and families of those with terminal illnesses should be questioned as to whether the patients are Hospice patients. For those with DNR requests or those withdrawing life support, staff should provide the patient palliative rather than curative measures, such as pain control and/or oxygen, and emotional support to the patient and family. Religious traditions and beliefs about death should be treated with respect.

HIPAA

The Health Insurance Portability and Accountability Act (HIPAA) and state laws govern **who may receive healthcare information** about a person, how permission is to be obtained, how the information may be shared, and patients' rights concerning personal information. HIPAA strives to protect the **privacy** of an individual's healthcare information. Facilities must prevent this information from being accessed by unauthorized personnel. Healthcare information is required to be protected on the **administrative**, **physical**, and **technical** levels. The patient must sign a release form to allow any sharing of patient information. There are stiff penalties for violation of these laws, ranging from $100 for an unintentional violation to nearly $70,000 for a willful violation. Facilities that violate HIPAA may also be subject to corrective actions. Penalties are governed by the Department of Health and Human Services' Office for Civil Right and the state attorneys general.

Application of HIPAA to Practice

As an integral member of the health care team, the nurse must always be aware of HIPAA regulations and apply this knowledge to practice. The nurse is responsible for the following efforts to protect and maintain patient privacy:

- The nurse must read and follow facility policies regarding the transfer of patient data.
- Communication between health care personnel about a patient should always be in a private place so that this information is not overheard by those who do not have the right to share the information.
- Access to charts must be restricted to only those health care team members involved in that patient's care.
- Patient care information for unlicensed workers cannot be posted at the bedside, but must be on a care plan or the patient chart in a protected area.
- The nurse must not give information casually to anyone (e.g., visitors or family members) unless it is confirmed that they have the right to have that information.
- Family members must not be relied upon to interpret for the patient; an interpreter must be obtained to protect patient privacy.
- Computers with patient information must have passwords and safeguards to prevent unauthorized access of patient information.
- The nurse should not leave voicemail messages containing protected healthcare information for a patient but should instead ask the patient to call back.

Review Video: HIPAA
Visit mometrix.com/academy and enter code: 412009

OSHA

The **Occupational Safety and Health Act (OSHA)** seeks to keep workers safe and healthy while on the job. OSHA mandates that employers maintain a safe environment, workers are made fully aware of any hazards, and that access to personal protective gear is made available to workers who come into contact with hazardous materials. By following these regulations, an employer keeps injury and illness of workers to an absolute minimum. This fosters productivity, since workers are not absent due to illness or injury, employee health costs are contained, and the turnover rate is decreased, saving money spent on hiring and training new employees. OSHA is concerned about healthcare employee exposure to radiation, as well as chemical and biological agents, when caring for patients. Information is available to help hospitals and other facilities write plans that comply with best practices to deal with this and other threats to employees. Cleaning procedures, decontamination, and hazardous waste disposal are all covered by OSHA and apply to everyday hospital operation as well as disaster situations.

Review Video: Intro to OSHA
Visit mometrix.com/academy and enter code: 913559

CMS

The **Centers for Medicare and Medicaid (CMS)**, part of the U.S. Department of Health and Human Service department, see to it that healthcare regulations are observed by healthcare facilities that receive federal reimbursement. They reimburse facilities for care given to Medicare, Medicaid, and the state Children's Health Insurance Program (CHIP) recipients. They also monitor adherence to HIPAA regulations concerning healthcare information portability and confidentiality. CMS examines documentation of patient care when deciding to reimburse for care given. CMS has regulations for all types of medical facilities, and these regulations have profoundly impacted nursing practice because nurses must ensure that they comply with regulations related to the quality of patient care and concerns regarding cost-containment. Each facility should provide guidelines to assist nursing staff in meeting the specific documentation requirements of CMS.

OBRA 1987

The **Omnibus Budget Reconciliation Act of 1987 (OBRA 1987)**, also known as the Nursing Home Reform Act, instituted requirements for nursing homes with the purpose of strengthening and protecting patient rights. These requirements are as follows: "a facility must provide each patient with a level of care that enables him or her to attain or maintain the highest practicable physical, mental, and psychosocial wellbeing." OBRA 1987 required that all nursing home patients receive an initial evaluation with yearly follow-ups. Every patient is required to have a comprehensive care plan. Patients were ensured the right to medical care and the right to be informed about and refuse medical treatment. OBRA 1987 requires each state to establish, monitor, and enforce its own licensing requirements in addition to federal standards. Each state is also required to fund, staff, and maintain investigative and Ombudsman units.

OBRA 1990 (PSDA)

The Omnibus Budget Reconciliation Act of 1990 included the amendment called the **Patient Self Determination Act (PSDA)**. The PSDA required healthcare facilities to provide written information about advanced healthcare directives and the right to accept or reject medical or surgical treatments to all patients. Patients who make an advanced directive are leaving instructions about what medical interventions they authorize or refuse if they are incapacitated by illness or injury. They can also nominate another person to make these decisions for them in this situation. The PSDA also protected the right of patients to accept or refuse medical treatments. Healthcare facilities and hospitals are legally required to communicate these rights to all patients, to respect these rights, and to educate staff and personnel about these rights.

EMTALA

The **Emergency Medical Treatment and Active Labor Act (EMTALA)** is designed to prevent patient "dumping" from emergency departments (ED) and is an issue of concern for risk management that requires staff training for compliance:

- Transfers from the ED may be intrahospital or to another facility.
- Stabilization of the patient with emergency conditions or active labor must be done in the ED prior to transfer, and initial screening must be given prior to inquiring about insurance or ability to pay.
- Stabilization requires treatment for emergency conditions and reasonable belief that, although the emergency condition may not be completely resolved, the patient's condition will not deteriorate during transfer.
- Women in the ED in active labor should deliver both the child and placenta before transfer.
- The receiving department or facility should be capable of treating the patient and dealing with complications that might occur.
- Transfer to another facility is indicated if the patient requires specialized services not available intrahospital, such as to burn centers.

AHRQ

The **Agency for Healthcare Research and Quality (AHRQ)** is part of the US Department of Health and Human Services. This agency is concerned about health care and primarily promotes scientific research into the safety, effectiveness, and quality of healthcare. It encourages evidence-based healthcare that produces the best possible outcome while containing healthcare costs. It makes contracts with institutions to review any published evidence on healthcare in order to produce reports used by other organizations to write guidelines. The agency operates a Patient Safety Network (PSNet), which digitally compiles the most recent research and evidence-based practices that support quality and patient safety initiatives, while also housing training and educational opportunities. This network can be browsed by clinical area or collection, or simply by key terms. The resources housed within PSNet are written by many different health-related professional organizations and are used by primary healthcare providers, nurses, and healthcare facilities to guide patient treatment and care.

Information Technology

Telehealth Nursing

Telehealth nursing is a process that provides nursing care for patients over the telephone or other medium of non-physical interaction. Through telehealth services, patients are able to call in and speak with nurses about their symptoms or current condition, and in turn, telehealth nurses can provide health information and guidance to patients without seeing them in person. In addition to phone calls, these visits may also be conducted through videoconferencing, the internet, or other types of media. Some nurses who perform case management services for clients may also utilize telehealth to contact patients and review their current states of health. This type of technology allows these nurses to make assessments with the information provided from the patient, and to then compare these data with former conversations or visits to determine if the patient is moving toward expected outcomes in management of illness.

Necessary Skills

The nurse must master certain skills in order to be able to provide quality care via telehealth:

- The nurse must have excellent **verbal skills** and be able to effectively communicate over the phone to meet patient needs.
- The nurse must have a knowledge of **cultural differences** and be competent in communicating by telephone with patients of different cultures.
- The nurse must be able to **prioritize** the needs of the patient, using the standards of care provided by the *Telehealth Nursing Standards of Practice*, most recently revised in 2017.
- The nurse must be able to **perform** telehealth nursing in a variety of environments, including, but not limited to, clinics, physician's offices, emergency departments, and call centers.
- The nurse must be able to **ask specific questions** that will lead to the optimum treatment plan for the patient and assist in triaging for both nonemergent and emergent states of health.

Telephone Triage

Telephone triage is the process in which the receiving nurse uses protocols and guidelines to assess and prioritize the needs of a patient as they describe their condition over the phone. Telehealth does not allow the nurse to physically see the patient, so the nurse must be skilled at asking the appropriate questions and prioritizing needs based on the patients responses. The nurse must develop a plan of care that may include education, wellness promotion, and preventative education. The telehealth nurse is an extension of the clinic; therefore, he or she must also advocate for the patient and provide additional emotional support. Telehealth nursing increases patient satisfaction by providing the patient with a reliable source of information, direction, and emotional support.

Algorithms

In the telehealth process, patients are guided through triage questions to help the nurse reach a decision for care. **Algorithms** may be used as part of protocol for this triage process. Algorithms are a set of rules designed to solve a certain problem. They are different than a guideline because algorithms direct the nurse toward the best line of treatment. Algorithms also provide a systematic way to evaluate a broad problem or issue. They cover six areas of evaluation, which include the following:

- Assessment and data collection.
- Classification of acuity.

- Degree of advice or intervention.
- Education of caller.
- Validation of the caller.
- Evaluation/Follow-up.

The process follows a chain of logic and relies on the nurse's ability to assess, analyze, and interpret the patient's responses to questions posed by the nurse. The nurse may use algorithms as a direct line of questioning with "yes or no" answers. Each answer directs the nurse to the next type of question, ultimately guiding the nurse to the appropriate way to manage the situation by ruling out other conditions. The use of algorithms in telehealth nursing helps nurses to effectively triage patients over the phone, thereby potentially reducing the frequency of unnecessary emergency department visits and elevated costs.

EFFICIENT USE OF PROTOCOLS OR GUIDELINES

Protocols and guidelines in telehealth provide structure to the assessment process tailored to the patient's symptoms. They help to promote quality care when followed universally by telehealth nurses. Universal guidelines ensure that no matter where a patient lives, he or she is getting information based on the universal nursing standards of care. Some guidelines may be used to educate the patient on upcoming procedures such as ocular exams or hearing tests. Preoperative instructions can also be given through telehealth using standardized guidelines, as are post-hospitalization follow-up instructions. Guidelines are symptom-based and do not require a confirmed medical diagnosis. For example, if a patient calls in with a suspected sprain or break to the leg, the telehealth nurse would refer to the guideline for care that applies to an injury to an extremity (more generally). The nurse must listen carefully to what a patient is saying, but also to what is not being said in order to carefully prioritize the symptoms the patient is describing.

NECESSARY PROFESSIONAL COMPETENCIES AND PROFESSIONAL DEVELOPMENT

As with nurses in any other specialty, telehealth nurses must demonstrate professional nursing competencies and an ongoing knowledge of health care practices. They must show clinical expertise with the populations they serve. **Professional competencies** for the telehealth nurse include the following:

- A knowledge of health and illness across all age groups.
- Assessment skills specific for telephone triage.
- Communication skills, both verbal and written.
- Assertiveness and excellent listening skills.
- Critical thinking skills and effectiveness at educating patients over the phone.
- Customer service skills, including the knowledge of how to refer patients to internal and external resources, and the use of guidelines and protocols.
- Skills in written documentation.
- Skills in electronic documentation (including computers, telephones, fax machines, and other electronic forms of communication).

FORMS OF DOCUMENTATION

The telehealth nurse must understand and use proficiently the nursing process. The process should be **documented** in the patient record regardless of whether the patient was seen in person or attended to by telephone. Included in the patient record is the assessment of complaint(s), allergies, a history of the present illness/injury, and a medical history. The nurse's categorization of the call as urgent, nonurgent, etc. should also be documented. The plan provided by the nurse should be documented, including a referral if one is made. An evaluation of the patient's understanding and acceptance of the plan of care should also be conducted and documented. It must be remembered that the telehealth nurse may not meet every need of the patient in a single call. Rather, the telehealth nurse's focus should be to prioritize what needs to meet first. Documentation is important to evaluate and ensure that follow-up is conducted.

Application of HIPAA Standards to Telemedicine

The Health Insurance Portability and Accountability Act (HIPAA) was passed in 1996 as a measure to protect private health information of patients. Health care centers have enacted protocols to protect this information by limiting those with access to protected health information and maintaining confidentiality standards set forth by the act. The same standards apply in telemedicine, although there is an additional component of needed safety measures because the information is passing through media or telecommunications. These systems may require increased security to prevent hacking or the transmission of data into the wrong hands. Additional security systems should be in place, such as antiviral software, encryption systems, and password-protected files. Patients should be educated about the security measures being used in order to instill confidence that their personal information is protected.

Hospital-at-Home Model of Care

The hospital-at-home model of care allows patients with acute illnesses to be cared for in their home environment rather than at the hospital. The hospital-at-home model uses all aspects of telehealth (e.g., videoconferencing, monitors, and mobile health devices) as well as at-home visits by physicians, nurses, and other healthcare providers as needed. Patients are screened for eligibility, must be stable, must have access to technology, and must live within a specified distance from the hospital. Healthcare providers must be available at all times to respond to emergencies. Advantages of this model include improved outcomes, lower risk of infections, reduced costs, and improved patient comfort.

Remote Patient Monitoring

Remote patient monitoring allows patients to be monitored outside of the healthcare setting either continuously or intermittently through various devices. Remote patient monitoring can improve access to care for those living in rural or underserved communities and can reduce the costs of care. Remote patient monitoring can also lead to earlier detection of abnormalities and interventions and increase patients' engagement in their healthcare. Many remote patient monitoring devices allow for collection of data. Different types of patient monitoring devices include the following:

- Wearable fitness trackers/smartwatches (their capabilities vary): May monitor the heart rate, heart rhythm, blood pressure (BP), electrical signals in the heart with an electrocardiogram (ECG), respirations, sleep patterns, and physical activity.
- Personal devices: These are used intermittently for a specific purpose and include weight scales, pulse oximeters, apnea monitors, fetal monitors, blood glucose meters, KardiaMobile (for remote ECG), and BP monitors.
- Heart monitoring: Wearable devices such as the Zio patch, cardiac event recorders, the Holter monitor, and surgically implanted devices such as the Reveal LINQ insertable cardiac monitor, which monitors the heart continuously for 3 years.

Delegation and Supervision

Five Rights of Delegation

Prior to delegating tasks, the nurse should assess the needs of the patients and determine the task that needs to be completed, assure that he/she can remain accountable and can supervise the task appropriately, and evaluate effective completion. The **5 rights of delegation** include:

- **Right task**: The nurse should determine an appropriate task to delegate for a specific patient. This would not include tasks that require assessment or planning.
- **Right circumstance**: The nurse has considered the setting, resources, time factors, safety factors, and all other relevant information to determine the appropriateness of delegation. A task that is usually in one's scope (such as feeding a patient) may require assessment that makes it inappropriate to delegate (feeding a new stroke patient).
- **Right person**: The nurse is in the right position to choose the right person (by virtue of education/skills) to perform a task for the right patient.
- **Right direction**: The nurse provides a clear description of the task, the purpose, any limits, and expected outcomes.
- **Right supervision**: The nurse is able to supervise, intervene as needed, and evaluate performance of the task.

Delegation of Tasks in Teams

On major responsibility of leadership and management in performance improvement teams is using delegation effectively. The purpose of having a team is so that the work is shared, and leaders can cripple themselves by taking on too much of the workload. Additionally, failure to delegate shows an inherent distrust in team members. Delegation includes:

- Assessing the skills and available time of the team members, determining if a task is suitable for an individual
- Assigning tasks, with clear instructions that include explanation of objectives and expectations, including a timeline
- Ensuring that the tasks are completed properly and on time by monitoring progress but not micromanaging
- Reviewing the final results and recording outcomes

Because the leader is ultimately responsible for the delegated work, mentoring, monitoring, and providing feedback and intervention as necessary during this process is a necessary component of leadership. Even when delegated tasks are not completed successfully, they represent an opportunity for learning.

Nursing Process

Purpose of Nursing Assessment

Nursing assessment evaluates patient data to help in diagnosis and treatment. The nurse assesses baseline health and medical history to be sure the patient will be safe. The nurse also determines what limitations the patient may have in terms of understanding or cooperation. Nursing assessment is an ongoing process, which includes baseline information, information on the patient's response and recovery to the intervention, and continued efforts to maintain the patient's health. The nurse can collaborate with other team members to help in this assessment.

Purpose of Nursing Diagnosis and Planning

Nursing diagnosis is directed at patient comfort and outcome. With a diagnosis, nurses establish nursing interventions that are needed for the patient to be safe and comfortable. The nurse uses the diagnosis to direct therapies and to anticipate potentially needed interventions.

Planning allows the nurse to outline the methods needed to achieve patient goals. This accounts for alternative therapies that may be needed, setting priorities, satisfactory outcomes to be achieved, and expectations for discharge. The nurse needs to document the plan. The plan outlines nursing responsibilities, possible interventions, and expected outcomes.

Implementation of Nursing Plan

Implementing the nursing plan requires a measure of fluidity. The original plan is based on initial data. As new data is accumulated, however, the original plan may be modified. There is a need to incorporate individual needs of the patient as the plan proceeds. Different interventions may be called for depending on individual responses or limitations. The nurse needs to continually monitor the patient's response and status to be able to offer appropriate nursing interventions. Documentation is essential at every step of the way. The information can be useful in further treatment of the individual. It can also be used to assess the process so that improvements or adjustments can be made. The documentation may also be used for research purposes to further the knowledge of nursing practice. The record may become necessary for legal purposes as well.

Evaluation Process

In order to provide the best care for the patient, the nurse must **evaluate** the process in effect. This entails reviewing procedures and interventions in relation to standards of care, quality of care, and patient outcomes. Critical evaluation of the nursing process can lead to changes that may improve the quality of care for patients and/or identify personnel issues that need to be addressed. Modifying care plans is important to maintaining effective patient care. Deficiencies may be noted and can, therefore, be addressed. This underscores the importance of adequate documentation. In order to evaluate the process, the nurse must have access to the documentation to assess the present process. This evaluation may lead to changes that improve the quality of care in the nursing unit.

Planning of Nursing Care for Patients

The patient's needs as defined by the **nursing diagnoses** are first prioritized with the help of the patient and family:

- **Critical needs** are met immediately and then other needs are ranked according to the patient's priorities and Maslow's Hierarchy of Needs.
- When diagnoses are prioritized, **desirable outcomes** for each diagnosis are defined. Outcomes include desirable changes in patient behavior and are the backbone of the care plan. Outcomes are used to determine whether the nursing care has met its objectives.
- **Goals** for each nursing diagnosis are devised with patient and family input. Immediate, intermediate, and long-term goals that combine to meet the desired outcome are defined along with a timetable. Intermediate and long-term goals usually pertain to the prevention of complications and patient and family teaching concerning self-care and rehabilitation needs.

Each goal is then completed by a list of specific **actions** needed to achieve the goal. These actions include nursing interventions and may also include coordination of actions by other healthcare personnel.

Review Video: Plan of Care
Visit mometrix.com/academy and enter code: 300570

Resources for Care Planning

Various resources provide lists of nursing diagnoses, interventions, and expected outcomes to help guide the nurse care planning process:

- The **North American Nursing Diagnosis Association (NANDA)** compiles a list of the most commonly used nursing diagnoses and refines them so that they are acceptable for study and nursing research. This list is updated biannually and is useful when developing care plans.
- **Nursing-Sensitive Outcomes Classification (NOC)** lists nursing outcomes for specific needs. Each outcome has an associated scale of achievement and can be used to evaluate patient progress in achieving the outcome desired.
- **Nursing Interventions Classification (NIC)** consists of interventions appropriate for specific nursing needs. These interventions can be individualized for each patient's needs.

NANDA, NIC, and NOC utilize the **Taxonomy of Nursing Practice** to classify nursing diagnoses, outcomes, and interventions. The Taxonomy of Nursing Practice divides patient problems into four domains:

- **The functional domain** includes classes consisting of patient movement, relief of symptoms, developmental status, nutrition, ADLs, sexuality, belief systems, and sleep.
- **The physiological domain** consists of bodily needs for proper functioning divided into classes concerning the cardiovascular, respiratory, gastrointestinal, genitourinary, neurological, metabolic, immune, reproductive, musculoskeletal, and integumentary systems. The effects of medications and other substances on system functioning are included.

- **The psychosocial domain** contains classes concerning emotional health (coping mechanisms, mental state, self-image, and self-esteem), mental health (knowledge and behaviors), and social status (communication with others, relationships, and support network).
- **The environmental domain** is concerned with patient populations, public and individual health and safety in the environment, healthcare delivery, and management of risks.

By using the taxonomy, all three tools describe the same problems in the same way in language that is specific and refined, yet universal.

Utilizing Clinical Pathways in Care Planning

Clinical pathways are written tools that direct the treatment of a specific group of patients according to diagnosis. They provide a way to standardize medical and nursing care according to evidence-based practice guidelines, predict the cost of the care, and ensure quality, timeliness, and cost-effectiveness of care. Each plan consists of the DRG or group that it addresses, time segments with specific activities, and desired outcomes for each time segment. They include a place to record activities that deviate from the pathway. Nursing care is charted according to the pathway, which serves as the patient's plan of care. Nurses are responsible for helping to formulate and change clinical pathways. They initiate the pathways when the patient presents for treatment and ensure that the care is given for each time segment. They also use the pathways to monitor patients as case managers for hospitals or insurance companies. The patient may receive a copy that the nurse then discusses to make the patient aware of the treatment course and desired goals.

Incorporating Patient and Family Rights into Plan of Care

In order for patient and family rights to be incorporated into the plan of care, the care plan needs to be designed as a **collaborative effort** that encourages participation of patients and family members. There are a number of different programs that can be useful, such as including patients and families on advisory committees. Additionally, assessment tools, such as surveys for patients and families, can be utilized to gain insight in the issues that are important to them. While infants and small children and sometimes the elderly cannot speak for themselves, the "patient" is generally understood to include not only the immediate family but also other groups or communities who have an interest in the care of the individual. Because many hospital stays are now short-term, programs that include follow-up interviews and assessments are especially valuable in determining if the needs of the patient were addressed in the care plan.

Psychosocial Factors That Affect Care Planning

There are many psychosocial factors that affect patient care. A patient's **psychological state** influences how that patient interacts with others, including nurses and hospital staff, and can also affect compliance and positive health outcomes. For instance, anxiety or depression can make a patient incapable of performing the instructions necessary for completing a full recovery; the psychological problem would need to be addressed in the patient's care plan.

Social and culture factors also shape a patient's **perception** of health and disease, communication style, and decision-making methods. It is important to understand that differences in ethnicity, race, sex, gender, religion, age, socioeconomic status, family dynamics, sexual orientation, and life experiences mean that patients experience illness and healing differently. Being sensitive to these differences can lead to more effective patient care across the spectrum.

Consideration of Comorbidities in Care Planning

Comorbidity, also known as multimorbidity, refers to the coexistence of multiple chronic or acute medical diseases within one patient. Comorbid conditions are associated with poorer outcomes, the need for more complex medical or surgical management, and elevated healthcare costs. It is now the norm, as opposed to the exception, that patients have multiple comorbid medical conditions. Some examples would be an obese patient with concomitant diabetes, heart disease, and osteoarthritis; a multi-system trauma patient with diabetes, chronic obstructive pulmonary disease, and cardiovascular disease; or a cancer patient with anxiety, depression, and multiple pulmonary emboli.

Implementation of a Nursing Plan

The patient's nursing care plan is implemented as soon as the patient has been stabilized. During stabilization, nursing care is guided by standards of practice and logarithms that define care for life-threatening situations. Once the patient is stabilized, **interventions** are guided by the patient's individualized plan of care:

- The nurse has the responsibility of performing the planned nursing interventions and of delegating and coordinating care given by others to meet the patient's needs.
- All care is documented along with patient response.
- Additional patient information, changes in condition, patient priorities, and needs guide the nurse in continuously modifying the care plan.
- Orders are analyzed, clarified, and questioned as needed to meet collaborative patient needs.
- Patient input is necessary to the evaluation of nursing care and revision of the care plan as needed. Patient response to interventions, treatments, and procedures is assessed and care is given accordingly.
- The results of labs and tests are also used to determine actions according to the care plan.

Critical Thinking and Judgment

Elements of Research

The following are elements of research:

- **Variable**: An entity that can be different within a population
- **Independent variable**: The variable that the researchers change to evaluate its effect
- **Dependent variable**: The variable that may be changed by alterations in the independent variable
- **Hypothesis**: The proposed explanation to describe an expected outcome in a study
- **Sample**: The selected population to be studied
- **Experimental group**: The population within the sample that undergoes the treatment or intervention
- **Control group**: The population within the sample that is not exposed to the treatment of intervention being evaluated

The nurse must be taught and must understand the process of critical analysis and know how to conduct a survey of the literature. **Basic research concepts** include:

- **Survey of valid sources**: Information from a juried journal and an anonymous website or personal website are very different sources, and evaluating what constitutes a valid source of data is critical.
- **Evaluation of internal and external validity**: Internal validity shows a cause-and-effect relationship between two variables, with the cause occurring before the effect and no intervening variable. External validity occurs when results hold true in different environments and circumstances with different populations.
- **Sample selection and sample size**: Selection and size can have a huge impact on the results, but a sample that is too small may lack both internal and external validity. Selection may be so narrowly focused that the results can't be generalized to other groups.

Validity, Generalizability, and Replicability

Many research studies are most concerned with **internal validity** (adequate unbiased data properly collected and analyzed within the population studied), but studies that determine the efficacy of procedures or treatments, for example, should have **external validity** as well; that is, the results should be **generalizable** (true) for similar populations. **Replication** of the study under different circumstances and with different subjects and researchers should produce similar results. For various reasons, some people may be excluded from a study so that instead of randomized subjects, the subjects may be highly selected so when data is compared with another population in which there is less or more selection, results may be different. The selection of subjects, in this case, would interfere with external validity. Part of the design of a study should include considerations of whether or not it should have external validity or whether there is value for the institution based solely on internal validation.

Hypothesis

A hypothesis should be generated about the probable cause of the disease/infection based on the information available in laboratory and medical records, epidemiologic study, literature review, and expert opinion. For example, a hypothesis should include the infective agent, the likely source, and the mode of transmission: "Wound infections with *Staphylococcus aureus* were caused by reuse and inadequate sterilization of single-use irrigation syringes used during wound care in the ICU."

Hypothesis testing includes data analysis, laboratory findings, and outcomes of environmental testing. It usually includes case-control studies, with 2–4 controls picked for each case of infection. They may be matched according to age, sex, or other characteristics, but they are not infected at the time they are picked for the study. Cohort studies, whose controls are picked based on having or lacking exposure, may also be instituted. If the hypothesis cannot be supported, then a new hypothesis or different testing methods may be necessary.

Critical Reading

There are several steps to critical reading to evaluate research:

- **Consider the source** of the material. If it is in the popular press, it may have little validity compared to something published in a peer-reviewed journal.
- **Review the author's credentials** to determine if a person is an expert in the field of study.
- **Determine the thesis**, or the central claim of the research. It should be clearly stated.
- **Examine the organization** of the article, whether it is based on a particular theory, and the type of methodology used.
- **Review the evidence** to determine how it is used to support the main points. Look for statistical evidence and sample size to determine if the findings have wide applicability.
- **Evaluate** the overall article to determine if the information seems credible and useful and should be communicated to administration and/or staff.

Major Study Types Utilized in Statistical Analysis

When conducting research, the nurse should be aware of the **types of studies** available and when each type of study is appropriate and most reliable:

- **Case-control studies** are simple. They use pre-existing cases with and without the disorder of interest. For example, case-control studies may be done with mesothelioma and exposure to possible pleural irritants. These are good for rare diseases to determine cause and effect.
- **Cross-sectional studies** utilize a cross-section of data from the population and analyze variables at one time point. They are not good for determining cause and effect, but they are useful for correlating characteristics with disorders.
- **Cohort studies** follow a cohort of a population for a period of time and attempt to make a link with diseases. As in the previous example, researchers could follow a group exposed to asbestos and study the incidence of mesothelioma.
- **Randomized controlled trial** is the gold standard, with patients assigned to the control or experimental group. This is a difficult type of test to design and implement but very useful, as the data is often well-controlled. It is the most expensive type of study.

Bias in Research

Selection bias occurs when the method of selecting subjects results in a cohort that is not representative of the target population because of inherent error in design. For example, if all patients who develop urinary infections are evaluated per urine culture and sensitivities for microbial resistance, but only those patients with clinically-evident infections are included, a number of patients with sub-clinical infections may be missed, skewing the results. Selection bias is only a concern when participants in studies are specifically chosen. Many surveillance studies do not involve the selection of subjects.

Information bias occurs when there are errors in classification, so an estimate of association is incorrect. Non-differential misclassification occurs when there is similar misclassification of disease or exposure among both those who are diseased/exposed and those who are not. Differential misclassification occurs when there is a differing misclassification of disease or exposure among both those who are diseased/exposed and those who are not.

Qualitative and Quantitative Data

Both qualitative and quantitative data are used for analysis, but the focus is quite different:

- **Qualitative data**: Data are described verbally or graphically, and the results are subjective, depending upon observers to provide information. Interviews may be used as a tool to gather information, and the researcher's interpretation of data is important. Gathering this type of data can be time-intensive, and it can usually not be generalized to a larger population. This type of information gathering is often useful at the beginning of the design process for data collection.
- **Quantitative data**: Data are described in terms of numbers within a statistical format. This type of information gathering is done after the design of data collection is outlined, usually in later stages. Tools may include surveys, questionnaires, or other methods of obtaining numerical data. The researcher's role is objective.

Classes of Evidence-Based Practice

Evidence-based practice is treatment based on the best possible evidence, including a study of current research. Literature is searched to find evidence of the most effective treatments for specific diseases or injuries, and those treatments are then utilized to create clinical pathways that outline specific multi-departmental treatment protocols, including medications, treatments, and timelines. Evidence-based guidelines are often produced by specialty organizations that undertake the task of searching and analyzing literature to produce policies, procedures, and guidelines that become the standard of care for the disease. These guidelines are then used when a patient fits the disease criteria for that guideline.

Evidence-based nursing aims to improve the quality of nursing care by examining the reasons for all nursing practices and determining those that have the most positive outcomes. Evidence-based nursing focuses on the individual nurse utilizing evidence-based observations to influence decision-making.

Evidence-Based Practice Guidelines

The creation of evidence-based practice guidelines includes the following components:

- **Focus on the topic/methodology:** This includes outlining possible interventions and treatments for review, choosing patient populations and settings, and determining significant outcomes. Search boundaries (such as types of journals, types of studies, dates of studies) should be determined.
- **Evidence review:** This includes review of literature, critical analysis of studies, and summarizing of results, including pooled meta-analysis.
- **Expert judgment:** Recommendations based on personal experience from a number of experts may be utilized, especially if there is inadequate evidence based on review, but this subjective evidence should be explicitly acknowledged.
- **Policy considerations:** This includes cost-effectiveness, access to care, insurance coverage, availability of qualified staff, and legal implications.
- **Policy:** A written policy must be completed with recommendations. Common practice is to utilize letter guidelines, with "A" being the most highly recommended, usually based on the quality of supporting evidence.
- **Review:** The completed policy should be submitted to peers for review and comments before instituting the policy.

Critical Pathways

Clinical/critical pathway development is done by those involved in direct patient care. The pathway should require no additional staffing and cover the entire scope of an illness. Steps include:

1. Selection of patient group and diagnosis, procedures, or conditions, based on analysis of data and observations of wide variance in approach to treatment and prioritizing organization and patient needs
2. Creation of interdisciplinary team of those involved in the process of care, including physicians to develop pathway
3. Analysis of data including literature review and study of best practices to identify opportunities for quality improvement
4. Identification of all categories of care, such as nutrition, medications, and nursing
5. Discussion and reaching consensus
6. Identifying the levels of care and number of days to be covered by the pathway
7. Pilot testing and redesigning steps as indicated
8. Educating staff about standards
9. Monitoring and tracking variances in order to improve pathways

Levels of Evidence in Evidence-Based Practice

Levels of evidence are categorized according to the scientific evidence available to support the recommendations, as well as existing state and federal laws. While recommendations are voluntary, they are often used as a basis for state and federal regulations.

- **Category IA** is well supported by evidence from experimental, clinical, or epidemiologic studies and is strongly recommended for implementation.
- **Category IB** has supporting evidence from some studies, has a good theoretical basis, and is strongly recommended for implementation.
- **Category IC** is required by state or federal regulations or is an industry standard.
- **Category II** is supported by suggestive clinical or epidemiologic studies, has a theoretical basis, and is suggested for implementation.

- **Category III** is supported by descriptive studies, such as comparisons, correlations, and case studies, and may be useful.
- **Category IV** is obtained from expert opinion or authorities only.
- **Unresolved** means there is no recommendation because of a lack of consensus or evidence.

Outcome Evaluation

Outcome evaluation is an important component of evidence-based practice, which involves both internal and external research. All treatments are subjected to review to determine if they produce positive outcomes, and policies and protocols for outcome evaluation should be in place. **Outcome evaluation** includes the following:

- **Monitoring** over the course of treatment involves careful observation and record-keeping that notes progress, with supporting laboratory and radiographic evidence as indicated by condition and treatment.
- **Evaluating** results includes reviewing records as well as current research to determine if outcomes are within acceptable parameters.
- **Sustaining** involves discontinuing treatment but continuing to monitor and evaluate.
- **Improving** means to continue the treatment but with additions or modifications in order to improve outcomes.
- **Replacing** the treatment with a different treatment must be done if outcome evaluation indicates that current treatment is ineffective.

Admissions, Transfers, and Discharge

Skills Needed for Collaboration

Nurses must learn the set of skills needed for collaboration in order to move nursing forward. Nurses must take an active role in gathering data for evidence-based practice to support nursing's role in health care, and they must share this information with other nurses and health professionals in order to plan staffing levels and to provide optimal care to patients. Increased and adequate staffing has consistently been shown to reduce adverse outcomes, but there is a well-documented shortage of nurses in the United States, and more than half currently work outside the hospital setting. Increased patient loads not only increase adverse outcomes but also increase job dissatisfaction and burnout. In order to manage the challenges facing nursing, nurses must develop the following skills needed for collaboration:

- Be willing to compromise
- Communicate clearly
- Identify specific challenges and problems
- Focus on the task
- Work with teams

Communication Skills

Collaboration requires a number of communication skills that differ from those involved in communication between nurse and patient. These skills include:

- **Using an assertive approach**: It's important for the nurse to honestly express opinions and to state them clearly and with confidence, but the nurse must do so in a calm, non-threatening manner.
- **Making casual conversation**: It's easier to communicate with people with whom one has a personal connection. Asking open-ended questions, asking about others' work, or commenting on someone's contributions helps to establish a relationship. The time before meetings, during breaks, and after meetings presents an opportunity for this type of conversation.
- **Being competent in public speaking**: Collaboration requires that a nurse be comfortable speaking and presenting ideas to groups of people. Speaking and presenting ideas competently also helps the nurse to gain credibility. Public speaking is a skill that must be practiced.
- **Communicating in writing**: The written word remains a critical component of communication, and the nurse should be able to communicate clearly and grammatically.

Communication and Hand Offs

The nurse is usually the primary staff member responsible for **external and internal hand off transitions of care**, and should ensure that communication is thorough and covers all essential information. The best method is to use a standardized format:

- **DRAW**: Diagnosis, recent changes, anticipated changes, and what to watch for.
- **I PASS the BATON**: Introduction, patient, assessment, situation, safety concerns, background, actions, timing, ownership, and next.
- **ANTICipate**: Administrative data, new clinical information, tasks, illness severity, contingency plans.
- **5 Rs**: Record, review, round together, relay to team, and receive feedback.

A reporting **form** or checklist may be utilized to ensure that no aspect is overlooked.

For external transitions, the nurse must ensure that the type of transport team and monitoring is appropriate for patient needs, and provide insight when determining the most appropriate mode of transportation: ground transfer for short distance, helicopter for medium to long distance, and fixed-wing aircraft for long distances.

SBAR Technique

The SBAR technique is used to hand-off a patient from one caregiver to another to provide a systematic method so that important information is conveyed:

- **(S) Situation**: Overview of current situation and important issues
- **(B) Background**: Important history and issues leading to current situation
- **(A) Assessment**: Summary of important facts and condition
- **(R) Recommendation**: Actions needed

Shift Reporting

Shift reporting should include bedside handoff when possible with oncoming staff members. The nurse handing off the patient should follow a specific format for handoff (such as I PASS the BATON) so that handoff is done in the same manner every time, as this reduces the chance of omitting important information. The shift report should include introduction of the oncoming staff to the patient, the triage category or acuity level of the patient, diagnosis (potential or confirmed), current status, laboratory and imaging (completed or pending) and results if available, and medications or treatments administered and pending. Any monitoring equipment (pulse oximetry, telemetry) should be examined. Any invasive treatments (Foley catheter, IV) should be discussed and equipment examined. The nurse should report any plans for admission, transfer, or discharge. It is essential that all staff be trained in shift reporting and the importance of consistency.

Collaboration Between Nurse and Patient/Family

One of the most important forms of collaboration is that between the nurse and the patient/family, but this type of collaboration is often overlooked. Nurses and others in the healthcare team must always remember that the point of collaboration is to improve patient care, and this means that the patient and patient's family must remain central to all planning. For example, including family in planning for a patient takes time initially, but sitting down and asking the patient and family, "What do you want?" and using the Synergy model to evaluate patient's (and family's) characteristics can provide valuable information that saves time in the long run and facilitates planning and expenditure of resources. Families, and even young children, often want to participate in care and planning and feel validated and more positive toward the medical system when they are included.

Collaboration with External Agencies

The nurse must initiate and facilitate collaboration with external agencies because many have direct impacts on patient care and needs:

- **Industry** can include other facilities sharing interests in patient care or pharmaceutical companies. It's important for nursing to have a dialog with drug companies about their products and how they are used in specific populations because many medications are prescribed to women, children, or the aged without validating studies for dose or efficacy.
- **Payers** have a vested interest in containing health care costs, so providing information and representing the interests of the patient is important.

- **Community groups** may provide resources for patients and families, both in terms of information and financial or other assistance.
- **Political agencies** are increasingly important as new laws are considered about nurse-patient ratios and infection control in many states.
- **Public health agencies** are partners in health care with other facilities and must be included, especially in issues related to communicable disease.

INTERDISCIPLINARY TEAMS

There are a number of skills that are needed to lead and facilitate coordination of **intra- and inter-disciplinary teams**:

- Communicating openly is essential. All members must be encouraged to participate as valued members of a cooperative team.
- Avoiding interrupting or interpreting the point another is trying to make allows free flow of ideas.
- Avoiding jumping to conclusions, which can effectively shut off communication.
- Active listening requires paying attention and asking questions for clarification rather than to challenge other's ideas.
- Respecting others' opinions and ideas, even when opposed to one's own, is absolutely essential.
- Reacting and responding to facts rather than feelings allows one to avoid angry confrontations and diffuse anger.
- Clarifying information or opinions stated can help avoid misunderstandings.
- Keeping unsolicited advice out of the conversation shows respect for others and allows them to solicit advice without feeling pressured.

LEADERSHIP STYLES

Leadership styles often influence the perception of leadership values and commitment to collaboration. There are a number of different leadership styles:

- **Charismatic**: Relies on personal charisma to influence people, and may be very persuasive, but this type leader may engage followers and relate to one group rather than the organization at large, limiting effectiveness.
- **Bureaucratic**: Follows organization rules exactly and expects everyone else to do so. This is most effective in handling cash flow or managing work in dangerous work environments. This type of leadership may engender respect but may not be conducive to change.
- **Autocratic**: Makes decisions independently and strictly enforces rules. Team members often feel left out of process and may not be supportive of the decisions that are made. This type of leadership is most effective in crisis situations, but may have difficulty gaining the commitment of staff.
- **Consultative**: Presents a decision and welcomes input and questions, although decisions rarely change. This type of leadership is most effective when gaining the support of staff is critical to the success of proposed changes.
- **Participatory**: Presents a potential decision and then makes final decision based on input from staff or teams. This type of leadership is time-consuming and may result in compromises that are not entirely satisfactory to management or staff, but this process is motivating to staff who feel their expertise is valued.

- **Democratic**: Presents a problem and asks staff or teams to arrive at a solution, although the leader usually makes the final decision. This type of leadership may delay decision-making, but staff and teams are often more committed to the solutions because of their input.
- **Laissez-faire ("free reign")**: Exerts little direct control but allows employees/teams to make decisions with little interference. This may be effective leadership if teams are highly skilled and motivated, but in many cases, this type of leadership is the product of poor management skills and little is accomplished because of this lack of leadership.

Identifying the Need for Patient Referral

Issues to consider when making patient referrals include:

- **Necessity**: The referral may be needed if the patient's needs are outside of the provider's scope or practice or field of expertise and if the provider cannot provide adequate assessment and treatment for the patient's condition.
- **Insurance requirements**: The provider should determine whether the patient's carrier requires preauthorization or other steps to make sure the patient's referral is covered.
- **Selection of specialist/therapist**: The specialist, in many cases, must be selected from a group of physicians who are participating in an insurance plan if the service is to be covered completely or at all by the insurance company. When possible, the patient should be given choice of referrals.
- **Submission**: The referral should be sent along with appropriate records and releases. The provider may need to make personal contact if specialists are selective, have waiting lists, and may not approve a referral.

Safe, Effective Care Environment: Safety and Infection Control

Medical and Surgical Asepsis

Pathogenic Organisms

Pathogenic organisms that cause infection are becoming increasingly resistant to antibiotics. Methicillin-resistant *Staphylococcus aureus* (MRSA) and Vancomycin-resistant *Enterococcus* (VRE) are two of the most common resistant strains of bacteria causing nosocomial infections in the hospital. The more resistance these organisms acquire to antibiotics, the more difficult they are to treat. Organisms with endotoxins in their outer cell membranes are more virulent than other organisms and thus cause an infection with fewer amounts of bacteria present than other organisms. Treatment for inoculation of these organisms becomes difficult, lengthy, and costly. Strict maintenance of aseptic technique prevents nosocomial spread of these bacteria and demonstrates the importance of maintaining this technique at all times.

Surgical Hand Antisepsis

The scrubbing procedure for surgical hand antisepsis is as follows:

1. All jewelry is removed from the hands and wrists, and a surgical mask is donned. A scrub sponge/brush is selected, the water is turned on, and the hands are first washed with **soap and running water**.

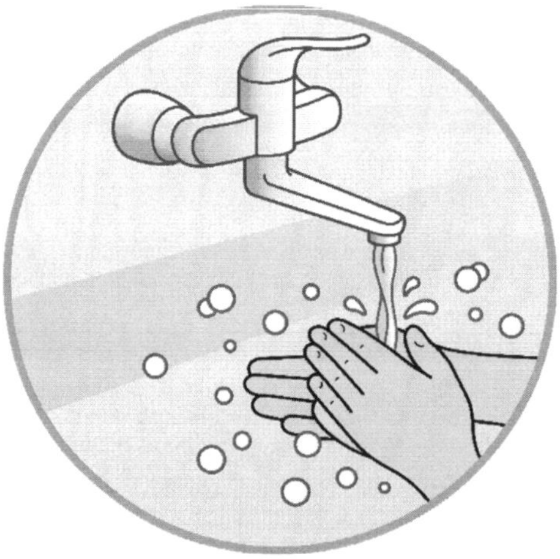

2. The scrub brush is opened, and the nail cleaner is used to clean in and around **nails** under running water and repeated on the other side. The hands are then rinsed.

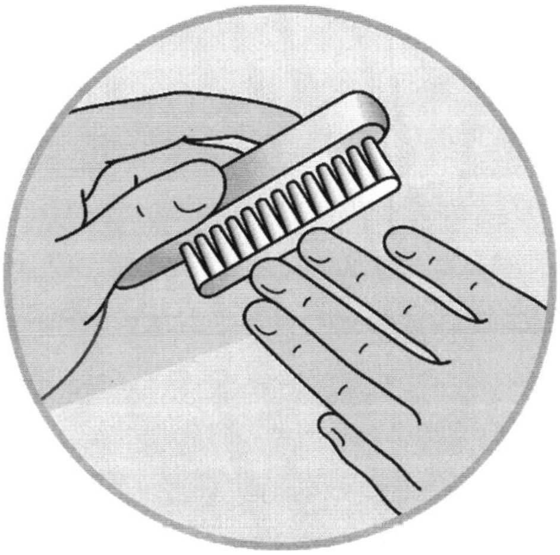

3. The scrub brush is moistened and the arms are held in the flexed position with hands held up above the elbows and water running toward the elbows. With the arms in this position, the nails, fingers, hands, wrists, and arms are scrubbed according to facility requirements (either timed or surface scrubbed a certain number of times) from the **fingertips** down to the **elbow**. The hands are then rinsed.

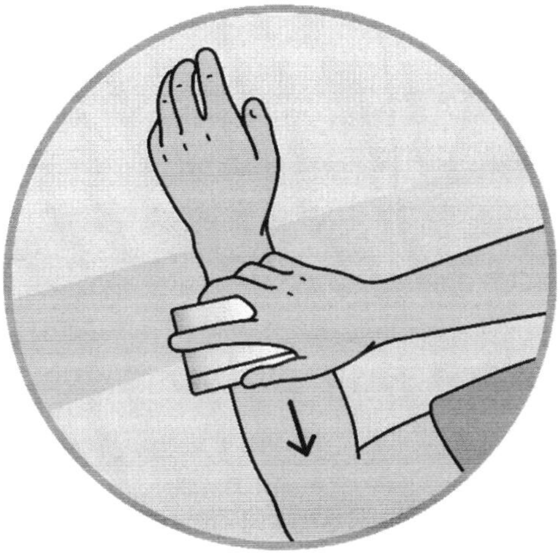

4. The sink is then turned off using the elbow. If an **alcohol-based rub** is to be used instead of scrubbing, hands are dried after washing on a clean towel, and then the rub is applied to hands and forearms, which are rubbed until the product and hands are dry.

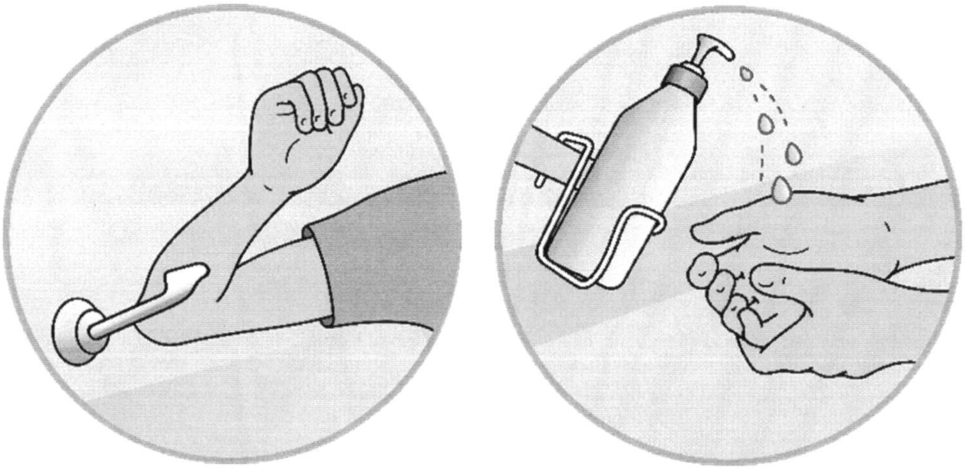

Gowning and Gloving Using Surgical Antiseptic Technique

When gowning and gloving using surgical antiseptic technique, the nurse must take into account the following considerations:

- Care is taken by the scrubbed person to maintain a **sterile field** while gowning and gloving.
- Reusable gowns must be **inspected** for wear as they lose protective qualities with repeated washings.
- If the gown does not have a removable pull-tab, a sterile instrument can be used by the scrubbed person and handed to the nonsterile person to wrap the **tie** around.
- One must use **latex-free gloves** when a patient has a latex allergy.
- Gloves should be free of **powders** as powders can cause inflammatory reactions if introduced under the skin.
- When using the open-gloving technique, the bare hands should only touch the **inside** of the glove. Unwrapping of the cuff should be done by the sterile, gloved hand.

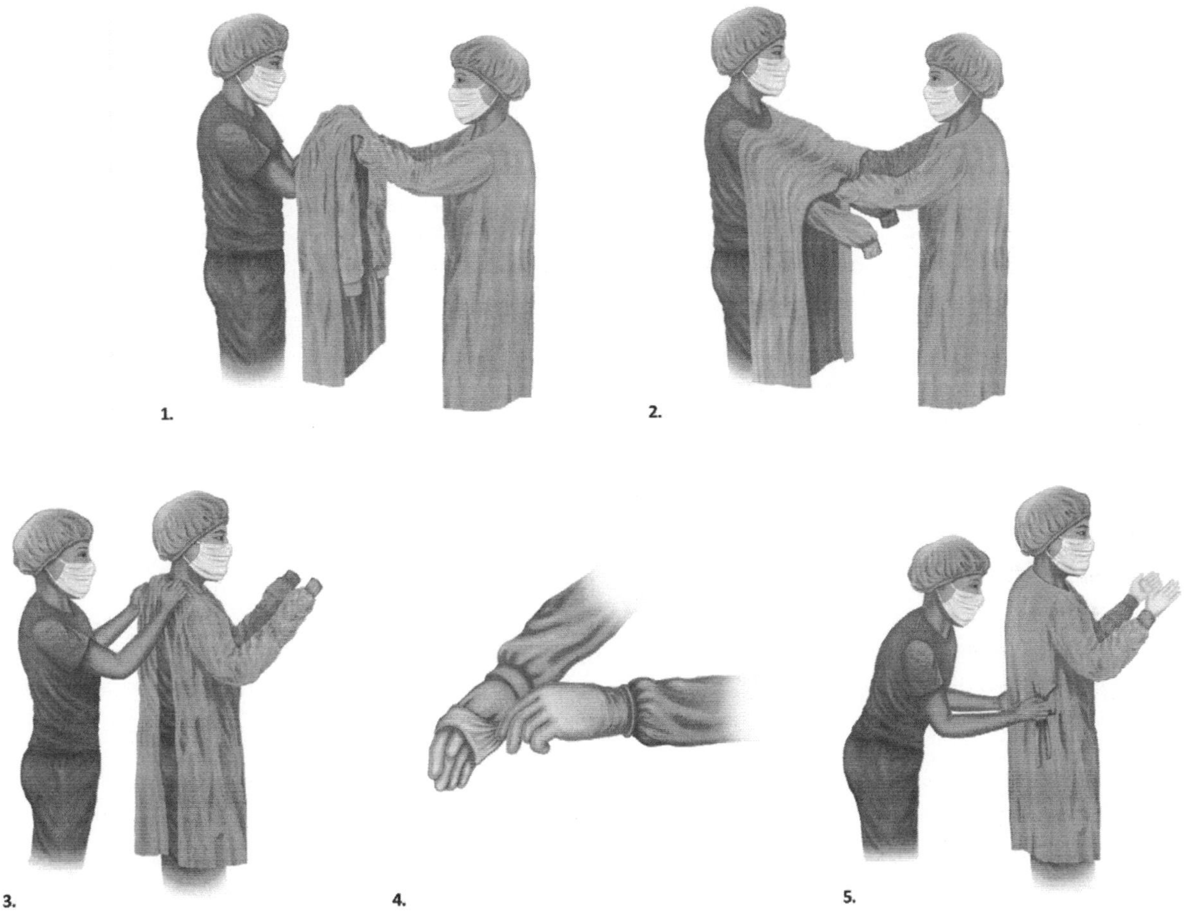

Gowning and Gloving Procedure

The gowning and gloving procedure, maintaining surgical asepsis, is as follows:

1. The gown is handled by the **neckline** by the **sterile scrub person**, lifted off and away from the sterile field, and allowed to unfold down.
2. The **armholes** are identified and both arms are inserted into the corresponding holes simultaneously to prevent dragging of the gown on the floor. The hands are inserted up to the cuff if a closed-gloving technique is required, through the cuff for open gloving.
3. A **nonsterile scrub person** fastens the gown at the neck and at the waist.
4. **Gloves** are donned in a sterile manner, pulling the gloves over the cuffs of the gown. Gloves can also be donned through **assistive gloving**, in which the scrub person holds the glove open and the sterile person inserts their hand into the glove, only touching the inside of the glove. The glove should completely cover the cuff of the sterile gown.
5. Using the pull-tab that is easily removed without contaminating the gown, a nonsterile member pulls the **tie** around the gown so the sterile person can grab the end and tie it around the waist.

Glove Contamination and Perforation

Specific protocol must be established and enforced with regard to glove contamination (with blood, bodily fluids, or hazardous material) and glove perforation. During invasive surgical procedures AORN guidelines recommend that gloves are changed under the following circumstances:

- After sterile draping
- After manipulating instruments/objects with sharp or rough edges (including body parts such as bones)
- After the procedure and every 90-150 minutes when relevant
- In the case of perforation, actual or suspected (If perforation occurs in the outer glove, it should be removed and the inner glove examined.)
- After touching contaminated objects (surgical helmet/hood/visor, fluoroscopes, or eye pieces of surgical microscopes)
- After touching hazardous materials (methyl methacrylate, specific medications)

Gloves should be changed away from the sterile field and with the helped of an unscrubbed team member (to remove the glove) and a scrubbed team member (to don the new glove)

Prepping and Maintaining Sterile Field

A new sterile field is prepped for each procedure, immediately prior to the patient's arrival at the procedure room. Hand antisepsis and sterile gown/glove donning should be performed prior to setup. In order to maintain a sterile field and prevent its contamination the following must be taken into consideration:

- **Basins** for holding solutions are held at the edge of the field to prevent splashing of the sterile field.
- Constant monitoring of a **sterile field** should take place to prevent potential contamination of the field without notice. Therefore, it is best and easiest to monitor when the field is created as close to surgery time as possible.
- **Furniture and equipment** that are part of the sterile field are often covered to prevent contamination.
- **Talking** is kept to a minimum to prevent droplet contamination of the field.
- **Movement** within the sterile field is done in a manner that preserves sterility of the field. Personnel pass each other back-to-back to prevent potential contamination of one's back to one's sterile front side. Standing persons should remain standing, and sitting persons should remain sitting.
- Only personnel who are **scrubbed** and who don hats, gowns, and gloves are to operate within a sterile field. Only the chest down to the sterile field of the person is considered sterile and the gloved hands to two inches above the elbow. Areas of potential perspiration and edges are not considered sterile.
- Sterile **drapes** establish and maintain the sterile field.
- Any **items introduced** to a sterile field must be sterile. Any items thought to be contaminated are not introduced and/or are removed to prevent contamination. Proper techniques are used to make sure that items are transferred to the sterile site appropriately. Packaging is thoroughly inspected for punctures or other threats to the sterility of the item. Wrapped items are unwrapped with the furthest item unwrapped first and the closest last. Items not able to be dropped or flipped onto the field are to be picked up by a sterile scrubbed person. Heavy items are to be carefully placed to prevent rolling, dropping, etc.

Maintaining Sanitation of Operating Room

Before and During the Procedure

The following are some standards the operating room personnel utilize to maintain sanitation of the operating room area **before and during the procedure:**

- All persons who may potentially come into contact with blood or body fluids must wear **personal protective equipment**.
- All furniture and equipment are **damp dusted** in the operating room before the first procedure to reduce dust and particulate matter in the room.
- Patients with **latex allergies** are often scheduled as the first case of the day as latex products used later in the day may deposit latex particles in the operating room.
- All contamination is **confined, cleaned, and disinfected** during the procedure as much as possible.
- **Large spills** are soaked up with a cloth, and the remaining residue cleaned with a germicidal agent.
- Soiled **disposable items** are thrown away. Soiled **reusable items** are wiped with an antiseptic agent and placed in a leak-proof container.
- All **tissue specimens** are placed in leak-proof containers and sealed. If indicated, the outside may be wiped with a germicidal agent.

After the Procedure

The following are some standards the operating room personnel utilize to maintain sanitation of the operating room **after the procedure**:

- All items on the sterile field after the procedure are considered **contaminated**.
- **Disposable items** are put into hazardous waste bags/receptacles.
- **Infectious waste fluids** can either be poured into a sewer drain or placed in appropriate leak-proof containers and placed in a hazardous waste bag/receptacle.
- All **sharps** are considered infectious waste and are put in appropriate sharps containers.
- All other **instruments that are reusable** are cleaned and processed for reuse. They are put in appropriate transportation containers to cleaning areas.
- All **furniture/equipment**, including the floor, in the operating room is wiped down with an appropriate germicidal agent after the procedure. At the end of the day, all furniture, equipment, and surfaces are terminally cleaned.
- Periodic cleaning of areas just **outside the operating room** takes place to prevent contamination into the operating room. Locker rooms, cabinets, walls, restrooms, etc. are included in these areas.

Infection Control

Nosocomial Infections

Nosocomial infections are those that are healthcare-associated or hospital-acquired. The following is a list of common nosocomial infections.

- *Enterococci* infections include urinary infections, bacteremia, endocarditis as well as infections in wounds and the abdominal and pelvic areas.
- *Enterobacteriaceae* cause about half of the urinary tract infections and a quarter of the postoperative infections.
- *Escherichia coli* primarily causes urinary tract infections (especially related to catheters), diarrhea, and neonatal meningitis but it can also lead to pneumonia, and bacteremia (usually secondary to urinary infection).
- Group B β-hemolytic *Streptococci* (GBS) has increasingly been a cause of infections in neonatal units, causing pneumonia, meningitis, and sepsis. GBS infections may occur as wound infections after Cesarean sections, especially in those immunocompromised.
- *Staphylococcus aureus* is a major cause of nosocomial post-operative infections, both localized and systemic, and from indwelling tubes and devices.
- Methicillin-resistant *Staphylococcus aureus (MRSA)* is a common cause of surgical infections.
- *Clostridioides difficile* causes more nosocomial diarrhea cases than any other microorganism.
- *Candida*, a yeast fungal pathogen, can overgrow and lead to mucocutaneous or cutaneous lesions and sepsis.
- *Aspergillus* spp., filamentous fungi, produce spores that become airborne and can invade the respiratory tract, causing pneumonia.

Catheter-Related Infections

Intravenous catheter-related infections are a significant cause of morbidity and mortality in the hospital setting. Usually, these infections are due to *Staphylococcus aureus*, *enterococcus*, or fungal infection such as *Candida*. These infections are important because they may progress and eventually lead to bacteremia, infective endocarditis, septic pulmonary emboli, septic shock, osteomyelitis, or superficial thrombophlebitis. Therefore, vigilance should be maintained to prevent these infections. The patient may exhibit fevers, chills, and discomfort around the catheter site. The site itself may show purulence or erythema. The subclavian vein is the preferred intravenous site and the femoral is the least-preferred site due to high infection rates. Infections are diagnosed with blood cultures and catheter tip cultures. Initial treatment includes removal of the catheter and antibiotic treatment. Antibiotics should be empiric at first, then directed toward culture results. Treatment duration should be 2 weeks at first, but 4–6 weeks if there is a complicated infection.

Infection Control Measures

Standard infection control measures are designed to prevent transmission of microbial substances between patients and/or medical providers. These measures are indicated for everyone and include frequent handwashing, gloves whenever bodily fluids are involved, and face shields and gowns when splashes are anticipated. For more advanced control with tuberculosis, SARS, vesicular rash disorders (such as VZV), and COVID-19, **airborne precautions** should be instituted to prevent the spread of tiny droplets that can remain suspended in the air for days and travel throughout a hospital environment. Therefore, negative pressure rooms are essential, and providers and patients should wear high-efficiency N95 masks and be fitted in advance. For disorders such as influenza or other infections spread by droplets (spread by cough or sneeze) basic surgical masks should be worn (**droplet precautions**). For **contact precautions** in the setting of fecally-transmitted infection or vesicular rash diseases, gowns/gloves should be used and contact limited. White coats are not a substitute for proper gowning. In the case of a *Clostridioides difficile* infection, contact precautions should be used in addition to washing hands with soap and water (rather than alcohol-based hand sanitizer) after patient contact.

Infection Control Plan

The purpose of an infection control/surveillance plan should be clearly outlined and may be multifaceted, including the following elements:

- **Decreasing rates of infection**: The primary purpose of a surveillance plan is to identify a means to decrease nosocomial infections, including a notification system and laboratory surveillance.
- **Evaluating infection control measures**: Surveillance can evaluate effectiveness of infection control measures. (Surgical checklists, handwashing, housekeeping, ventilation).
- **Establishing endemic threshold rates**: Establishing threshold rates can help to enact control measures to reduce rates.
- **Identifying outbreaks**: About 5–10% of infections occur in outbreaks, and comparing data with established endemic threshold rates can help to identify these outbreaks if analysis is done in a regular and timely manner.
- **Achieving staff compliance**: Objective evidence may convince staff to cooperate with infection control measures.
- **Meeting accreditation standards**: Some accreditation agencies require reports of infection rates.
- **Providing defense for malpractice suits**: Providing evidence that a facility is proactive in combating infections can decrease liability.
- **Comparing infection rates with other facilities**: Comparing data helps focus attention and resources.

Protocol for Needlestick Injury and Postexposure Prophylaxis

If the healthcare provider experiences a **needlestick injury**, the individual's initial response should be to irrigate the wound with soap and water. As soon as possible, the incident must be reported to a supervisor and steps taken according to established protocol. This may include testing and/or prophylaxis, depending on the patient's health history. In some cases, the patient may also be tested for communicable diseases, such as HIV, in order to determine the risk to the healthcare provider. PEP (post-exposure prophylaxis) is available for exposure to HIV (human immunodeficiency virus) and hepatitis B virus (hepatis B immune globulin). However, no PEP is available for HCV (hepatitis C virus) although the CDC does provide a plan for management. PEP should be initiated within 72 hours of exposure. All testing and treatments associated with the needlestick injury must be provided free of cost at a hospital or medical facility.

Immunization vs. Vaccination

Immunization refers to the body's buildup of defenses (antibodies) against specific diseases. It has an important role in preventing the spread of infection. Immunization prevents the individual from contracting a disease or lessens the severity of the disease, and can also prevent the complications (encephalitis, hearing loss, paralysis) associated with the infectious diseases. **Vaccination** is one method of creating immunity through the introduction of a small amount of the virus's or bacteria's antigen to the body, which then stimulates the body's creation of antibodies against that disease. Vaccination prevents the spread of infection to infants who are too young to have developed immunity and to those who are immunocompromised (cancer patients, transplantation recipients). Herd immunity results from a majority of the population being immune to a disease, therefore minimizing transmission. It is defined in terms of the percentage of the population that must be immunized in order to prevent outbreaks. This percentage may range from 80-85% for some disorders, but those that are highly contagious, such as measles, may require a herd immunity of 93-95%. Herd immunity can be obtained via widespread vaccination or widespread infection, though it is not recommended that individuals avoid immunization and rely on herd immunity for protection, as rates of immunization vary from one community to another.

Types of Vaccines

There are a number of different types of vaccines:

- **Conjugated forms**: An organism is altered and then joined (conjugated) with another substance, such as a protein, to potentiate immune response (such as conjugated Hib).
- **Killed virus vaccines**: The virus has been killed but can still cause an immune response (such as inactivated poliovirus).
- **Live virus vaccines**: The virus is live but in a weakened (attenuated) form so that it doesn't cause the disease but confers immunity (such as measles vaccine).
- **Recombinant forms**: The organism is genetically altered and, for example, may use proteins rather than the whole cell to stimulate immunity (such as Hepatitis B and acellular pertussis vaccine).
- **Toxoid**: A toxin (antigen) that has been weakened by the use of heat or chemicals so it is too weak to cause disease but stimulates antibodies.

Some vaccines are given shortly after birth; others begin at 2 months, 12 months, or 2 years and some later in childhood.

DTaP and Tdap Vaccines

Diphtheria and pertussis (whooping cough) are highly contagious bacterial diseases of the upper respiratory tract. Cases of diphtheria are now rare in the United States, although they still occur in some developing countries. There have, however, been recent outbreaks of pertussis in the United States. Tetanus is a bacterial infection contracted through cuts, wounds, and scratches. The **diphtheria, tetanus, and pertussis (DTaP) vaccine** is recommended for all children. DTaP is a newer and safer version of the older DTP vaccine, which is no longer used in the United States. **Tdap** is the DTaP booster shot meant to continue immunity to these diseases through adulthood, given every 10 years starting at age 11.

DTaP requires 5 doses:

- 2 months
- 4 months
- 6 months
- 5-18 months
- 4-6 years (or at 11-12 years if booster missed between 4-6)

According to recent ACIP recommendations, DTaP may now also be administered to children ages 7-9 as part of a catch-up series, but children will then require their routine Tdap dose at age 11-12. If DTaP is administered to children ages 10-18 it can be counted as their adolescent Tdap booster. Adverse reactions can occur, but they are usually mild soreness, fever, and/or nausea. About 1 in

100 children will have high fever (>105 °F) and may develop seizures. Severe allergic responses can occur.

HPV Vaccine

Human papillomavirus (HPV) comprises >100 viruses. About 40 are sexually transmitted and invade mucosal tissue, causing genital warts, which are low risk for cancer, or changes in the mucosa, which can lead to cervical cancer. Most HPVs cause little or no symptoms, but they are very common, especially in those 15-25. Over 99% of cervical cancers are caused by HPV and 70% are related to HPVs 16 and 18. The HPV vaccine, Gardasil, protects against HPVs 6 and 11 (which cause genital warts), along with 16 and 18, which can cause cancer. Protection is only conveyed if the female has not yet been infected with these strains. The vaccine is currently recommended for females under 26 but studies have determined that those not adequately covered over the age of 26 and up to 45 can benefit. A series of 3 injections is required over a 6-month period:

- Initial dose 11-12 years (but may be given as young as 9 or ≥18)
- 2 months after first dose
- 6 months after first dose

PPV

Pneumococcal polysaccharide-23 vaccine (PPV) (Pneumovax and Pnu-Immune) is a vaccine that has been available since 1977 to protect against 23 types of pneumococcal bacteria. It is given to adults ≥65 and children ≥2 years in high-risk groups that include:

- Children with chronic heart, lung, sickle cell disease, diabetes, cirrhosis, alcoholism, and leaks of cerebrospinal fluid
- Children with lowered immunity from Hodgkin's disease, lymphoma, leukemia, kidney failure, multiple myeloma, nephrotic syndrome, HIV/AIDS, damaged or missing spleen, and organ transplant

Children ≤2 may not respond to this vaccine and should take PCV-7. Administration is as follows:

- One dose is usually all that is required although a second dose may be advised for children with some conditions, such as cancer or organ/bone marrow transplantations.
- If needed, a second dose is given 3 years after the first for children ≤10 and 5 years after the first for those ≥10.

Hepatitis A Vaccine

Hepatitis A is a contagious virus that causes liver disease and can cause serious morbidity and death. It is spread through the feces of a person who is infected and often causes contamination of food and water. The **Hep A vaccine** is now recommended for all children at one year of age. It is not licensed for use in younger infants. Two doses are needed:

- 12 months (12-23 months)
- 18 months (or 6 months after previous dose)

Older children and teenagers may receive the two-injection series if they are considered at risk, depending upon lifestyle, such as young males having sex with other males or those using illegal drugs. It is also recommended if outbreaks occur. Adverse reactions are mild and include soreness, headache, anorexia, and malaise although severe allergic reactions can occur as with all vaccines.

Hepatitis B Vaccine

Hepatitis B is transmitted through blood and body fluids, including during birth; therefore, it is now recommended for all newborns as well as all those <18 and those in high-risk groups >18. Hepatitis B can cause serious liver disease leading to liver cancer. Three injections of **monovalent HepB** are required to confer immunity:

- Birth (within 12 hours)
- At 1-2 months
- ≥24 weeks

Note: If combination vaccines are given after the birth dose, then a dose at 4 months can be given.

If the mother is Hepatitis B positive, the child should be given both the monovalent HepB vaccination as well as HepB immune globulin within 12 hours of birth. Adolescents (11-15) who have not been vaccinated require 2 doses, 4-6 months apart. Adverse reactions include local irritation and fever. Severe allergic reactions can occur to those allergic to baker's yeast.

Rotavirus Vaccine

Rotavirus is a cause of significant morbidity and mortality in children, especially in developing countries. Most children, without vaccination, will suffer from severe diarrhea caused by rotavirus within the first 5 years of life. The new **rotavirus vaccine** is advised for all infants but should not be initiated after 12 weeks or administered after 32 weeks, so there is a narrow window of opportunity. Three doses are required:

- 2 months (between 6 and 12 weeks)
- 4 months
- 6 months

An earlier vaccine was withdrawn from the market because it was associated with an increase in intussusception, a disorder in which part of the intestine telescopes inside another. Rates of intussusception in those receiving the current (RotaTeq) vaccine have been investigated and incidence of intussusception was within the range of normal occurrences with no evidence linking the occurrences to the vaccine.

Inactivated Poliovirus Vaccine

Poliomyelitis is a serious viral infection that can cause paralysis and death. Prior to introduction of a vaccine in 1955, there were >20,000 cases of polio in the United States each year. There have been no cases of polio caused by the poliovirus for >20 years in the United States, but it still occurs in some third world countries, so continuing vaccinations is very important. Oral polio vaccine (OPV) is no longer recommended in the United States because it carries a very slight risk of causing the disease (1:2.4 million). Children require 4 doses of injectable polio vaccine (IPV):

- 2 months
- 4 months
- 6-18 months
- 4-6 years (booster dose)

IPV is contraindicated for those who have had a severe reaction to neomycin, streptomycin, or polymyxin B. Rare allergic reactions can occur, but there are almost no serious problems caused by this vaccine.

Varicella Vaccine

Varicella (chickenpox) is a common infectious childhood disease caused by the varicella zoster virus, resulting in fever, rash, and itching, and it can also cause skin infections, pneumonia, and neurological damage. After infection, the virus retreats to the nerves by the spinal cord and can reactivate years later, causing herpes zoster (shingles), a significant cause of morbidity in adults. Infection with varicella conveys immunity, but because of associated problems, it is recommended that all children receive varicella vaccine. Two doses are needed:

- 12-15 months
- 4-6 years (or at least 3 months after first dose)

Children ≥13 years and adults who have never had chickenpox or previously received the vaccine should receive 2 doses at least 28 days apart. Children should not receive the vaccine if they have had a serious allergic reaction to gelatin or neomycin. Most reactions are mild and include soreness, fever, and rash. About 1:1000 may experience febrile seizures. Pneumonia is a very rare reaction.

MMR Vaccine

Measles is a viral disease characterized by fever and rash but can cause pneumonia, seizures, severe neurological damage, and death. Mumps is a viral disease that causes fever and swollen glands but can cause deafness, meningitis, and swelling of the testicles. Rubella, also known as German measles) is also a viral disease that can cause rash, fever, and arthritis, but the biggest danger is that it can cause a woman who is pregnant to miscarry or deliver a child with serious birth defects. The **measles, mumps, and rubella (MMR) vaccine** is given in 2 doses:

- 12-15 months
- 4-6 years

Children can get the injections at any age if they have missed them, but there must be at least 28 days between injections. Children with severe allergic reactions to gelatin or neomycin should not get the injection. Severe adverse reactions are rare, but fever and mild rash are common. Teenagers may have pain and stiffness in joints. Occasional seizures (1:3000) and thrombocytopenia (1:30,000) occur.

PCV-7

Heptavalent pneumococcal conjugate vaccine (PCV-7) (Prevnar) was released for use in the United States in 2001 for treatment of children under 2 years old. It provides immunity to 7 serotypes of *Streptococcus pneumoniae* to protect against invasive pneumococcal disease, such as pneumonia, otitis media, bacteremia, and meningitis. Because children are most at risk ≤1, vaccinations begin early:

Administration is in 4 doses:

- 6-8 weeks
- 4 months
- 6 months
- 12-18 months

Although less effective for older children, PCV-7 has been approved for children between 2 and 5 years of age who are at high risk because of the following conditions:

- Chronic diseases: sickle cell disease, heart disease, lung disease, liver disease
- Damaged or missing spleen
- Immunosuppressive disorders: diabetes, cancer
- Drug therapy: chemotherapy, steroids

PCV-7 may also be considered for all children ≤ 5, especially those ≤3 and in group day care and in some ethnic groups (Native American, Alaska Natives, and African Americans).

Meningococcal Vaccine

Meningitis is severe bacterial meningitis that can result in severe neurological compromise or death. A number of different serotypes of *meningococci* can cause meningitis and current vaccines protect against 4 types although not against subtype B, which causes about 65% of meningitis cases in children. However, the vaccines provide 85-100% protection against sub-types A, C, Y, and W-135. There are 2 types of vaccine:

- **Meningococcal polysaccharide vaccine (MPSV4)** is made from the outer capsule of the bacteria and is used for children 2-10.
  - One dose is given at 2 years, although those at high risk may receive 2 doses, 3 months apart.
  - Under special circumstances, children 3-24 months may receive 2 doses, 3 months apart.
- **Meningococcal conjugate vaccine (MCV4)** is used for children ≥11 (who have not received MPSV4). One dose is required:
  - Ages 11-12, all children should receive the vaccine.
  - If not previously vaccinated, high school and college freshmen should be vaccinated.
- Side effects are usually only local tenderness.

Hib Vaccine

***Haemophilus influenzae* type b (Hib) vaccine** (HibTITER and PedvaxHIB) protects against infection with *Haemophilus influenzae,* which can cause serious respiratory infections, pneumonia, meningitis, bacteremia, and pericarditis in children ≤5 years old. *Administration* is as follows:

- 2 months
- 4 months
- 6 months (may be required, depending upon the brand of vaccine)
- 12-15 months (this booster dose must be given at least 2 months after the earlier doses for those who start at a later age than 2 months)

Children over age 6 usually do not require Hib, but it is recommended for older children and adults. Here are some conditions that place them at risk:

- Sickle cell disease
- HIV/AIDS
- Bone marrow transplant
- Chemotherapy for cancer
- Damaged or missing spleen

Some chemotherapy drugs, corticosteroids, and other immunosuppressive drugs may interact with the vaccine.

Infant Immunization Schedule Summary

The recommended schedule for immunizations for the infant is summarized below:

- All newborns receive **ophthalmic drops or ointment**, to prevent blindness from possible gonorrhea infection, and an injection of vitamin K to prevent hemorrhagic disease.
- Before discharge, newborns are tested for **phenylketonuria** and **hypothyroidism**, and will possibly have their **hematocrit** and **hemoglobin** checked.
- **Hepatitis B vaccine** is given at birth, 1-2 months, and 6-18 months.
- **Diphtheria/tetanus/pertussis vaccine** is administered at 2 months, 4 months, 6 months, and 15-18 months.
- **Hib (Haemophilus influenza type b) vaccine** is given at 2 months, 4 months, and 12 months or later.
- **Poliovirus vaccine** is given at 2 months, 4 months, and 6-18 months.
- **MMR vaccine** is given at 12-18 months.
- **Varicella (chickenpox) vaccine** can be given at 12 months.

Review Video: Child Immunizations and Schedule
Visit mometrix.com/academy and enter code: 167190

Required Immunization History for Children up to 6 Years of Age

According to the Centers for Disease Control and Prevention, by 6 years of age, children in the United States should receive a three-part series of hepatitis B, three doses of rotavirus prevention; four injections protecting against diphtheria, tetanus, and pertussis; four doses of *Haemophilus influenzae* type b; four doses of pneumococcal vaccine; four doses of polio vaccine; two injections that protect against measles, mumps, and rubella; two varicella vaccinations; one hepatitis A vaccination; and a yearly influenza prevention injection.

Vaccination of Children with Uncertain Immunization Histories

Children who have uncertain immunization histories may need vaccinations to meet guidelines. The number of vaccinations needed depends on the child's history. For children who are not up-to-date on immunizations, the necessary injections must be determined. These vaccinations can then be given on a schedule so that the child can catch up. For children with no immunization history or uncertain status, such as refugees or internationally adopted children, restarting the immunization series may be necessary to ensure adequate coverage with all vaccines, particularly measles, mumps, and rubella; varicella; hepatitis B; *Haemophilus influenzae* type b; and polio.

Possible Side Effects

Immunization reactions can be minimized and the child made more comfortable by giving acetaminophen prior to the immunizations. Common reactions to immunizations include irritability, decrease in appetite, fever less than 102 °F, and swelling, redness and tenderness at injection site. These may last for the first 1-2 days and can be treated with acetaminophen every 4-6 hours for the first day. If more severe reactions occur, such as fever greater than 102 °F, severe prolonged irritability, or high-pitched crying, or the symptoms last more than 2 days, the parents should call the healthcare provider immediately.

Important Considerations When Giving Immunizations

Every time a child comes into contact with the healthcare system, his **immunization status** should be assessed. Children are required, by all states, to be immunized before entering a licensed school or day care. Specific requirements will vary from state to state. Vaccines must be handled and stored according the manufacturers guidelines. Immunizations must be documented according to specific guidelines and parents must sign a consent form every time a vaccine is administered. Common illnesses such as colds, ear infections and diarrhea will not usually preclude giving vaccines. The MMR and varicella vaccines should not be given during pregnancy. There are two situations in which immunizations are contraindicated: a previous severe allergic reaction to a vaccine or one of its components and encephalopathy occurring within 7 days of giving a DTP or DTaP vaccine.

The Anti-Vaccination Movement

While **opposition to vaccination** is not a new concept, it is a movement that has gained momentum with the power of information sharing via social media. Opposers to vaccination, often referred to as "Anti-Vaxxers," believe that vaccinations can cause complications such as autism and SIDS, especially when administered in infancy and early childhood, and believe that these risks far outweigh the benefits. There are also those who oppose such medical interventions due to religious beliefs.

While the therapeutic effects of vaccinations have been supported by evidence for both individuals and communities, it is important that healthcare professionals be equipped to respectfully inform and care for those that oppose vaccinations. Individuals should be educated regarding the evidence supporting vaccinations and the vaccinations required by law. The CDC offers a wealth of resources for healthcare workers and for individuals regarding vaccinations. The most notable resource is the CDC's Vaccine Information Statement, a living document that outlines the benefits and risks of vaccines, that healthcare workers can use to inform individuals and parents. If, despite efforts to educate, the individual or caregiver still refuses vaccination, there are ICD codes that providers are required to use to document this refusal (for example, ICD-10-CM: Z28.82: Immunization not carried out because of caregiver refusal). The healthcare worker must also document that preventive medical counseling was provided.

Client Safety, Home Safety, and Ergonomics

Joint Commission's Patient Safety Goals

The Joint Commission has a set of **goals that impact patient safety** for each type of healthcare facility. Within the hospital environment, there are several goals that pertain:

- Each facility must have a way to identify patients that will avoid errors of identification.
- Caregivers are to give careful, accurate communications about patients and their care so that mistakes are not made.
- A system to avoid medication errors must be in place.
- Medications must be reconciled when the patient moves from place to place within the hospital or is discharged to other caregivers.
- The risk of infection must be decreased so that patients are at less risk for hospital-related infections.
- The facility must have a fall prevention program and evaluate its effectiveness.

All patients and family must be encouraged to be active in their own care to help to avoid errors. They must also know how to make sure their concerns for safety of care are heard and acted upon.

Environmental Aspects of Patient Safety in the Hospital

Deliberate decisions by the health care providers/facility can help create an environment conducive for patient safety. Some of those aspects include:

- **Educating the patient on signaling staff**: The patient must be educated about the use of the call light, and the call light placed within easy reach. If the patient is unable to use the call light, then an alternative means of calling for help, such as a handheld bell, should be available. If the patient is unable to manage any type of signaling system, then the nurse should check on the patient at least every hour.
- **Protecting from falls and electrical hazards**: All clutter should be removed from floors and cords secured away from walkways. All electrical appliances should be checked to ensure they are working properly and have no frayed cords. Patients should be provided assistive devices, such as walkers, if necessary, to improve stability.
- **Making appropriate room assignments**: Patients with the greatest need for supervision should be placed closest to the nursing desk and within the line of sight whenever possible. In environments such as critical care, each nurse should be able to visualize their patient assignment from their nursing station.

Medication Errors

There are about 7,000 deaths yearly in the United States attributed to **medication errors.** Studies indicate that there are errors in 1 in 5 doses of medication given to patients in hospitals. Patient safety must be ensured with proper handling and administering of medications:

- **Avoid error-prone abbreviations or symbols**. The Joint Commission has established a list of abbreviations to avoid, but mistakes are frequent with other abbreviations as well. In many cases, abbreviations and symbols should be avoided altogether or restricted to a limited approved list.
- **Prevent errors due to illegible handwriting or unclear verbal orders**. Handwritten orders should be block printed to reduce chance of error; verbal orders should be repeated back to the physician.
- **Institute barcoding and scanners** that allow the patient's wristband and medications to be scanned for verification.
- **Provide lists of similarly-named medications** to educate staff.
- Establish an **institutional policy** for the administration of medications that includes protocols for verification of drug, dosage, and patient, as well as educating the patient about the medications.

Assessing Patients for Non-Drug Allergies

When assessing patients for **allergies** it's important to determine the type of symptoms they have, when the initial reaction occurred, and what type of treatment they have used in the past to manage this complication (including antihistamines). Allergies of particular interest include:

- **Food**: Ask patients about any specific foods that cause an adverse reaction as some foods may have cross-reactivity to latex (such as kiwi, papaya, avocado, and bananas), so patients may be at risk of developing latex allergy and should avoid contact with latex. Some medications may contain substances derived from food, such as eggs, fish, gelatin, lactose, and soy.
- **Latex**: Sensitivity to latex can result in mild reactions, such as itching and rash, to severe anaphylactic reactions, and is common among those with repeated contact with healthcare environments, such as those with spina bifida or multiple surgeries, so it should be suspected with these clients. While non-latex options are more readily available in most hospitals (non-latex gloves and Foley catheters, for instance), latex continues to be used in hospital materials, therefore this allergy must be assessed immediately upon arrival so that appropriate materials can be substituted if necessary.
- **Environmental**: The most common environmental allergies include pollens, dust mites, animals, cigarette smoke, cockroaches, and mold/mildew, so the nurse should be sure to ask about these as well as any other environmental allergies. Some patients are sensitive to strong colognes and perfumes, so the use of these is often regulated by hospital dress codes on units with immunocompromised patients.

Non-Pharmacologic Prescription Precautions

Some non-pharmacologic prescriptions may contribute to accident or injury, including the following:

- **Oxygen supplies**: Oxygen may be administered at the wrong level of liters (too much or too little), and the oxygen supply may be inadvertently obstructed or disconnected. Oxygen concentrators may not have backup batteries and may fail to function if electricity goes off. If people smoke around oxygen, this increases the risk of fires. Nasal cannulas and face masks that delivery oxygen, when used over prolonged periods of time, can cause pressure injuries, therefore appropriate assessment and skin care is also necessary.
- **Assistive devices**: If equipment, such as canes and walkers, are improperly fitted, they may increase risk of falls.
- **Dialysis equipment**: Contamination of equipment is always a concern and can result in peritonitis (peritoneal dialysis) and sepsis (hemodialysis). If the lines become separated, the client may exsanguinate.
- **Hot/cold compresses**: If cold compresses are placed directly on the skin, they may damage the tissue, especially if left in place for too long. Hot compresses may cause burns if temperature is too high and may damage wounds if placed directly over them.

Seizure Precautions

Seizure disorders are broadly categorized as partial seizures (which begin locally) or generalized seizures (which are bilateral and symmetrical and may be convulsive or non-convulsive):

- **Partial seizures** include *simple partial* (with motor, sensory, and/or autonomic symptoms but without impaired consciousness), *complex partial* (with cognitive, affective, psychosensory, and/or psychomotor symptoms, as well as impaired consciousness), or *partial secondarily generalized.*
- **Generalized seizures** include seizures that are bilateral and symmetric without local onset and may be convulsive or non-convulsive. These seizures include *tonic-clonic, tonic, clonic, absence* (petit mal), *atonic*, and *myoclonic seizures*, as well as *unclassified seizures*.

Seizure precautions are a standard set of safety protocol that ensure patient safety in those patients with a high risk or history of seizures. Generally, these precautions include padding the siderails, keeping the bed at the lowest position, and maintaining suctioning at the bedside. Precautions also include ensuring privacy and providing supportive care in the event of a seizure, such as easing the patient to the floor and providing padding to protect the head. Side rails should be raised and pillow removed if the patient is in bed. The patient should be placed on one side with the head flexed so the tongue does not block the airway. The patient should *not* be restrained or a padded tongue-blade inserted between the teeth. Seizure start and stop time should be noted.

PATIENT DEFICITS THAT IMPEDE CLIENT SAFETY

Certain patient deficits can inherently impede client safety, including the following:

- **Visual impairment**: Patients are at risk of trips, slips, falls, burn injuries, poisoning (mistaken containers, ingredients), and medication errors because of taking the wrong medication or wrong dosage.
- **Hearing impairment**: Patients are at increased risk of falls and may not hear danger signals, such as fire alarms, smoke detectors, police/fire sirens, and tornado warning sirens, and may, therefore, not be aware that they are in danger. Most smoke detectors emit a high-frequency alarm that cannot always be detected by those with high-frequency hearing loss.
- **Sensory/perceptual impairment**: Patients (such as those with stroke or brain injury) may exhibit a wide variety of impairments so safety concerns may vary. For example, those with one-sided neglect may have injuries to the neglected side, such as from running into doors or other things. Those with face blindness may easily get lost if away from familiar places or people.

R.A.C.E. ACRONYM FOR FIRE SAFETY

RACE is an acronym used for fire safety on the hospital unit:

- **R**escue: Remove all patients from area of danger
- **A**ctivate alarm: Pull fire alarm/call 911
- **C**onfine the fire: Close doors to unit/place
- **E**vacuate/Extinguish (NFPA/OSHA fire safety): Use **PASS** for fire extinguisher
    - **P**ull
    - **A**im at the base of the flames
    - **S**queeze the trigger
    - **S**weep: Use a sweeping motion across the flames

ERGONOMICS

Ergonomics is the study of preventing workplace injury and stress. In nursing, it refers to the way in which a nurse can prevent injury to self and others due to the stressors and strains required in the nursing field. Some important **ergonomic principles** include:

- **Body mechanics:** The body should be kept in proper alignment during tasks, with a wide base of support and center of gravity low. Use larger muscles (buttocks, thighs, shoulders) for activities rather than smaller when possible. Avoid twisting or jerking movements. Maintain 90° angle in elbows and knees when sitting, elbows at the side, with back straight and looking straight ahead.
- **Lifting:** Use appropriate transfer devices; use as many people as necessary. Manual lifting should be avoided. Bend at the knees, tighten core, and keep weights close to the body – *never* bend or twist when lifting.
- **Repetition**: Avoid repetitive movements/stressors and use proper safety equipment when needed (earplugs for loud noises, etc.).

CONTINUOUS QUALITY IMPROVEMENT

Continuous quality improvement is a multidisciplinary management philosophy that can be applied to all aspects of an organization, whether related to such varied areas as the cardiac unit, purchasing, or human resources. The skills used for epidemiologic research (data collection, analysis, outcomes, action plans) are all applicable to the analysis of multiple types of events, because they are based on solid scientific methods. Multi-disciplinary planning can bring valuable insights from various perspectives, and strategies used in one context can often be applied to another. All staff, from housekeeping to supervising, must be alert to not only problems but also opportunities for improvement. Increasingly, departments must be concerned with cost-effectiveness as the costs of medical care continue to rise, so the quality professional in the cardiovascular unit is not in an isolated position in an institution but is just one part of the whole, facing similar concerns as those in other disciplines. Disciplines are often interrelated in their functions.

NURSE'S INVOLVEMENT IN QUALITY IMPROVEMENT

The following are ways in which nurses can be involved in quality improvement in their facility:

- **Identify situations** in the nursing unit that require improvement and might benefit patient outcomes (cost containment, incident reporting, etc.) if changed.
- **Identify potential items** that can be measured to be able to test the problem or to be able to monitor patient outcomes.
- **Collect data** on those measurements and determine current patient outcomes.
- **Analyze the data** and identify procedures, methods, etc., that can be utilized to potentially make positive changes in patient outcomes, doing research if necessary.
- **Make recommendations for changes** to be implemented to determine the effect on patient outcomes.
- **Implement recommendations** after approval from administrative personnel.
- **Collect data** using the same measurements and determine if the changes improved patient outcomes or not.

RISK MANAGEMENT

Risk management attempts to prevent harm and legal liability by being proactive and by identifying a patient's **risk factors**. The patient is educated about these factors and ways that they can modify their behavior to decrease their risk. Treatments and interventions must be considered in terms of risk to the patient, and the patient must always know these risks in order to make healthcare decisions. Much can be done to avoid mistakes that put patients at risk. Patients should note medications and other aspects of their care so that they can help prevent mistakes. They should feel free to question care and to have their concerns heard and addressed. When mistakes are made, the actions taken to remedy the situation are very important. The physician should be made aware of the error immediately, and the patient notified according to hospital policy. Errors must be evaluated to determine how the process failed. Honesty and caring can help mitigate many errors.

NURSING MALPRACTICE, NEGLIGENCE, UNINTENTIONAL TORTS, AND INTENTIONAL TORTS

- **Malpractice** is unethical or improper actions or lack of proper action by the nurse that may or may not be related to a lack of skills that nurses should possess.
- **Negligence** is the failure to act as any other diligent nurse would have acted in the same situation.

- Negligence can lead to an **unintentional tort**. In this case, the patient must prove that the nurse had a duty to act, a duty proven via standards of care, and that the nurse failed in this duty and harm occurred to the patient as a result of this failure.
- **Intentional torts** differ in that the duty is assumed and the nurse breached this duty via assault and battery, invasion of privacy, slander, or false imprisonment of the patient.

Review Video: Medical Negligence
Visit mometrix.com/academy and enter code: 928405

Security and Disaster Plans

Disaster

A disaster is an event where many people are exposed to hazards that result in injury, death, and damage to property. There are a number of hazards that have the potential to lead to a disaster situation. In general, they can be **classified** as natural, technological, or caused by human conflict. Some specific examples of each are as follows:

- **Natural**: Firestorms, flood, land shift, tornado, epidemic, earthquake, volcano, hurricane, high winds, blizzard, heat wave
- **Technological**: Hazmat spills, explosions, utility failure, building collapse, transportation accident, power outage, nuclear accident, dam failure, fire, water loss, ruptured gas main
- **Human conflict**: Riots, strikes, suicide bombings, bomb threat, employee violence, mass shootings, equipment sabotage, hostage events, transportation disruption, weapons of mass destruction, computer viruses/worms

Disaster Management Plan

Development

There are many different types of disaster management plans. Regardless of the type, there are several basic steps for its **development**. To begin with, a **planning team** must be established that includes representatives from all levels within the organization. The planning team is responsible for creating a timeline for completion of the plan as well as an estimation of the costs, fees, and resources necessary to complete the plan. Once this is done, an **analysis of potential disasters** can begin. In this step, potential hazards are identified and vulnerability of the organization to disasters is assessed. A **disaster response plan** is established that includes the reduction/removal of hazardous situations. The final steps are **plan implementation and review**. The plan can be tested for efficacy through drills and mock disaster situations. It is critical to review and update the plan yearly.

Types

There are several different **types of disaster management plans**, some more specific than others. They are listed and briefly described below:

- **Emergency action plan**: OSHA required, evacuation plans and emergency drills
- **Business continuity plan**: Business operation-specific, aimed at reducing losses and resuming productivity
- **Risk management plan**: Off-site effects of chemical exposures
- **Emergency response plan**: Immediate response to disasters
- **Contingency plan**: General, designed to handle events not covered in other plans
- **Federal response plan**: Coordinates federal resources
- **Spill prevention, control, and countermeasures plan**: Deals with the prevention, control, and clean-up of oil spills
- **Mutual aid plan**: Plan for shared resources between other companies/firms
- **Recovery plan**: Deals with repair and rebuilding post-disaster
- **Emergency management plan**: Plan for healthcare facilities
- **All-hazard disaster management plan**: General plan that is not hazard-specific

Emergency Response Plans

Emergency response plans must include plans for communication, resources and assets available, safety and security measures, responsibilities of staff, utilities, and measure to support clinical activities.

Bomb Threats

The response to a **bomb threat** depends on the type of bomb threat and the information gleaned from the threat. The first response is to notify the police and designated staff via landlines (avoiding cell phones, which can trigger some devices) or overhead paging. An initial search may be carried out by staff in each area to try to locate possible bombs. Administration should make the decision about evacuation, and plans for evacuation should be in place. With terrorist bombing and improvised explosive devices (IEDs), situational awareness is critical because multiple explosive devices (some undetonated) may be at the scene. IEDs may be inside backpacks, suitcases, and packages left unattended. Additionally, people wearing suicide vests or belts may mix in with other victims or people escaping the blast area.

Active Shooters

Medical facilities can be targets of active shooters given their accessibility to a large number of people combined with the possibility of trauma experienced within a medical facility that may motivate a shooter. Every medical facility, particularly hospitals, must have a plan for responding to an active shooter due to the amount of damage that may be done in the small amount of time before local law enforcement can respond to the distress call. Plans should begin with education to all employees of the facility, often using the Run (evacuate the space, helping others if possible), Hide (if unable to evacuate, find a spot to hide that is out of view and ideally can be locked or blocked), Fight (if unable to evacuate or hide, take action against the shooter) method. The Department of Homeland Security also recommends the formation of an Emergency Action Plan (EAP) for active shooters, which include the preferred method(s) for reporting a shooter to authorities, evacuation plans, training, and prevention/monitoring measures.

Natural Disasters

Plans vary according to type of **natural disaster**. If anticipated, extra food, clothing, and supplies should be stockpiled for both clients and staff (who may be required to stay at the facility for extended periods). A command structure should be in place. With a hurricane or tornado, clients may need to be moved away from windows and to more secure areas, such as interior hallways, during the storm. The hospital must prepare plans to evacuate clients if necessary (such as with flooding, earthquakes, or storm damage) and transfer them to other facilities and must also be prepared for an influx of clients.

Community Planning

Healthcare providers, such as hospitals, should work closely with the community to identify community resources that are available for emergency response and the needs that may arise in response to disasters, including the number of people who may depend on the hospital for care.

Review Video: Emergency Response, Business Continuity, and Disaster Planning
Visit mometrix.com/academy and enter code: 678024

ICS

The **Incident Command System** (ICS) was developed by the Department of Homeland Security as a part of the **National Incident Management System**. It is a highly organized, hierarchical disaster management system that focuses on planning and organization, communication and delegation of responsibility, as well as response evaluation so that any disaster or emergency response effort runs as smoothly as possible. An **Incident Commander (IC)** is established as the person in charge. Safety officers, operations section officers, planning officers, and logistics officers are all appointed. These different officer positions are responsible for reporting back to the IC.

Multiple-Casualty Incidents Versus Mass-Casualty Incidents

Multiple-casualty incidents involve more than one person, but different jurisdictions may quantify the total number of persons differently. It usually refers to the following:

- An incident involving at least three patients
- An incident involving only one jurisdiction and only one to three agencies (ambulance, fire department, and police)
- An incident requiring triage, but generally only primary triage
- Standards of care are maintained, and all patients not coded black (deceased) are transported for care

Mass-casualty incidents also involve more than one person, but may involve much larger numbers—dozens, if not hundreds to thousands.

- Often involves multiple jurisdictions and agencies
- Requires triage but may also involve separate waiting areas for color-coded individuals and secondary triage
- Standards of care may be modified, and patients coded black (expectant) and not expected to live may be left in the field and/or receive delayed care if they are still living after the red- and yellow-coded individuals are transported

Principles of Triage During Mass Casualty Events

Primary triage is a rapid method (30-60 seconds) of prioritizing clients based on severity of condition and carried out at the scene of multiple casualty incidents. All clients are triaged and tagged according to international color-coding priority (P) guidelines on foot or wrist (not clothing):

- **P1—Red**: Immediate care needed for urgent systemic life-threatening conditions, such as airway/breathing problems, severe bleeding, severe burns (especially with breathing problems), decreased mental status, shock, and severe medical problems, Glasgow Coma Score ≤13.
- **P2—Yellow**: Delayed care and able to wait 45-60 minutes for treatment. Conditions include burns (without breathing problems), multiple bone/joint injuries, back and/or spinal cord injuries (unless in respiratory distress).
- **P3—Green**: Hold, able to wait hours for treatment of minor injuries.
- **P4—Black**: Deceased or with injuries so extensive that they are not survivable.

Resource management involves identifying a triage officer, who remains at the scene during the event, and identifying the need for additional personnel and equipment and providing those to the clients with the highest priority.

Identifying Clients to Discharge in Disaster Situations

In the event of a **disaster situation**, the surge capacity of a hospital may need to increase markedly with a large influx of clients in need of emergency care and hospitalization, so appropriate clients must be quickly identified for possible discharge. All elective admissions and procedures should be cancelled and non-critical clients, such as those with non-life-threatening conditions or those near discharge, should be discharged or transferred to other facilities if possible. Generally, hospitalists, charge nurses, or team leaders may be in the best position to identify clients for discharge as well as the person tasked with monitoring length of stay. If an acuity-based model of client care is utilized, then those already categorized as the least acute should be quickly assessed for discharge. Ideally, each unit should have plans in place for rapid discharge so that assessment and discharge can be carried out quickly and safely.

Terrorism

Terrorism is defined as the use of violence (or threat of violence) to frighten and coerce governments or societies into accepting the instigator's (terrorists) **demands**. The demands and goals of terrorists are often extreme and focused on areas with high population densities. This means that large companies can become potential targets of a terrorist attack. For this reason, when developing an emergency preparedness/disaster management plan, terrorist attacks should be included as a potential disaster. There are many different possible ways that terrorists can strike. Some examples are weapons of mass destruction, biological agents (i.e., bacteria, viruses, or toxins), nuclear and radiological incidents, incendiary devices, chemicals, and explosive devices.

Organizational Plan for Bioterrorism

The ICP and the infection control team should develop specific plans for dealing with different **bioterrorism** agents, and training should be provided to staff. An organized approach should include the following:

- Be on the alert for possible bioterrorism-related infections, based on clusters of patients or symptoms.
- Use personal protection equipment, including respirators when indicated.
- Complete thorough assessment of patient, including medical history, physical examination, immunization record, and travel history.
- Provide a probable diagnosis based on symptoms and lab findings, including cultures.
- Provide treatment, including prophylaxis, while waiting for laboratory findings.
- Use transmission precautions as well as isolation for suspected biologic agents.
- Notify local, state, and federal authorities per established protocol.
- Conduct surveillance and epidemiological studies to identify at-risk populations.
- Develop plans to accommodate large numbers of patients:
    - Restricting elective admissions
    - Transferring patients to other facilities

B-NICE Hazardous Material Incidents Associated with Terrorist Attacks

Category	Response
B—Biological (bacteria, viruses, fungi, toxins)	Inhalation type—evacuate for 80 feet, shut down air-handling systems, wear appropriate PPE and SCBA, and avoid contamination. Visible agent—decontaminate with soap and water. Symptoms may vary but are usually delayed.
N—Nuclear/ Radiological	Inhalation type (most common)—Isolate/Secure the area, avoid smoke/fumes, stay upwind, and use PPE and SCBA. Isolate victims and decontaminate as appropriate. Symptoms are usually delayed.
I—Incendiary	Be on alert for multiple devices and sabotaged fire suppression equipment. Symptoms include burns, pain, and trauma.
C—Chemical	Isolate/Secure the area, decontaminate victims with soap and water, and be on alert for chemical dispersal devices. Approach toward uphill and upwind. Isolate symptomatic patients from others. Symptoms vary but may include burns, blistering, vomiting, breathing difficulty, and neurological damage.
E—Explosives	Be alert for secondary devices, undetonated devices, and secondary hazards (unstable buildings and debris). Remove victims from the area, secure the perimeter, and stage away from the incident area. Decontaminate as necessary. Symptoms include burns, amputations, cuts, and penetrating and blunt trauma.

All-Hazards Safety Approach to Mass-Casualty Incidents

The all-hazards safety approach to mass-casualty incidents aims to provide plans that can be used to deal with all types of hazards (natural disasters, terrorist attacks, and mass-casualty incidents) as well as encompassing the four components of emergency management: mitigation, preparedness, response, and recovery. Organizations in an area coordinate to develop joint action plans that can be activated in response to incidents, with the chain of command clearly outlined. This approach lowers costs to individual organizations and provides for faster and more effective response. However, although the basic structure may be the same for responding to all hazards, there are inevitable differences between (for example) a terrorist attack with active shooters and a natural disaster, such as a hurricane, which can be anticipated and mitigated to some degree. For this reason, modifying existing incident action plans to meet the needs of a situation is essential.

Disaster Recovery Aspect of Disaster Planning and Management

Disaster recovery is the final stage of any disaster response and deals with the actions necessary to return the disaster site to normal. The recovery effort can be divided into **two different periods**:

- The **restoration period** is an immediate recovery step in which the area is made safe, utilities repaired, wreckage removed, and evacuees are allowed to return.
- The **reconstruction/replacement period** is a longer process where the disaster area is rebuilt and returned to its pre-disaster condition, both physically and economically. The reconstruction period can take many years, and is dependent on the degree of damage and availability of resources for reconstruction efforts.

As a part of the disaster recovery process, steps should be taken to prevent a recurrence of the disaster in the future.

Security Plan

A security plan is a plan that is set in place to help guide the actions of employees in case of a breach in security at a healthcare facility. All employees must be educated and comfortable with their facilities plan, in order to facilitate the safety of staff and patients alike. The security plan usually has several components:

- **Security workers**: Most facilities have securities guards who patrol the campus and help maintain patient and visitor safety. If a patient/visitor threatens violence or becomes combative, security should be called immediately.
- **Silent alarms**: Most units have "silent alarms," which are usually buttons or switches underneath the secretary's desk or in some other discreet location. These are pushed in the case of a threat to security in which a call cannot safely be made.
- **Locked units**: Certain units in the hospital (such as mother/baby, critical care units, psychiatric floors, etc.) are locked and require an access code to enter.
- **Do not acknowledge**: Certain patients may be deemed as "do not acknowledge," meaning that the nurse cannot give out any information regarding these patients, including acknowledging the patients' presence in the facility. Examples include psychiatric patients, victims of crime, celebrities, and others. If someone calls asking about the patient, it is appropriate and ethical for the nurse to state, "I do not have any information regarding a patient with that name."
- **Overhead announcements**: Many facilities have different codes that they may call overhead to alert staff of emergences/safety threats without overt language.
- **Newborn nursery security**: Measures include matching ID bands for infant and parents/caregivers, foot-printing and photographing the infant after birth, transporting infants in bassinets rather than carrying them, utilizing a tracking and security alarm system that can trigger automatic lockdown, limiting access to obstetrics and nursery areas, having staff wear easily-identifiable ID badges, and utilizing video surveillance.
- **Violence prevention**: Measures include educating staff about de-escalation techniques, having an alarm system in place, providing adequate security, utilizing video surveillance, limiting access, identifying clients who may be at risk for behaving violently, and requiring visitors' badges.
- **Controlled access**: Measures include locked areas that require a password, biologic ID (fingerprint, eye scan), access card for entry, turnstiles at entry and/or metal detectors, security personal stationed at entry points, and video surveillance of entries, exits, stairwells, hallways, elevators, and storage areas.

Principles of Evacuation in a Security Plan

Principles of evacuation in a security plan, according to OSHA, should include:

- Conditions that would trigger an evacuation
- Chain of command for decision making
- Procedures for evacuation, including methods of evacuation and preferred routes. Exits should be clearly identified
- Procedures for assisting clients who are disabled and those who do not speak English
- Procedures for determining who are responsible for terminating critical operations
- Procedures for tracking personnel and clients
- Transportation plans for transferal of clients to other facilities

The path of least resistance is an important concept to understand for evacuation, especially if they involve fire and any products of combustion (smoke, heat, gas). Fire's path of least resistance is usually vertical, although fire also spreads horizontally, especially if a vertical path is not available. Water, on the other hand, also flows vertically, but downward and then horizontally if the downward flow is blocked. Clients should be evacuated according to the path of least resistance; that is, the route that is the easiest and safest.

INFECTIONS WITH BIOLOGICAL WEAPONS

ANTHRAX

A number of different infections could be part of a bioterrorism attack. The type of barrier/isolation needed is dependent upon the symptoms and the mode of transmission. Knowledge of typical presenting symptoms and prompt precautions are essential to prevent spread of disease. **Anthrax (Bacillus anthracis)** usually occurs from contact with animals, but as a bioterrorism weapon, anthrax would most likely be aerosolized and inhaled. It is not transferred from person to person. There are 3 types:

- **Inhalation**: Fever, cough, shortness of breath, and general debility
- **Cutaneous**: Small non-painful sores that blister and ulcerate with necrosis at the center
- **Gastrointestinal**: Nausea, vomiting, diarrhea, and abdominal pain

The inhaled form of anthrax is the most severe with about a 50% mortality rate. The vaccine for anthrax is not yet available to the public.

Precautions are as follows:

- Prophylaxis with antibiotics after exposure
- Standard precautions
- Contact precautions for wounds if there are cutaneous lesions

PNEUMONIC PLAGUE

Yersinia pestis causes **pneumonic plague**, which is normally carried by fleas from infected rats but can be aerosolized to use as a biologic weapon. There are 3 forms of plague, but they sometimes occur together and bubonic and septicemic plague can develop into pneumonic, which is the primary concern related to bioterrorism:

- **Bubonic** occurs when a person is bitten by an infected flea.
- **Pneumonic** occurs with inhalation and results in pneumonia with fever, headache, cough, and progressive respiratory failure.
- **Septicemic** occurs when *Y. pestis* invades the bloodstream, often after initial bubonic or pneumonic plague.

Pneumonic plague can spread easily from person to person. There is no vaccine available. Precautions include the following:

- Immediate antibiotics within first 24 hours are necessary, so early diagnosis is critical.
- Prophylaxis with antibiotics may protect those exposed.
- Droplet precautions should be used with appropriate barriers, such as surgical mask.

Botulism

Clostridium botulinum produces an extremely poisonous toxin that causes botulism. The organism can be aerosolized or used to infect food. There are 3 primary forms of botulisms:

- **Foodborne botulism** results from contamination of food. This type poses the greatest threat from bioterrorism. Symptoms usually appear 12-36 hours after ingestion but may be delayed for 2 weeks, and include nausea, vomiting, dyspnea, dysphagia, slurred speech, progressive weakness, and paralysis.
- **Infant botulism** results from *C. botulinum* ingested into the intestinal tract. Constipation, poor feeding, and progressive weakness are presenting symptoms.
- **Wound botulism** results from contamination of open skin, but symptoms are similar to foodborne botulism.

Botulism is not transmitted from person to person, but contaminated food has the potential to infect many people, especially if the contaminated food is manufactured and widely distributed.

Precautions include the following:

- Antitoxin after exposure and as early in disease as possible
- Standard precautions
- Do not feed honey to infants, as there is a risk of spore ingestion

Tularemia

Francisella tularensis causes tularemia, which is usually transmitted from small mammals to humans through insect bites, ingestion of contaminated food or water, inhalation, or handling of infected animals. Although there is no evidence of person-to-person transmission, *F. tularensis* has the potential to be aerosolized for use in bioterrorism because it is highly infective and requires only about 10 organisms to infect. Flu-like symptoms appear in 3-5 days after exposure and progress to severe respiratory infection and pneumonia. A vaccine for laboratory workers was available until recently, but the FDA is currently reviewing it, and it is unavailable in the United States.

- Prophylaxis with antibiotics within 24 hours may prevent disease.
- Standard precautions are sufficient.
- Biologic safety measures should be used for laboratory specimens.
- Autopsy procedures that may cause tissue to be aerosolized should be avoided.

Smallpox

The variola virus causes **smallpox**, which has been eradicated worldwide since 1980, but has the potential for use as a biological weapon because people are no longer vaccinated. Smallpox is extremely contagious and has a high mortality rate (about 30%). Flu-like symptoms appear about 7-17 days after exposure with fever, weakness, vomiting, and rash that begins on the face and arms and spreads. The rash becomes pustular, crusts, scabs over, and then sloughs off, leaving scars. People remain infective from the first rash until all scabs are gone. The disease can spread through contact with infective fluid from lesions or from contact with clothes or bedding. Aerosol spread is theoretically possible. Precautions are as follows:

- Vaccination must be done before symptoms appear and as soon as possible after exposure as vaccination after rash appears will not affect the severity of the disease; vaccination is done by scratching the skin with a small needle on the upper arm, leaving a characteristic pox scar.
- Contact precautions should be used, which includes the use of gowns and gloves to enter the room and keeping the patient in a private or cohorted room.

Viral Hemorrhagic Fevers

Viral hemorrhagic fevers are zoonoses (spread from animals to humans) and comprise a number of different diseases: Ebola, Lassa, Marburg, yellow, Argentine and Crimean-Congo. Some hemorrhagic fevers can spread person to person, notably Ebola, Marburg, and Lassa, through close contact with body fluids or contaminated items. Hemorrhagic fevers are extremely contagious multi-system diseases, and those in contact with infected patients are at risk of infection. Symptoms vary somewhat according to the disease but present with flu-like symptoms that progress to bleeding under the skin and internally, and some people develop kidney failure and central nervous system symptoms, such as coma and seizures. Treatment is supportive and mortality rates are high. Only yellow fever and Argentine have vaccines.

Precautions are as follows:

- **Maximum precautions** must be used with full barrier precautions, with care used in any handling of blood and body fluids or wastes.
- **Screening**: ask patient if they have been out of the country in the last 3-6 months.

Pandemic Management

Since the COVID-19 pandemic and its subsequent overwhelming burden on health care workers and health care systems, pandemic-management has become paramount as a component of disaster management. Pandemic management must consider the healthcare facility's capacity to manage a surge of patients in terms of available staffing, equipment, and beds. Each facility must also have a plan prepared to prioritize the care of critical patients over those scheduled for elective procedures, and healthcare workers may be deployed from their usual unit or specialty to assist in the management of critical patients.

Containment and prevention measures must also be in place in the case of a pandemic. Containment includes efforts to screen and identify infected individuals so that they can be appropriately quarantined and staff can be appropriately protected with PPE. Prevention measures include vaccination efforts, masking, and education on hand hygiene and quarantine protocols. Containment and prevention measures must also be carried out on the national and international level to include the tracking of outbreaks and recommended travel bans to prevent the spread of disease.

Health Promotion: Nursing Throughout the Lifespan

Health Promotion and Disease Prevention

Health Promotion

Nurses promote health when they assist individuals to change behavior in ways that help them to attain and maintain the highest level of wellbeing possible. Health promotion is a very popular way to control healthcare costs and reduce illness and early death. Health is increasingly the topic of newscasts and literature. The public is demanding more information pertinent to the maintenance of health and to the ways in which the average person can act independently to do so. Health promotion is centered on ideal personal habits, lifestyles, and environmental control that decrease the risk for disease. The US Public Health Service periodically identifies national health goals and most recently published a program called ***Healthy People 2030***, with measurable goals to increase the general quality and years of life for all and to increase the health status of all groups to an equal level of wellness. Health promotion programs in the community are now offered by workplaces, clinics, schools, and churches, not just by hospitals as in the past.

Healthy People 2030

The 5 **main goals** of *Healthy People 2030* are

- Attaining healthy, thriving lives free of preventable disease, disability, injury, and premature death
- Eliminating health disparities, achieving health equality, and increasing health literacy
- Creating environments conducive to health-promotion
- Improving health in all life stages
- Collaborating with leadership and key stakeholders in policy design that improves the health and well-being of all

Healthy People 2030 has 62 topic areas with 355 total objectives divided across five sections:

- Health Conditions
- Health Behaviors
- Populations
- Settings and Systems
- Social Determinants of Health

Main Components of Health Promotion

Health promotion efforts are concentrated in four areas:

- Individuals must be educated to realize that their **lifestyle and choices** have a large impact on their health. They must then be motivated to choose to modify their personal risk factors and take the responsibility to do so.
- The emphasis on **good nutrition** as the biggest factor that impacts health and the length of life must be brought into general awareness. This is occurring via the media through numerous books and articles educating people about the essential nutrients needed to maintain health.
- **Stress** is a constant in a production-driven society. Individuals must learn ways to manage and decrease stress to achieve and maintain health and to decrease the effects of stress upon chronic illness, risk of infections, and trauma.
- **Physical fitness** helps cardiovascular status, relieves stress, controls weight, delays aging, promotes strength and endurance, and improves appearance and performance. Individuals must have programs that increase activity gradually to prevent injury and are designed to meet individual needs.

Health Self-Management

Health self-management includes health maintenance, disease prevention, and health promotion. Health maintenance is defined as strategies that help maintain and/or improve health over time. Health maintenance is dependent on three factors, which include health perception, motivation for behavioral change, and compliance to set goals. Disease prevention is an effort to limit the development or progression of lifestyle-related illness. **Disease prevention** can be categorized into primary, secondary, and tertiary prevention.

- **Primary prevention** measures are employed prior to disease onset and are used in health populations.
- **Secondary prevention** measures are used to screen, detect, and treat disease in earlier stages to prevent further progression or development of other complications.
- **Tertiary prevention** measures are used to prevent the worsening of a disease and the onset of other complications or comorbid conditions secondary to that disease.

Health promotion strategies include risk reduction strategies applied to the general population.

Influences on Decision to Modify Behavior to Achieve and Maintain Health

Many factors have an influence on people's efforts to change behavior in a way that improves and maintains their health status. These factors include age, ethnicity, gender, lifestyle, level of education, self-esteem, motivation, and self-image. The patient's support network and the availability of health promotion programs and healthcare systems also have an influence on healthcare behaviors. Some people may be prevented from accessing health promotion programs because of lack of medical insurance. Financial status and employment are important as well. The presence of addictions and diseases, the length of illness, and the severity of disabilities are all factors to be considered. The value placed on health, the threat of potential losses, and the perceived benefits of behavior modification are important motivating factors.

Strategies to Encourage Smoking Cessation

The **health impact associated with smoking** varies among smokers and can be affected by the number of cigarettes used daily, exposure to smoking-associated stimuli, and educational level. The presence of stress and depression, psychosocial problems, lack of coping mechanisms, low income, and long-term habitual behavior are problematic for the quitter. Nurses can promote smoking cessation by taking every opportunity to bring up the subject, educating about the dangers of smoking and benefits of quitting, and providing **resources** to help patients quit. Strategies include:

- Educating about the personal effects of smoking upon that individual
- Encouraging patients to set a quit date
- Referring to programs and smoking cessation information
- Educating about the use of nicotine replacements including nicotine gum, lozenges, inhalers, transdermal patches, and nasal sprays
- Educating about the use of medications such as Zyban, Catapres, and Chantix
- Providing support via phone calls or office visits
- Discovering the reason for relapses
- Praising and rewarding any success in the quitting process

Healthy Nutrition Principles

Healthy nutrition principles include the following:

- Eating a range of different kinds of foods, and eating increased amounts fruits, vegetables, whole grains, poultry, and fish.
- Diets should consist of 55–60% **carbohydrates**, less than 30% **fat**, and the rest should be **protein** (0.8–1.0 g/kg).
- Restrict **saturated fat** to <10%. Restrict **cholesterol** to 300 mg/day.
- Utilize moderate amounts of sugar, salt, and sodium.
- Take a **multivitamin** including folic acid if the patient is female and able to have children. Get 200–800 IU/day of vitamin D in order to absorb calcium.
- **Calcium** intake should be: 1,300 mg/day for women age 13–18 or those who are pregnant/nursing; 1,000 mg/day for women age 19–50 years; 1,500 mg/day for age 51 years and older.
- **Weight loss** may improve diabetes, joint pain, inflammation, cardiovascular disease, hypothyroidism, or renal disease.

Young Adult Health Screenings

Health screening is encouraged for conditions that are very likely to occur and diseases that are likely to kill if they are not identified early. The assessment should be supported by evidence using standardized techniques and proper follow-up.

Young adult (ages 20-39 years) screenings, according to the US Preventive Services Task Force (USPSTF), should include:

- A full head-to-toe physical (every 5-6 years)
- Routine blood pressure screening
- Cholesterol screening (every 5 years; more frequently when total cholesterol is higher than 200 mg/dL)
- PPD test for tuberculosis when patient has had known contact with TB or is at increased risk (health care workers, prisoners, homeless, or immunocompromised)
- Dental check-up (annually)
- Thyroid palpation (every 3 years)
- Depression screening (at every visit)
- Men perform self-testicular exam every month
- Women conduct a self-breast exam every month; should receive a clinical breast exam every 3 years
- Pap smear and pelvic assessments every 3 years (or up to 5 years in conjunction with HPV testing)
- Screening for gonorrhea and chlamydia for all sexually active individuals
- Health education and promotion (every time patient is seen)
- Influenza vaccination (annually)
- Td immunization every 10 years

Adult Screenings

Adults (age 40 and older) screenings, according to the USPSTF, should maintain the same schedule as young adults (unless indicated below) in addition to the following:

- A full head-to-toe physical (annually)
- Blood pressure screening (annually)
- ECG (over 40, annually; only when there are cardiac risks)
- Clinical breast exam (annually in women over 40)
- Mammogram (biennially in women over 40)
- General colorectal cancer screening for risks (annually), and colorectal cancer screening via colonoscopy (every 10 years starting at age 45 until age 75)
- Prostate-specific antigen screening (men over 50 with average risk, or younger if higher risk; upon the patient's informed request only)

Disease Prevention for the Elderly

Although life spans are longer, **ongoing (chronic) diseases** are still the primary reason patients die. Elderly patients have more of an absolute chance of getting a disease, but they also react well to prevention. Keep good records of the elderly patient's history, including updating every year and following advice for patients over the age of 65 years. Evaluate nutrition, functional ability, alcoholic beverage intake (more than 2 alcoholic beverages a day constitutes abuse), smoking, illegal drugs, misuse of prescriptions, and exercise level.

- **Preventative measures** include a physical, screening assessments, and immunizations.
- Some **routine screenings** include: fasting glucose, papanicolaou smear, dipstick urinalysis, mammography, PPD, fecal occult blood/sigmoidoscopy, electrocardiogram, thyroid function, glaucoma and sight, hearing, and cholesterol.
- **Immunizations** include yearly flu shot, pneumococcal vaccine, and tetanus; respiratory syncytial virus (RSV) vaccination at age 75.

The following screens are controversial: depression for someone with no symptoms, dementia for someone with no symptoms, osteoporosis including bone densitometry for postmenopausal females (counsel females regarding hormone prophylaxis), colon and prostate cancer, and cholesterol for someone with no symptoms.

Client Education

Bandura's Theory of Social Learning

In the 1970s, Bandura proposed the theory of social learning, in which he posited that learning develops from observing, organizing, and rehearsing behavior that has been modeled. Bandura believed that people are more likely to adopt the behavior if they value the outcomes, if the outcomes have functional value, and if the person modeling the behavior is similar to the learner and is admired because of status. Behavior is the result of observation of behavioral, environmental, and cognitive interactions. There are **four conditions** required for modeling:

- **Attention**: The degree of attention paid to modeling can depend on many variables (physical, social, and environmental).
- **Retention**: People's ability to retain models depends on symbolic coding, creating mental images, organizing thoughts, and rehearsing (mentally or physically).
- **Reproduction**: The ability to reproduce a model depends on physical and mental capabilities.
- **Motivation**: Motivation may derive from past performances, rewards, or vicarious modeling.

Transtheoretical Model of Change

The transtheoretical model of change puts forth concepts applicable to the process of educating patients and their family members. The **stages** of the transtheoretical model of change include the following:

- The first stage is **precontemplation**. At this point, the patient is not aware of any need for a change in the health behavior.
- In the next stage, **contemplation**, the patient begins to realize why the change may be necessary after recognizing that the health behavior in question is unhealthy and weighing the consequences of continuing this behavior.
- During the stage of **preparation**, the patient imagines making the change at a future time and starts to formulate a plan to do so.
- The **action** stage occurs when the patient makes specific modifications in health behavior and begins to note the resulting positive changes.
- During the **maintenance** stage, the patient is able to implement the change over time by utilizing strategies to prevent a return to previously unhealthy behaviors.
- **Termination** is the stage at which a patient has incorporated the changed behavior into daily functioning, and the patient will not resume the previous unhealthy behavior.

Kurt Lewin

Force Field Analysis

Force field analysis was designed by Kurt Lewin, a social psychologist, to analyze both the driving forces and the restraining forces for change:

- **Driving forces** instigate and promote change, such as leaders, incentives, and competition.
- **Restraining forces** resist change, such as poor attitudes, hostility, inadequate equipment, or insufficient funds.

The educator can use this force field analysis diagram to discuss variables related to a proposed change in process:

- Write the proposed change in the center column.
- Brainstorm and list driving forces and opposed restraining forces. Score the forces. (When driving and restraining forces are in balance, this is a state of equilibrium or the status quo.)
- Discuss the value of the proposed change.
- Develop a plan to diminish or eliminate restraining forces.

Lewin's Model of Change Theory

Lewin's model of change theory may be used to help some patients make decisions for change. Patients can be educated about the need for change and can be assisted with making alterations in behavior or thoughts in order to better facilitate change; however, only the patient can truly implement the change permanently. Lewin's concept of change theory involves a three-part process:

- **Unfreezing** is the part of the model in which the patient becomes open to change, sees a need for it, and removes the boundaries inhibiting change.
- The patient then makes the **actual change** according to expected outcomes and goals.
- Finally, **refreezing** is the process of maintaining the change so that it becomes a habit, and one that the patient is likely to uphold for a long period of time.

Lewin's theory also involves either driving forces or restraining forces. Driving forces are those outside measures that support the change, while restraining forces inhibit success in implementing the change.

Principles of Adult Learning

Adults have a wealth of life and/or employment experiences. Their attitudes toward education may vary considerably. There are, however, some **principles of adult learning** and typical characteristics of adult learners that an instructor should consider when planning strategies for teaching parents, families, or staff.

- Practical and goal-oriented:
  - Provide overviews or summaries and examples.
  - Use collaborative discussions with problem-solving exercises.
  - Remain organized with the goal in mind.
- Self-directed:
  - Provide active involvement, asking for input.
  - Allow different options toward achieving the goal.
  - Give them responsibilities.
- Knowledgeable:
  - Show respect for their life experiences/education.
  - Validate their knowledge and ask for feedback.
  - Relate new material to information with which they are familiar.

- Relevancy-oriented:
  - Explain how information will be applied.
  - Clearly identify objectives.
- Motivated:
  - Provide certificates of professional advancement and/or continuing education credit for staff when possible.

Review Video: Adult Learning Processes and Theories
Visit mometrix.com/academy and enter code: 638453

Learning Styles

Every individual learns differently, some better through listening and talking, others through seeing, and others through interacting. More commonly, learners are most enriched when a combination of teaching styles are utilized to ensure maximum retention across all learning types. A range of teaching materials and methods that relate to all three major learning preferences (visual, auditory, and kinesthetic) and that are appropriate for different ages should be available. Below are various methods through which education can be provided to ensure it is accessible to diverse learning preferences.

- Provide written directions or picture guides, or demonstrate procedures.
- Use charts and diagrams, and provide photos/videos when useful.
- Explain procedures while demonstrating them.
- Plan extra time to discuss and answer questions when possible.
- Provide audio recordings when relevant to the education being provided.
- Provide hands-on experience throughout teaching.
- Encourage handling of supplies and equipment when educating specific skills.
- Allow the learner to demonstrate/practice the skill.

Approaches to Teaching

There are many approaches to teaching, and the educator must prepare, present, and coordinate a wide range of educational workshops, lectures, discussions, and one-on-one instructions on any chosen topic. All types of classes will be needed, depending upon the purpose and material:

- **Educational workshops** are usually conducted with small groups, allowing for maximal participation. They are especially good for demonstrations and practice sessions.
- **Lectures** are often used for more academic or detailed information that may include questions and answers but limits discussion. An effective lecture should include some audiovisual support.
- **Discussions** are best with small groups so that people can actively participate. This is a good method for problem solving.
- **One-on-one instruction** is especially helpful for targeted instruction in procedures for individuals.
- **Online learning modules** are good for independent learners.

Participants should be asked to evaluate the presentations in the forms of surveys or suggestions, but ultimately the program is evaluated in terms of patient outcomes.

Readiness to Learn

The patient/family's readiness to learn should be assessed because if they are not ready, instruction is of little value. Often, readiness is indicated when the patient/family asks questions or shows an interest in procedures. There are a number of factors related to readiness to learn:

- **Physical factors:** There are a number of physical factors that can affect ability. Manual dexterity may be required to complete a task, and this varies by age and condition. Hearing or vision deficits may impact a person's ability to learn. Complex tasks may be too difficult for some because of weakness or cognitive impairment, and modifications of the environment may be needed. Health status, age, and gender may all impact the ability to learn.
- **Experience:** People's experience with learning can vary widely and is affected by their ability to cope with changes, their personal goals, motivation to learn, and cultural background. People may have widely divergent ideas about what constitutes illness and/or treatment. Lack of English skills may make learning difficult and prevent people from asking questions.
- **Mental/emotional status:** The external support system and internal motivation may impact readiness. Anxiety, fear, or depression about one's condition can make learning very difficult because the patient/family cannot focus on learning, so the nurse must spend time to reassure the patient/family and wait until they are emotionally more receptive.
- **Knowledge/education:** The knowledge base of the patient/family, their cognitive ability, and their learning styles all affect their readiness to learn. The nurse should always begin by assessing what knowledge the patient/family already has about their disease, condition, or treatment and then build from that base. People with little medical experience may lack knowledge of basic medical terminology, interfering with their ability and readiness to learn.

Teaching Elderly Patients

The elderly patient's level of functioning must be assessed before teaching. Cognitive abilities and mental functioning may be affected by illness and aging:

- Short-term memory loss can affect the amount of material retained.
- Concentration may be decreased.
- Reaction time is delayed.
- Color discrimination, general vision, and hearing may be decreased.

The nurse should **pace** the teaching accordingly and **tailor** materials for any deficits. Family should be present for teaching if possible, to help the patient to remember key points after discharge. Large print on non-glare paper that is easy to read should be used. The nurse should use color-coding cues only if colors are easily perceived. The learning environment must be quiet and comfortable with no distractions or interruptions.

- Repeat information numerous times and allow the patient as much practice time as needed.
- Use audio-visual aids to reinforce information given verbally.
- Face the patient when speaking and encourage him/her to use hearing devices if used.
- Make sure the lighting in the room is adequate.

Teaching Patients with Learning Disabilities

Determine the type of learning disability in order to design teaching:

- When a patient has a **visual problem**, the nurse should use **verbal teaching**, repeated several times as needed and record the session for the patient to hear later if possible or use prepared audiotapes or CDs containing the information. The patient should verbalize learning to show attainment of the learning goal.
- When **auditory perception** is a problem, learning materials should be **visual** with as few words as possible. Demonstration, role-playing, and practicing the procedure will be useful to the patient. Printed materials should employ pictures, and computer use can be useful.
- If the patient has an **expressive problem**, he/she needs time to process the input and to ask questions. **Hand gestures, demonstrations, and the senses** should be utilized for teaching when appropriate.

A developmental disability will require information presented in a format that is appropriate for the person's developmental level. The nurse should keep explanations simple, and use gestures, demonstrations, activities, and repetition to teach.

Teaching to Disabled Patients and Families

The teaching of disabled patients and their families begins with an assessment of the family's willingness and preparation for the heavy duty of care that will be required. The nurse must teach information about diseases or disabilities as well as medications, procedures, diet, and physical therapies. The patients must be taught to perform ADLs as well as possible and caregivers taught how to assist when needed:

- Give patients enough information to understand and manage the disabilities and to empower them with a sense of control and coping.
- Don't overwhelm them with information.
- Plan the teaching to provide information according to learning readiness and priorities but be flexible and change the plan if needed.
- Utilize checklists of skills to help keep track of all that has been learned.
- Give praise, continued feedback, support, and empathy with every teaching session.
- Provide resources that patients and family can use after discharge and refer to home health for continuing support and teaching.

Importance of Patient's Culture in Design of Teaching Plan

The nurse must always assess the individual's cultural beliefs and values and not assume that they are the same as the culture on a whole. These beliefs determine what information the patient feels that they can pursue. Teaching that conflicts with these beliefs will be rejected. The patient's perception of health and the healthcare system must be determined because a lack of confidence in the teacher can impair motivation to learn. The nurse must **assess the patient's beliefs** about the following to develop a personalized teaching plan:

- Body image, self-esteem
- Abilities and level of knowledge
- Principles of living
- Diet, activity, health practices
- Involvement of family and support persons
- Physical and mental health and disease
- Causes of disease

- Aging
- Gender issues
- Spirituality, customs, rituals, religious precepts

Human Growth and Development

Issues of Human Development

Several issues of human development that are addressed by theory are described below:

- **Universality vs. context specificity**: Universality implies that all individuals will develop in the same way, no matter what culture they live in. Context specificity implies that development will be influenced by the culture in which the individual lives.
- **Assumptions about human nature** (3 doctrines: original sin, innate purity, and tabula rasa):
    - Original sin says that children are inherently bad and must be taught to be good.
    - Innate purity says that children are inherently good.
    - Tabula rasa says that children are born without good or bad tendencies and can be taught right vs. wrong.
- **Behavioral consistency**: Children either behave in the same manner no matter what the situation or setting, or they change their behavior depending on the setting and who is interacting with them.
- **Nature vs. nurture**: Nature is the genetic influences on development. Nurture is the environment and social influences on development.
- **Continuity vs. discontinuity**: Continuity states that development progresses at a steady rate and the effects of change are cumulative. Discontinuity states that development progresses in a stair-step fashion and the effects of early development have no bearing on later development.
- **Passivity vs. activity**: Passivity refers to development being influenced by outside forces. Activity refers to development influenced by the child himself and how he responds to external forces.
- **Critical vs. sensitive period**: The critical period is that window of time when the child will be able to acquire new skills and behaviors. The sensitive period refers to a flexible time period when a child will be receptive to learning new skills, even if it is later than the norm.

Developmental Tasks According to Erikson

The developmental tasks according to Erik Erikson:

- **Trust vs. mistrust (Birth to 1 year)**: Trust, faith, and optimism develop if the needs of warmth, food, and love are met. If not, this can result in mistrust.
- **Autonomy vs. shame/doubt (Ages 1-3)**: The child desires independence in basic self-care tasks and wants choice. If independence is not encouraged, this can lead to doubt and shame. Independence develops self-control and willpower.
- **Initiative vs. guilt (Ages 3-6)**: The child engages in self-directed play and starts activities without outside influence. Imaginative play and competition are introduced. This can lead to guilt or direction and purpose based on how this initiative is supportive.
- **Industry vs. inferiority (Ages 6-12)**: The child values feeling capable and competent and develops a sense of pride and self-worth. They desire to do what is right and good. Social interactions between peers become more important, and comparing achievements can result in feelings of pride or feelings of inferiority if not properly guided.
- **Identity vs. role confusion (Ages 12-18)**: Parents, teachers, peers, family members, church, culture, and ethnicity all role model and pressure youth to adopt certain behaviors. The task of adolescents is to discover their own identity.

- **Intimacy vs. isolation (Ages 18-40)**: Young people learn to commit to another person in a love or family relationship. They learn the behavior required to maintain this relationship.
- **Generativity vs. stagnation (Ages 40-65)**: Adults have many tasks when they try to find their own interests and niche in the work world. Family, community, and work roles are defined.
- **Integrity vs. despair (Ages 65+)**: Older people ponder their life experiences to put them into perspective. They learn to accept the aging process and begin to think about their own death.

Sigmund Freud's Stages of Psychosexual Development

Sigmund Freud's stages of psychosexual development are listed and described below:

- **Oral stage (Birth to 1 year)**: obsessed with oral activities and must have these needs met for proper psychosocial development, very attached to mother.
- **Anal stage (Ages 1-3)**: masters toilet training.
- **Phallic stage (Ages 3-6)**: child focuses on childbirth and differences between the sexes, develops sexual obsession with parent of opposite sex (Oedipal complex-boy drawn to mother, Electra complex-girl drawn to father).
- **Latency stage (Ages 6-11)**: Oedipal or Electra complex wanes, focus is now socialization, begins to gravitate toward the same-sex parent to learn appropriate gender roles.
- **Genital stage (Ages 12 and older)**: puberty, attracted to opposite sex, learns to relate to opposite gender and control sexual drive.

Piaget's Theory of Cognitive Development

Piaget believed that development was progressive and followed a set pattern. He believed the child's environment, his interactions with others in that environment, and how the environment responds help to shape his cognitive development. There are **four stages to Piaget's theory:**

- The **sensorimotor stage (birth to age 2)** is when the child learns to work toward a goal, the relationship between cause and effect, that objects still exist even though they cannot see them, and a sense of self.
- In the **preoperational stage (ages 2-7)**, language skills develop, the child only sees his point of view, he does not think abstractly, and has a difficult time telling fact from fantasy.
- The **concrete operations stage (ages 7-11)** is when children begin to understand relationships between objects and events, learn to classify and use patterns, understand that some occurrences are reversible, and see others' points of view.
- The **formal operations stage (ages 12 years and older)** is the stage of abstract thinking, better reasoning skills, and forward-thinking.

Review Video: Piaget's Cognitive Development Theory
Visit mometrix.com/academy and enter code: 100376

Maslow's Hierarchy of Needs

Maslow defined human motivation in terms of needs and wants. His **hierarchy of needs** is classically portrayed as a pyramid sitting on its base divided into horizontal layers. He theorized that, as humans fulfill the needs of one layer, their motivation turns to the layer above. The layers consist of (from bottom to top):

- **Physiological**: The need for air, fluid, food, shelter, warmth, and sleep.
- **Safety**: A safe place to live, a steady job, a society with rules and laws, protection from harm, and insurance or savings for the future.
- **Love/Belonging**: A network consisting of a significant other, family, friends, co-workers, religion, and community.
- **Esteem or self-respect**: The knowledge that you are a person who is successful and worthy of esteem, attention, status, and admiration.
- **Self-actualization**: The acceptance of your life, choices, and situation in life and the empathetic acceptance of others, as well as the feeling of independence and the joy of being able to express yourself freely and competently.

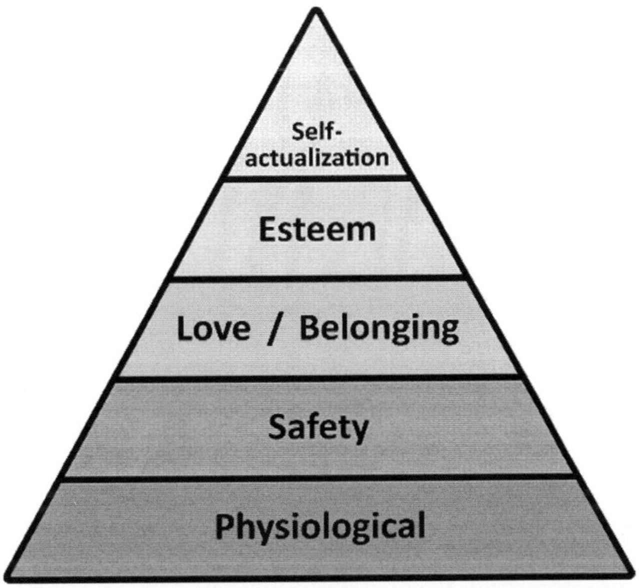

Review Video: Maslow's Hierarchy of Needs
Visit mometrix.com/academy and enter code: 461825

Behavioral Theories

Pavlov demonstrated **classical conditioning** when he found that a dog that would salivate when presented with food would also salivate when the person who normally fed him was present. He paired a bell ringing with the feeding and found that after a time, the dog would also salivate to the ringing of the bell. Consequently, his theory was that learning takes place when a behavior can be produced in response to something totally unrelated to that behavior.

Skinner demonstrated **operant conditioning** when he found that behavior can be changed depending on the response given to the behavior. If the response to the behavior was positive (praise, a hug), then the behavior would continue or increase in frequency. If the response was negative (a frown, words of criticism), then the behavior would decrease in frequency or cease altogether.

Biopsychosocial Theory of Patient Care

The biopsychosocial theory of patient care recognizes that **biology, psychology, and social circumstances** all interact in the development of an illness, the patient's perception of the illness, and the patient's ability to make a good recovery. In the biopsychosocial care model, a multidisciplinary healthcare team, including nurses, mental health professionals, social workers, and physicians, work together to address all aspects of a patient's health issue—the medical problem, psychological state, and social, cultural, and economic situation—in order to find an integrated solution. For example, adding stress-reduction, exercise, and nutritional programs to the standard medical treatment protocol for cardiovascular disease patients has been shown to be more effective. Many patients with chronic diseases or conditions may benefit from support groups that provide social and psychological benefits that may enhance the effects of drug therapy and surgery.

Biological Theories of Aging

There are a number of biological theories of aging:

- **Wearing down**: The body is compared to a machine that begins to wear down over time because of the damage caused by years of use.
- **Autoimmune reaction**: The body develops an autoimmune reaction against itself with aging, causing damage and destruction to tissues.
- **Free radical accumulation**: Chemicals that bring about aging accumulate in the body.
- **Cellular programming**: The cells of every organism have a predetermined programmed life expectancy beyond which one cannot survive.
- **Mutation**: Mutations within the organism occur over time, and these eventually make changes that are incompatible with life.
- **Homeostasis**: Over time, the body is unable to maintain stable levels of necessary chemicals in the body.

Selye's Theory of Adaptation

Selye developed a theory of adaptation concerning a person's physiologic response to stress called the general adaptation syndrome. This syndrome starts with the classic "fight or flight" response of the body to physiologic stress. Catecholamines are released and the adrenal cortical response begins. This is called the **alarm response** and is short-lived. This immediate response allows the person to respond quickly to stress. Since the alarm response cannot be sustained without resulting in death, the body next shifts into the **resistance stage**. Some cortisol is still being released as the body begins to adapt to the stressor. If the stressor persists, the body becomes exhausted. Changes then occur to the cardiovascular, gastrointestinal, and immune systems, and death can occur. The **exhaustion stage** does not always occur in response to most life stressors. As the body ages, it loses some of its resistance and ability to adapt to stress. This results in exhaustion and death in the elderly more easily than it does in younger people.

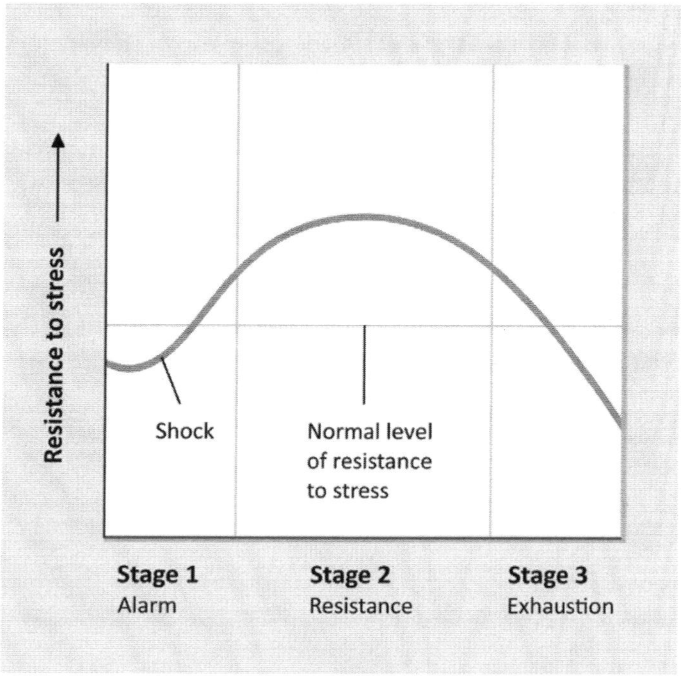
Resistance to stress
Shock
Normal level of resistance to stress
Stage 1
Alarm
Stage 2
Resistance
Stage 3
Exhaustion

Illness and Injury Prevention

Risk Analysis as Part of Disease Prevention

Risk analysis is an important part of health promotion and disease prevention because it can help to identify those factors (normed for age and sex) that put a child at risk for current or future disease. Typically, risk analysis uses observations, interviews, and questionnaires to gain information about a child and their family so that interventions and diagnostic testing can be targeted to areas of increased risk. Risk factors may be controllable (diet and exercise) or non-controllable (genetic), but once identified, a plan of care can be formulated. Risk analysis is an important component of cost-containment because early identification and treatment or intervention can reduce future costs of care. **Areas for risk analysis** may include:

- Nutrition
- Exercise
- Cardiovascular
- Diabetes
- Hypertension
- Cancer
- Osteoporosis
- Vision
- Behavior and lifestyle

Results of risk analysis are not diagnostic, but they indicate if the child is at a low, medium, or high risk of developing a disease or health problem.

Components of Risk Analysis

Risk analysis can be used to assess individual risks or to assess the risk and effectiveness of different treatments and programs in a broader sense. Risk analysis should be carried out for all new treatments and procedures to determine if the benefits outweigh the risks and if they are cost-effective. Risk analysis should be an ongoing part of the nurse's role. There are three primary **components** to risk analysis:

- **Assessing** requires gaining information by questioning, observing, or analyzing data, which may be derived from active study or review of the research.
- **Intervening** involves taking information from the assessment and making changes in management, treatments, or procedures to reflect the risk analysis with the aim of providing the most beneficial and cost-effective care.
- **Communicating** requires publishing the results or sharing those with the organization, family, child, or the general public, depending on the scope of the risk analysis.

Risk Factors for Neonates Associated with Maternal Disease

There are a number of **maternal factors** that put the infant at increased risk:

- **Diabetes mellitus**: Both gestational and pre-existing diabetes put the infant at risk of stillbirth, hypoglycemia, and macrosomia (larger size than normal) as well as birth injury. Maternal pre-existing diabetes is also associated with birth defects, including abnormal development of the cardiovascular and gastrointestinal systems, neurological and spinal cord disorders, and urinary tract abnormalities.
- **HIV/Hepatitis B**: Infectious diseases may be transmitted during pregnancy or delivery.

Implications of Fetal Drug Exposure

There are many drugs that can profoundly affect the growing fetus. Some are prescribed drugs, such as Accutane, but the greatest numbers are illicit drugs, such as crack, heroin, or cocaine. Increasing numbers of children are born to addicted mothers. While each drug has specific effects, there are many effects that are common with any type of fetal drug exposure:

- Premature weight and low birth weight with infants who are small for gestational age (SGA)
- Failure to thrive often related to poor sucking and dysphagia
- Increased risk of congenital infectious disease (HIV, hepatitis, CMV)
- Increased risk of SIDS
- Withdrawal symptoms typically manifest within 72 hours of birth:
    - Tremors, excitability, seizures
    - Vomiting, diarrhea, diaphoresis
    - Dry, red, irritated skin
- Developmental and cognitive problems that vary with age. Initial problems often subside within the first couple of years, but in a small number of children learning disabilities and behavioral problems persist.

Implications of Fetal Alcohol Syndrome

Fetal alcohol syndrome (FAS) is a syndrome of birth defects that develop as the result of maternal ingestion of alcohol. Despite campaigns to inform the public, women continue to drink during pregnancy, but no safe amount of alcohol ingestion has been determined. FAS results in:

- **Facial abnormalities**: Hypoplastic (underdeveloped) maxilla, micrognathia (undersized jaw), hypoplastic philtrum (groove beneath the nose), and short palpebral fissures (eye slits between upper and lower lids).
- **Neurological deficits**: May include microcephaly, intellectual disability, motor delay, and hearing deficits. Learning disorders may include problems with visual-spatial and verbal learning, attention disorders, and delayed reaction times.
- **Growth retardation**: Prenatal growth deficit persists with slow growth after birth.
- **Behavioral problems**: Irritability and hyperactivity. Poor judgment in behavior may relate to deficit in executive functions.

Indication of brain damage without the associated physical abnormalities is referred to as alcohol-related neurodevelopmental disorder (ARND).

Infant Withdrawal from Fetal Exposure to Drugs

Fetal exposure to drugs, such as opioids, methadone, cocaine, crack, and other recreational drugs causes **withdrawal symptoms** in about 60% of infants. There are many variables, which include the type of drug, the extent of drug use, and the duration of maternal drug use. For example, children may have withdrawal symptoms within 48 hours for cocaine, heroin, and methamphetamine exposure, but there may be delays of up to 2-3 weeks for methadone. Short hospital stays after birth make it imperative that children who are at risk are identified so that they can receive supportive treatment, particularly since they often feed poorly and can quickly become dehydrated and undernourished. Polydrug use makes it difficult to describe a typical profile of **symptoms**, but they usually include:

- Tremors
- Irritability
- Hypertonicity
- High-pitched crying
- Diarrhea
- Dry skin
- Seizures (in severe cases)

Treatment is supportive, but children with opiate exposure may be given decreasing doses of opiates, such as morphine elixir, with close monitoring until the child is weaned off of the medication.

Fetal Nicotine/Carbon Monoxide Exposure

About 25% of women who smoke regularly before becoming pregnant continue to smoke throughout pregnancy, and others are exposed to second-hand smoke, putting the fetus at risk for a number of abnormalities from **exposure to nicotine and carbon monoxide**:

- Fetal growth retardation with damage to neurotransmitters accompanied by nervous system cell death with concomitant damage to peripheral autonomic nervous system
- Vasoconstriction from nicotine and interference with oxygen transport caused by carbon monoxide can lead to fetal hypoxia
- Vasoconstriction leading to increased risk of spontaneous abortion, prematurity, and low birth weight
- Increased risk for perinatal death and SIDS
- Cognitive deficiency and learning disorders, such as auditory processing defects (Children of mothers who smoke have a 50% increase in idiopathic intellectual disability.)
- Increased cancer risk, especially for acute lymphocytic leukemia and lymphoma

Cardiovascular Risk Reduction

Some children, specifically those with diabetes mellitus, Kawasaki disease, and familial hypercholesterolemia, are at increased risk of developing **cardiovascular disease**, which can lead to severe coronary artery disease in less than ten years from onset. Screening children who are at risk should begin at age 2 and include cholesterol levels to assess for an elevation of low-density lipoprotein (LDL):

- Total cholesterol <170 and LDL <110: Normal level
- Total cholesterol 170-199 and LDL 110-120: Borderline elevation
- Total cholesterol >200 with LDL >130: Elevated

Early dietary intervention to reduce cholesterol and prevent further increase in LDLs can significantly reduce morbidity and mortality. Dietary recommendations to reduce LDLs include guidelines provided in the *Therapeutic Lifestyle Changes* diet created by the National Institutes of Health for those at risk or with elevated cholesterol.

- 25–30% of diet should be from fat and <7% from saturated fat
- 10–25 g of soluble fiber per day
- <200 mg dietary cholesterol per day
- ≥2 g of plant sterols or stanols per day (found in vegetables, fruits, and nuts)
- 30 minutes of moderate to vigorous exercise per day

ENVIRONMENTAL ASSESSMENT

ENVIRONMENTAL HEALTH HISTORY

The environmental health history is important to determine potential hazards in the child's surroundings that may contribute to poor health or injuries. Examples of potential exposures that should be considered when taking a pediatric environmental health history include air pollution, including industrial exposure, cigarette smoke, carbon monoxide from furnaces or machinery; lead exposure through paint or plumbing in older homes; allergen exposure, such as pet dander, pollen, or mold; exposure to ultraviolet radiation during outdoor activities; water quality; and nutrition.

ENVIRONMENTAL INFLUENCES ON THE PEDIATRIC PATIENT'S HEALTH

Safety in the home environment is a big influence on the health of the child. Accidental injuries in and around the home can include burns from scalding liquids or cooking appliances, drownings in pools or bathtubs, falls from climbing or from bicycles, and motor vehicle accidents or pedestrian-car accidents. Children who spend a great deal of time watching TV or playing video games are at risk for obesity and health issues that accompany obesity. Some children may try to be like characters they see on TV shows or other media, which can lead to aggressive behavior and risk-taking.

CONSIDERATION OF ENVIRONMENTAL FACTORS PRIOR TO A CHILD'S RETURN HOME

Environmental factors should be assessed within the **actual environment** if at all possible. If not, careful questioning and drawing of diagrams and approximate floor plans with the patient (or the patient's parent)—or asking for a drawing—can be useful, especially when showing the patient needed modifications. Family members may also assist with the assessment, providing useful information. Some patients or their parents, may be reluctant to admit that the home is cluttered or that they are unable to maintain the home environment in a sanitary condition. Brochures and handouts about home safety and assistive devices should be provided to the patient and caretaker as well as contact names and numbers for equipment needed in the home. A checklist should be compiled of all necessary changes or additions, with specific details, such as "Install 18-inch grab bar across from toilet." In some cases, a social worker or occupational therapist should visit the home.

GENERAL ELEMENTS OF ENVIRONMENTAL SAFETY

Some elements of an environmental assessment are not specific to rooms in the house but are **general needs** that must be met in order for individuals, especially the disabled child and their caregivers, to remain safe:

- **Environmental hazards** such as piles of papers or junk on the floors, loose carpet or rugs, and cluttered pathways can cause falls and must be cleared, organized, or repaired.
- **Lighting** should be adequate enough for reading in all rooms and stairways.

- **Heat and air conditioning** must be adequate. The young and the elderly are especially susceptible to heat and cold injury.
- **Sanitation** should ensure that health hazards do not exist, such as from rotting food or infestations of cockroaches or rodents.
- **Animals** should be cared for adequately with access to food, water, toileting, and routine veterinary care.
- **Smoke/chemicals** in the environment may pose a hazard, such as exposure to cigarette smoke or cleaning materials.

Dangerous Weapons and Toys

Parents should be advised that any guns kept in the home must be secured, with the guns unloaded and with the ammunition separately secured in a different location. All children, from an early age, should be taught to never pick up a gun or point it at anyone, even in play, and to immediately tell a trusted adult if they see anyone with a gun or know of anyone, such as a peer, who is carrying a gun or intends to harm someone with a gun.

Children should be protected from **dangerous toys**, which can include toys with small parts that may cause choking, especially for infants and toddlers. Toys that shoot projectiles, have cords or strings attached, or have sharp edges may pose a risk as well. Some products, such as some types of slime, have been found to contain toxins, so parents should regularly check with the US Consumer Product Safety Commission for alerts and should always read and adhere to warning labels. Smart toys and electronic devices that connect to the internet may provide identifying information about the child to unauthorized individuals.

Recommendations for Parents and Children Regarding Social Situations

Recommendations for social situations include:

- **Strangers**: Parents should stress the importance of going places and playing outside with a friend or an adult and not being alone. Children should know to run and yell if a stranger asks them to carry something, help get something out of a car, or to help look for or see a puppy or kitten. Parents should stress that children should never get into a car with a stranger or an acquaintance who says that the child's parent has sent the person unless this person uses a password. Children should know to yell what is happening ("This woman is taking me!") and should know their full name, address, and phone number as soon as they are old enough to learn them.
- **Violence**: Parents should limit children's exposure to violent media content (TV, movies, video games) and use blocking tools when appropriate. Parents should encourage children to talk about their feeling if they've experienced or observed violence and to reassure them. If violence is common, children should play only in safe areas and learn safety rules, such as dropping to the ground if they hear gunshots.
- **Bullying**: Parents should recognize the signs that a child is being bullied (depression, withdrawal, dislike of school, change in affect, lack of friends, change of sleep patterns, bruises) and teach children the impact that bullying has on others. Advise parents to teach children to tell an adult if they are being bullied and to respond assertively, act unimpressed, make a joke out of mean comments, and get involved in activities, such as clubs, where they feel safe. If children are cyberbullied, they should block the senders, change passwords, and report it to an adult.

- **Automobile safety/distracted driving**: Children should be seated and secured properly for their age and size and should be taught to avoid yelling, throwing things, and scuffling while in the car as this may distract the driver. Teenage drivers should be taught safe driving (including never driving while drinking), should have clear consequences for unsafe driving (such as a loss of driving privileges), and should have an app on their phones that prevents texting while driving and provides their location to their parents.

Recommendations for Sports and Recreation

Recommendations regarding sports and recreation include:

- **Concussion risks**: Greatest risks are from sports activities (football, hockey, soccer, lacrosse) and accidents (fall, car/bicycle). Parents should ensure that any sports team a child participates in has adequate safety rules (limits to tackling, for example) and that coaches carefully monitor the children. Children should always wear appropriate safety gear, such as helmets, when engaged in sports activities and should never continue playing if exhibiting any signs of head injury (headache, dizziness, confusion).
- **Helmet use**: Helmets (the appropriate type) should be worn for sports activities that may involve falls or blows to the head (hockey, football, skateboarding, baseball, bicycling). Helmets should fit snuggly so that they don't move if they are rotated, turned, or tilted, and the helmet should be pressed down at the crown to check for fitting of the jaw pads and chin straps. Football helmets may be air/fluid filled or padded.

Vehicle Safety

Boat Safety

According to the US Coast Guard's recommendations for **boat safety**, infants who are not of the appropriate weight and size to wear approved personal flotation devices (PFDs) should not be taken on recreational boats (rowboats, motorboats, kayaks, sailboats). All other children should wear life jackets that are properly fitted and secured. PFDs do not include swimming aids intended for play, such as water wings or pool noodles. If an infant is on a boat, a caregiver wearing a life jacket should hold the infant at all times and should not place the child in a car seat (which will not float). Infants and young children are more likely to develop hypothermia, so they should be wrapped with a dry blanket or towel if cold and shivering. Children by about age 3 should be taught safety rules, such as keeping hands and feet inside the boat and walking instead of running. All children should take swimming lessons. Older children should take a boat safety course if possible. Adolescents should be cautioned to never engage in drinking or recreational drug use while boating.

Car Seats

All infants, regardless of age, must be placed properly in an **infant car seat** during transit. Holding an infant while the car is in motion is not safe. Car seats should be new or in very good condition and fastened according to manufacturer's guidelines to ensure safety:

- Place the car seat in the back seat and away from any side airbags.
- Always securely buckle the child into the seat.
- Face the infant seat toward the rear of the car.
- Recline the seat so that the infant's head does not fall forward.
- Place padding around (not under) the infant if the infant slouches to one side.
- Place blankets OVER the straps and buckles, not under.

The infant/toddler should be placed in the rear-facing seat to the maximum weight and height allowed by the seat (some accommodate up to 65 pounds). Once transitioned to front-facing seats, children should be placed in belt-positioning booster seats until the vehicle's seat/shoulder belts fit properly (usually until 4' 9" and 8-12 years old). Until age 13, children should sit secured in the back seat and not the front.

Leading Causes of Death By Age Group

Birth to 10-Year Age Group

For the **birth to 10-year** age group, the US Preventive Services Task Force has assembled a list of the **five leading causes of death**. The number one cause of death in this age group is actually a group of conditions that arise in the time period surrounding birth (the "**perinatal period**"). There are a number of conditions that arise surrounding birth that are fatal, including placental problems (premature separation, abruption), umbilical cord problems (cord prolapse, nuchal cord, single umbilical artery), infections (chorioamnionitis, congenital pneumonia), trauma during the birthing process (nerve damage, intracranial hemorrhage), and hemolytic disease of the newborn. The second leading cause of death is attributed to **congenital defects**, including tetralogy of Fallot, transposition of the great arteries, spina bifida, and anencephaly. Other leading causes of death include **sudden infant death syndrome (SIDS)**, **motor vehicle injuries**, and **other unintentional injuries**.

Injury Prevention Counseling

Injury prevention counseling is a strong recommendation for the **birth to 10-year** age group, owing to the fact that motor vehicle accidents and other unintentional accidents are leading causes of death for this population. Children and their parents should be advised to use car safety seats until the age of 5 (this is subject to state law, however, as some states require the use of booster seats until a certain height or age is reached). After the age of 5, standard safety belts should always be used. When biking, skating, or skateboarding, a helmet should always be worn; these activities should not take place in the street. Parents should be advised to become CPR certified. They should also be advised to keep drugs, poisons, guns, other weapons, and matches out of the reach of children; to install smoke detectors and plan an escape route in the event of fire; and to make sure that stairs, windows, and pools are safe for children.

11- to 24-Year Age Group

The list of the top five leading causes of death in the **11-24** age population differs significantly from the leading causes of death in the birth to 10-year age population. Leading the list for ages 11-24 are deaths caused by either **motor vehicle accidents or other unintentional accidents**. Second on the list is **homicide**, followed by **suicide**. The fourth leading cause of death in the 11-24 age population is **cancer**. The most common fatal cancers in this age group include leukemia (acute lymphocytic leukemia and acute myeloid leukemia), brain tumors (medulloblastoma, astrocytoma, and brainstem glioma), rhabdomyosarcoma, neuroblastoma, Wilms tumor, Ewing sarcoma, and Hodgkin's lymphoma. The fifth leading cause of death in this age population is due to **general heart diseases**, which may include cardiomyopathies and faulty valves.

Youth Risk Behavior Surveillance System

The **Youth Risk Behavior Surveillance System** (YRBSS) is a program conducted through the CDC that monitors eight different categories of health-risk behaviors of adolescents:

- Unintentional injuries and violence
- Tobacco use
- Alcohol and other drug use

- Sexual behaviors
- Dietary behaviors
- Physical activity
- Obesity, overweight, and weight control
- Other health topics

The YRBSS gathers data from participating states and local surveys (such as large cities) from grades 9-12 and then compiles the information, assessing for trends. Current results reflect data collected in 2021 and released in 2023. Responses are either weighted (≥60% participation) or unweighted (relates only to those completing survey). Weighted results can be generalized to the teenage population at large in the area of the survey. The data obtained in the YRBSS is used to determine progress in national health objectives for health promotion.

YRBSS 2021 Results

Tobacco Use

The CDC conducts the Youth Risk Behavior Surveillance System to determine health-risk behaviors that contribute to significant morbidity in adolescents. **Tobacco,** often thought of as an adult issue, is a cause of concern for children and teenagers. Tobacco use is one of the leading preventable causes of death in the United States, but 2021 results showed that about 6.3% of children (down from 9.5% in 2019) have tried smoking before high school, often beginning by age 12, putting themselves at risk for heart and lung disease as adults. Almost 18% of children have tried smoking in total according to 2021 results, which is a downward trend. A newer trend is the use of electronic vapor products, with 36% of children reporting having tried this product at some point, and 18% reporting current use. Those most at risk are males in low-income families with parents who smoke. Male adolescents may smoke to be rebellious, but females often smoke to lose weight. Other factors include the desire to be part of a group, lack of supervision, and accessibility of tobacco. Intervention includes identifying those smoking, providing information about the dangers of smoking, beginning with children at about 9 years old, and providing programs to help teenagers quit smoking.

Drug Use

Drug use continues to be a serious problem for children and teenagers, with some starting as young as 9 or 10, using a wide variety of drugs, including marijuana, crack, prescription drugs, cocaine, inhalants (such as glue and lighter fluid), hallucinogens, and steroids. Marijuana is the most reported drug in the high school data, with about 28% of children reporting having used marijuana in their lifetime. Approximately 13% of children reported having used illicit drugs (e.g., cocaine, heroin, inhalants, methamphetamines, ecstasy, or hallucinogens) at least once in their lifetime. Risk factors for drug use include aggressive behavior, poor social skills, and poor academic progress coupled with lack of parental supervision, poverty, and availability of drugs. Small children who use drugs are often reacting to circumstances within the family, while teenagers are more likely to use drugs in response to peer pressure from outside the family. Studies have shown that early intervention to teach children better self-control and coping skills is often more effective than trying to change behavior patterns that are established, so family-based programs often show positive results. Teenagers may need help with basic academic skills and social skills to improve communication. Methods of resisting drugs must be provided and reinforced. Drug recovery programs can be helpful but are often too expensive or not available for those who need them.

Alcohol Use

Alcohol use is a significant problem in adolescence and even in younger children. It is the most-commonly abused substance. Of high schoolers who responded to the survey question in 2021, about 23% reported having had at least one drink within the past 30 days (down from 30% in 2019). While alcohol can impair development of almost all body systems in a growing child, it is of particular concern for the effects on the neurological system and liver. Additionally, because it interferes with impulse control, adolescents who drink are often involved in violence, abuse, and at-risk sexual behavior. Drinking should be suspected if a child has memory problems, changes in behavior, poor academic progress, emotional lability, and physical changes, such as slurring of speech, general lethargy, or lack of coordination. Intervention includes teaching children from around age 9 about the dangers of drinking, identifying those who are drinking, identifying underlying problems, and providing programs to help teenagers stop drinking, such as counseling or Alcoholics Anonymous.

High-Risk Sexual Behavior

High-risk sexual behavior in teenagers is often coupled with other health-risk behaviors, such as drinking and drug use. In 2021, about 30% of high school students reported having previously had sex (a significant decline from the 38.4% reported in 2019), with around 3% becoming sexually active before the age of 13. Risk factors include poverty, single-family homes, lack of supervision, and siblings or peers who are sexually active. Those who have sex before age 15 are especially vulnerable, often having multiple partners and unprotected sex, leading to sexually transmitted infections (STIs) and pregnancy. They are often emotionally vulnerable and unable to deal effectively with relationships. Intervention should begin early with age-appropriate honest sex education. Abstinence education, while the ideal, has not been successful in changing the sexual behavior of teenagers, with studies showing that many of those signing pledges to remain virgins are already sexually active. Teenagers who are sexually active should be advised regarding the use of condoms, birth control, and protection from STIs in a non-judgmental manner.

Prevention of STIs

The **CDC** has developed five strategies to prevent and control the spread of STIs:

- **Educate** those at risk about how to make changes in sexual practices to prevent infection.
- **Identify** symptomatic and asymptomatic infected persons who might not seek diagnosis or treatment.
- **Diagnose** and treat those who are infected.
- **Prevent infection** of sex partners through evaluation, treatment, and counseling.
- Provide pre-exposure **vaccination** for those at risk.

Practitioners are advised to inquire of patients' **sexual histories** and to assess risk. The 5-P approach to questioning is advocated. Practitioners should ask about:

- **Partners**: Gender and number
- **Pregnancy prevention**: Birth control
- **Protection**: Methods used
- **Practices**: Type of sexual practices (oral, anal, vaginal) and use of condoms
- **Past history of STIs**: High-risk behavior (promiscuity, prostitution) and disease risk (human immunodeficiency virus [HIV]/ hepatitis)

The CDC recommends a number of specific preventive methods as part of the clinical guidelines for prevention of sexually transmitted infections:

- **Abstinence or reduction** in number of sex partners.
- Pre-exposure **vaccination**: All those evaluated for STIs should receive hepatitis B vaccination, and men who have sex with men (MSM) and illicit drug users should receive hepatitis A vaccination.
- **Male latex (or polyurethane) condoms** should be used for all sexual encounters with only water-based lubricants used with latex.
- **Female condoms** may be used if a male condom cannot be used properly.
- Condoms and diaphragms should not be used with spermicides containing **nonoxynol-9 (N-9)**, and N-9 should not be used as a lubricant for anal sex.
- **Non-barrier contraceptive measures** provide no protection from STIs and must not be relied on to prevent disease.

Measures to Prevent Injury/Illness of Toddlers

Home and Auto Safety

Toddlers are curious and very mobile, so accidents can occur easily in and outside the home. **Auto safety** includes using the appropriate size child-safety seat in the back seat, and buckling the child up every time they are in a moving vehicle. Toddlers need to be supervised closely when playing outside, to prevent them from running into the street in front of moving vehicles. Parents can begin to teach them how to stop, look, and listen before crossing a street.

The home environment needs to be child-proofed, moving all poisonous substances well away from the toddler's reach (keeping in mind that toddlers will learn to climb). Poisons should be stored in a locked or inaccessible location to the child. Medication should be stored up high and children should not be told that medication is candy when they are taking it.

Water, Toy, and Gun Safety, and Burns

The following are some measures the parents can take to prevent injury and illness of their toddler, focusing on burns and water, toy, and gun safety:

- Never leave a toddler alone in or near water, as they can drown in as little as one inch of water. Toddlers are still unstable and prone to falling, possibly into a puddle or bucket.
- When appropriate, life jackets should be worn by toddlers (in a boat or near a lake, pond, or pool).
- Toddlers should wear helmets when riding tricycles.
- Make sure any toys given to toddlers are appropriate for their age and safe. Balloons, small toys, and plastic bags are potential choking hazards.
- A big concern today is guns kept in the home. Toddlers don't know the difference between a toy gun and a real gun, so all guns kept in the home must be properly secured.
- Teach the toddler the meaning of "hot," while using safety plugs on appliances, keep matches and lighters up high, turn pot handles toward the back of the stove, and don't use tablecloths in the home (toddlers can pull on these and topple hot food/liquids on themselves).

Measures to Prevent Injury/Illness of Preschoolers

Home and Auto Safety

Preschoolers are aware of potential dangers and can be taught safety rules. Poisonous substances, including medicines, need to have safety caps and be locked up. Watch for unsafe areas at playgrounds. Enforce the wearing of safety equipment when playing sports. Use the appropriate safety seat (booster) in the back seat until the child weighs 80 lb. After 80 lb, use a seat belt in the back seat. Do not leave a child alone in a car or home. Use close supervision when playing outside and near streets. Have the child wear a bike helmet when riding and teach him the rules for safe riding. Parents should have the poison control number saved to their phones or written down somewhere it can be quickly accessed.

Auto, Sports, and Water Safety

School age children are especially prone to accidents, due to their mobility and participation in sports and other physical activities. The following rules should be taught to children and enforced by the parents/caregivers:

- Children should always wear a seatbelt, and sit in the backseat, in a moving vehicle.
- When riding anything with wheels, the child should always wear a helmet and elbow and knee pads.
- The child must obey traffic signals when walking on or across streets.
- The school-aged child should participate in swim lessons and be taught to swim with a buddy, wear a life jacket when in a boat, and not dive into shallow water.

Measures to Prevent Injury/Illness of School Age Children

The following are some measures parents can take to prevent injury/illness of their school age child, focusing on drug, fire, stranger, and gun safety:

- Keep medicine locked and teach children the dangers of taking any medicine without adult supervision.
- Begin teaching the child about illegal drug use and smoking.
- Use sunscreen when playing outside.
- Establish an escape route for each member of the family in case of fire and practice the route monthly.
- Don't allow the child to use the stove without adult supervision.
- Teach the child to stay away from guns. Parents should keep guns unloaded and in a locked location with ammunition stored in a separate location.
- Teach the child to not talk to strangers or approach strange vehicles.
- Make sure the child knows their phone number, their address, and how to call 911.
- Find a neighbor's house that can serve as a safe place for the child if needed.

Measures to Prevent Injury/Illness of Adolescents

Adolescents think they are invincible, which can contribute to risk-taking behaviors.

- Motor vehicle accidents claim many teenagers' lives every year. Teens should take driver's education courses, wear seat belts at all times, obey traffic laws, and refrain from drinking and driving.
- If an adolescent legally uses firearms, they need to be taught safety rules and how to use and store firearms.
- Adolescents should be taught the risks of using drugs, alcohol, and nicotine.
- Sports teams should focus on safety, proper equipment, and appropriate conditioning.
- Adolescents should know proper swimming and water safety and use sunscreen when outside.
- Sexual activity is a high-risk behavior that should be addressed on a family level. If appropriate, the adolescent should be taught sexual responsibility.

Appropriate Sunscreen Use

While children need some exposure to the sun, sunscreen protects against harmful ultraviolet rays that can cause burns, sun damage, premature aging, and skin cancer. Sunscreen should be generously applied before children go out in the sun, covering the parts of the body that are exposed, including the face, lips, tops of the ears, and back of the neck. It should be reapplied at least every 2 hours, and if children are going to be around water, the sunscreen should be waterproof. The sun protection factor (SPF) should be a minimum of 30 for children older than 6 months, as recommended by the American Academy of Dermatology. The American Academy of Pediatrics recommends that children under the age of 6 months be kept out of direct sunlight. If they must be in direct sunlight, children should be covered by clothing and hats. A small amount of SPF 15 sunscreen is allowed on children under the age of 6 months, but only to small areas such as their face and the backs of their hands.

Guidelines for Using Insect Repellant

Insect repellant may be used on children to prevent insect bites, but it should be used with caution. Many insect repellants contain N,N-diethyl-meta-toluamide (DEET), which has been shown to be safe for limited use with children over 2 months of age. Repellants used on children should have less than a 30% concentration of DEET and should only be applied once a day. It should be sprayed on a caregiver's hand and then put on the child, rather than spraying the child directly. This decreases the likelihood of the child ingesting the repellant. Insect repellant can also be applied to clothing to provide some protection without applying it directly to the skin.

Geriatric Syndromes

Geriatric syndromes represent a category of illnesses that is comprised of the most common non-disease conditions that are seen amongst the geriatric community. It is the responsibility of the nurse to be competent in these critical areas:

- **Falls**: As individuals age, their senses dull, leaving them vulnerable to falls due to a combination of sensory decline and chronic disease. Patients and caregivers should be provided with recommendations for fall prevention, and health care providers should create safe inpatient environments with proper fall prevention protocols.
- **Frailty**: A syndrome characterized by decreased stamina, strength, weight, and speed. This combination of issues results from the natural decline of aging and presents specific risks (falls, confusion, and depression) that must be assessed amongst the geriatric population.

- **Incontinence**: Urinary incontinence is an especially common ailment amongst the elderly population due to neurological conditions, physical limitations, and cognitive decline. This particular ailment is not only physically limiting and introduces risks for skin breakdown and infection, but it is socially limiting and can lead to psychological issues as well.
- **Delirium**: Confusion is the most common manifestation of any physical ailment amongst the elderly, along with the prevalence of dementia amongst the elderly. Delirium should never be cast aside in an elderly individual. Though common, it may be an indication of other more serious issues.
- **Functional Decline**: Functional decline is the diminished ability of an individual to carry out the activities of daily living to sustain independence and perform self-care. With this, comes the consideration for additional support, be it live-in care, nursing homes, or assisted living communities.

Additional Health Issues for the Elderly

The following are additional health issues for the elderly:

- **Antibodies and Immunity**: An elderly patient can react to an infection with antibodies that have been created by the body before, but if the infection is new, it is more difficult for the body to respond appropriately. Cells in the immune system cannot proliferate as easily in an older patient as in a younger one. The number of T-cells is stable, but they do not work as well and can have less cytotoxicity. Additionally, there is not as much thymus-gained immunity because the thymus gland is smaller. This also means it is harder for an older patient to make antibodies.
- **Allergies**: Identify the type of allergic response the patient has and to what allergens, especially when getting the patient history. Determine if the response is actually an allergy to a medication or an adverse effect of it.
- **Driving**: An elderly patient senses change with age. A decreased ability to hear does not mean a patient cannot drive, but sight is very important, including binocular sight, ability to see color, and ability to see in the dark.
- **REM**: Rapid eye movement starts approximately 120 minutes after going to sleep, and happens again in 3–4 evenly spread out increments that last 10–15 minutes. It is linked to skeletal muscle atonia, rapid eye movements, and dreaming. REM sleep occurs less frequently as one gets older. With aging, the patient is more likely to wake up, which affects their sleep quality.

Urinary Incontinence

Urinary incontinence (UI) is the involuntary loss of urine. Incidence increases with age and is more common in women. There are several **types of urinary incontinence**:

- **Transient**: Adverse medication reaction, urinary tract infection, severe constipation, immobility, mental disorders.
- **Urge or Reflex**: Detrusor muscle spasms cause an urgent desire to urinate because of neurological impairment in Parkinson's, stroke, Alzheimer's, and sitting. Can be triggered by drinking, or hearing or seeing running water.
- **Stress (SUI)**: Increased intra-abdominal pressure from sneezing, coughing, laughing, pregnancy, childbirth damage to the detrusor muscle and pelvic floor fascia, and menopausal hormone changes. Twice as common in women as men.
- **Enuresis**: Bedwetting while asleep.

Decreased bladder strength, diminished ability to concentrate urine, and decreased urethral closing pressure following menopause are common causes of incontinence in the elderly. Incontinence is also influenced by depression, less mobility, decreased vision, and less awareness of feeling a full bladder. Voiding routines are helpful in managing incontinence among the elderly. The typical voiding routine for a fully-grown adult patient is as follows: The initial urge to go to the bathroom happens at the point of the bladder having 200-300 mL in it. Grown patients generally void 4-6 times daily, and most will not need to go during the night except when there is a condition that makes it so or if the patient is using diuretic medication. The sensation of the bladder beginning to fill up begins at 90-150 mL, and the need to go starts at 200-300 mL. Usually, an hour or two will elapse between the first feeling of needing to go and the bladder being at full capacity. Full, easy capacity is around 300-600 mL. There should not be any leaking if going to the bathroom has to be postponed.

Age-Related Changes in Respiratory System

As a patient ages, the respiratory system changes in the following ways:

- **Rib cage becomes more rigid**. There will be more width measured across the anteroposterior chest. When a patient gets old, the number of alveoli decreases. They get inflexible and can no longer draw back. This means that the patient cannot breathe out as well, leading to more residual volume. There is less basilar inflation and the patient cannot get foreign bodies out as well. This condition also happens to someone who has kyphosis.
- **Decreased ability for the chest wall to work** so that it is harder to take a deep inhalation.
- **Trachea and bronchi increase in measurement** so that there is more unused area and lessened air volume that gets to the alveoli. Small airway shutting means there is less vital capacity and more residual volume.
- **Lung parenchyma is not as elastic** so that the alveoli do not function as effectively.
- **Breaths are not as deep and coughs are not as forceful** because the muscles are not as strong.

Chronic Diarrhea

Chronic diarrhea is more than three bowel movements per day, with watery stools lasting more than two weeks. It is more common and potentially more serious for the elderly population. The most common cause is infectious, but **chronic diarrhea** in the elderly population can also be caused by inflammatory bowel disease, diverticulitis, colon cancer, medication side effects, and irritable bowel syndrome. Take a careful history, including a list of travel destinations. Look for these signs and **symptoms of dehydration** in the physical exam:

- Flushed, dry skin
- Dark, scanty urine
- Fast pulse and respiration
- Fever
- Vomiting or nausea
- Head rushes
- Thirst
- Dry mouth
- Anorexia
- Chills
- Tingling
- Cramps

- Exhaustion
- Confusion
- Seizures
- Unconsciousness

Send stools to the lab for culture, ova and parasites, occult blood, fecal leukocytes, and *C. difficile* toxin, especially if the patient was recently hospitalized. Collect blood for a CBC and electrolytes. Order an abdominal x-ray, and follow up with a barium enema or colonoscopy, if indicated. Treat the underlying cause. Significantly dehydrated patients require hospital admission for IV therapy.

Fractures

Fractures are a common cause of disability in the elderly population. The elderly population is at higher risk for sustaining **fractures** due to decreased bone mass and strength, and increased risk for falls due to poor vision and balance. The most common locations for fractures in the elderly are the distal radius, proximal humerus, proximal femur and tibia, vertebrae, hip, and pubic ramus. Most fractures are the result of minor trauma. Fractures are slightly more common in women. Make the diagnosis based on the history, physical exam, and x-ray results. Immobilize the fracture above and below the break. Administer analgesics. Refer the patient to a physiotherapist, an orthopedic surgeon, and a PSW. The goal of treatment is as rapid a return to normal activity as is possible. The elderly population is more vulnerable to complications, such as permanent functional impairment, bedsores, and pulmonary embolism. The aide, nurse, or caregiver must turn the patient every two hours to minimize complications.

Age-Related Cataracts

The lens is the clear part of the eye behind the pupil that focuses light on the retina. **Cataracts** are categorized by gradual clouding or opacification of the lens. One or both eyes can be affected, and cataracts can be congenital. Incidence increases with age and affects 70% of people over the age of 75. Risk factors include trauma, radiation, diabetes, family history, smoking, alcoholism, sun exposure, steroid use, and previous eye surgery. Signs and symptoms for cataracts include gradual lens clouding; blurry vision; decreased night vision; brown tint or color fading; halo or glare around lights; diplopia (double vision); trouble distinguishing blue and purple. An ophthalmologist makes the diagnosis by slit lamp exam and retinal exam. Cataracts are followed until they cause significant visual loss and then are treated by surgical removal of the clouded lens and replacement with a permanent intraocular or removable external lens.

Review Video: Glaucoma vs. Cataracts
Visit mometrix.com/academy and enter code: 279024

Hearing Loss

Approximately 25% of adults over the age of 65 have varying degrees of hearing loss. Risk factors for hearing loss include:

- A positive family history
- Chronic exposure to loud noises, especially if hearing protection was not worn
- Use of ototoxic drugs, like Gentamicin, NSAIDs, loop diuretics, or cancer chemotherapy

Hearing loss can be either peripheral or central. **Peripheral hearing loss** results when the ear canal is obstructed by impacted wax, a foreign object, or damage to the middle or inner ear. **Central hearing loss** is the result of damage to the portions of the brain that are needed for hearing: Vestibulocochlear nerve, brain stem, contralateral inferior colliculus, superior olivary nucleus, inferior colliculi, ipsilateral medial geniculate nucleus of the thalamus, and primary auditory cortex below the superior temporal gyrus in the temporal lobe.

Common Comorbidities Seen Amongst the Elderly Population

Geriatric comorbidities are combinations of chronic or acute illnesses that significantly increase the mortality rate amongst this population and are also associated with faster rates of disability exacerbation and functional decline. Understanding these comorbidities not only help the nurse manage these specific comorbidities, but also aid in the guidance of health promotion and disease prevention efforts to decrease the rates of comorbidity amongst their elderly patients. A 2010 study clustered comorbidities most commonly found in the elderly population into 3 groups (Ross, 2010). The three most common comorbidity patterns amongst the geriatric population include:

- **Cardiovascular/metabolic disorders**: Heart disease, MI, coronary artery disease and congestive heart failure often coincide with metabolic issues such as hypertension, diabetes, obesity, and gout.
- **Anxiety/depression/somatoform disorders and pain**: Pain (systemic, localized, or joint related) often coincide with psychological conditions such as anxiety, depression, and cognitive decline. Gastrointestinal issues also seem to coincide with these psychological conditions.
- **Neuropsychiatric disorders**: Psychiatric conditions such as Parkinson's and dementia, are often tied to neurological issues such as incontinence, vascular issues, and/or nerve pain.

Common Psychological Responses to Chronic Illness

Chronic illness not only effects the physical health of individuals, but often has many **psychological manifestations** as well. This psychological stress is tied to the most basic needs that are engrained in individuals as children, and therefore can cause the regression of the patient to adapt more childlike responses to chronic illness over time. Often these psychological responses to chronic illnesses are based on general concepts of fear, self-esteem, and loss of control.

- **Fear**: Chronic illness, when debilitating with possibly severe consequences, forces patients to face common fears of death, loss, and pain. Remaining in a constant state of fear (stress) can lead to depression, anxiety, and anger.
- **Self-esteem**: While in the early stages of chronic illness many patients find strength and determination to conquer the disease. But, after time, the inability to do so wears on the individual's sense of strength and capability. With a loss of self-esteem, can come feelings of despair and hopelessness, which often result in an increasing rate of decline. Patients with strong support systems and positive outlooks often fare better with chronic disease.
- **Loss of control**: When chronic disease dictates an individual's life and abilities, the patient loses a sense of control over their own life. Losing one's independence can be extremely difficult mentally and emotionally, especially when the patient was previously active and healthy. By providing the patient with treatment options and educating the patient on self-care the nurse can attempt to return some elements of control to the patient, which can motivate them to own their fight against disease and find a new normal in their life that is manageable and fulfilling.

Patient Interview

The **interview of an elderly patient** focuses on care vs. cure: is the patient ailing from something they can recover from, or are they ailing from conditions of old age that simply need to be managed? The nurse should collect a total and truthful account of the patient's medical history in the form of a personal account. A lot of the data gathered can be used to identify what the problem is and what the medical treatment will be. The nurse can develop a trusting relationship with the patient by creating an atmosphere of openness and compassion. Nursing considerations and focuses during the patient interview include the following:

- Find out what the main grievance of the patient is, which may not be the initial reason for seeking care.
- Keep the interview focused because the patient might come in with a lengthy, complicated medical past or struggle focusing or keeping track of long conversations.
- Control the dialogue and avoid close-ended (yes or no) questions.
- Review each matter separately.
- The patient's gender and age can be a factor in the relationship.
- Other family members can help with the interview, and the patient might depend on them to help answer queries. Conversely, the patient may be suffering from neglect by caregivers, an issue that the health care provider must always be assessing for.
- Additional delicate matters such as incontinence, abuse, failing mental ability, or sexual difficulties should be discussed appropriately. It is important to make the patient know that the discussion is confidential.

Putting Older Adults at Ease

It is important to regulate the **environment** in which the nurse collects information about the health history. The older adult may have difficulties hearing the conversation or may suffer from vision-related impairments such as glare intolerance. The nurse can have greater success during the history-taking period by reducing environmental noise and avoiding harsh light. Because of their increasing age, older adults may have developed more symptoms of illness, they may be on larger amounts of medications, and they have longer medical histories to discuss. The nurse should allow for extra time to cover all aspects of the history. The nurse's stance may make an impact on how comfortable the patient feels talking about their history. An open and friendly attitude that is respectful conveys a welcome message. If possible, the nurse should sit to speak with the patient instead of standing over him/her.

Observations Related to Appearance

The **initial impression** of the older adult is the nurse's opportunity to make observations about his/her overall appearance and mannerisms. Sometimes, this rapid observation will provide many clues about the patient's state of well-being, and the nurse can incorporate this information into the history and physical exam. Some initial observations that the nurse may make include the following:

- The patient's posture (slumped, evidence of kyphosis, sitting up erect)
- The patient's response to initial greeting (guarded, friendly, pleasant)
- The patient's overall affect (flat, animated, dull)
- The patient's appearance and personal grooming (hair that is not combed, foul breath, dirty clothing, or a clean and well-kept appearance)
- The appearance of injuries that may indicate an unsafe environment (bruises, scrapes, or guarding of extremities)

Information Needed for Health History of Elderly Patients

The health history of an elderly patient requires biographical information, family background regarding medical histories, job/career history and status, medications being used, cigarette use, use of banned substances, allergies, issues with drugs or foods, psychiatric/cognitive impairments or disorders, diet, sleep, physical activity, leisure activities, overview of systems, and prevention being done (such as screenings). The nurse must collect an account of the prior medical treatment, including any time the patient had to go to the hospital, surgeries, vaccinations, accidents, harm done, falling down, medical conditions from the past (including as a child), communicable diseases from the past, health practices, and religious elements that influence the body (such as fasting). Investigate safety concerns including work, home, and other places, the ability to drive, or any abuse. Discuss the Patient Self-Determination Act from 1990, including any advance directives, a living will, power of attorney, and doctor-assisted suicide. Find out where and with whom the patient lives, including who the main caregiver is. Talk about how a disability will affect income, and discuss help that can be found in the area.

Prior Health Issues

The first element of the **health assessment** involves the collection of an account of prior health issues that patient has had, which is the foundation of the patient's clinical picture, in combination with their lifestyle, demographics and biographical information (family history, etc.). With these elements, patients can also be evaluated for risk and education needs. Next, the health assessment should address current health problems, including the **OPQRST assessment**:

- **O**nset
- **P**rovocative/palliative (getting well or problem going downhill)
- **Q**uality/quantity
- **R**egion/radiation
- **S**etting
- **T**iming

Inquire about prior health issues/concerns/questions, including how the patient feels about their own health, prior conditions or hospital visits, injuries or surgeries (including when, what medical attention was required, and what follow up visits were done afterwards), emotional well-being, sexual well-being, allergies to food or drugs (and severity of the allergic reaction), current medications (prescribed and over-the-counter), immunization history, sleep routines, and prior physical assessments. Discuss individual routines, including the utilization of tobacco, alcohol, drugs, caffeine, nutrition, physical activity, hobbies, athletics, and contact sports.

Additional aspects of the health assessment include the following:

- **Familial health issues**: Discuss relatives, including their age (or age of death), well-being, and experiences with disease. Discuss health of children if relevant, and any conditions that are hereditary within the family.
- **Activity level**: Discuss any restrictions from activity/exercise, rapid heart rate or chest hurting upon physical activity, seizure, concussion, prior loss of consciousness, and whether the patient can run for a half- mile (or higher).
- **Psychosocial factors**: Find out about the patient's psychosocial influences, including where he or she currently lives, what level of schooling he or she has finished, religious and spiritual beliefs (as it relates to wellbeing and medical attention), a summary of a normal day, optimistic or pessimistic prospects for what is to come, stress and coping mechanisms, and signs of depression, anxiety, or thoughts of suicide. Ask about the social network.

- **Work and surroundings**: Collect an account of the patient's current and former work experience and the atmosphere where they spend time. Discuss any dangerous contact with anything (toxics, equipment, loud noise) at home or on the job, time in the military or in a war (when applicable), where the patient lives and how long they have lived there, whether the home is anywhere near a factory, shipyard, or another thing that could have harmful elements, and find out about leisurely pursuits and any other possible contact with unsafe elements.

Home Environment

Interviewing the patient about their **home environment** is very helpful when developing a care plan to provide for care and safety. Rooms should be assessed according to their function:

- The **entryway** should be free of obstacles and surfaces even. Handrails and/or ramps may be needed for those who are unsteady or wheelchair bound.
- **Stairs/steps** should have handrails, non-skid surfaces, and contrast markings for each step.
- The **living area** should be comfortable and furniture arranged for convenience. Chairs should be firm enough for people to stand from easily.
- **Bedrooms** should have a night light and phone near the bed. The bed should be positioned close to the nearest bathroom if possible and at the appropriate height for easy access and appropriate firmness.
- **Bathrooms** may require grab bars, a hand-held shower, an elevated toilet seat, and a tub seat.
- **Kitchen** items may need to be moved for convenient access. A sturdy step stool may be required. Unsafe equipment/tools should be removed.

Some elements of interviewing and assessing the patient's home environment are not specific to rooms in the house but are general needs that must be met in order for people, especially the elderly or disabled, to remain safe:

- **Environmental hazards** such as piles of papers or junk on the floors, loose carpet or rugs, and cluttered pathways can cause falls and must be cleared, organized, or repaired.
- **Lighting** should be adequate enough for reading in all rooms and stairways.
- **Heat and air conditioning** must be adequate. The young and the elderly are especially susceptible to heat and cold injury.
- **Sanitation** should ensure that health hazards do not exist, such as from rotting food or infestations of cockroaches or rodents.
- **Animals** should be cared for adequately with access to food, water, toileting, and routine veterinary care.
- **Smoke/chemicals** in the environment may pose a hazard, such as exposure to cigarette smoking or cleaning materials.

Environmental factors should be assessed within the actual environment if at all possible. If not, careful questioning and drawing of diagrams and approximate floor plans with the patient—or asking the patient to do drawings—can be useful, especially when showing the patient needed modifications. Family members may also assist with the assessment, providing useful information. Some patients, especially the elderly, may be reluctant to admit that the home is cluttered or that they are unable to maintain the home environment in a sanitary condition. Brochures and handouts about home safety and assistive devices should be provided to the patient as well as contact names and numbers for equipment needed in the home. A checklist should be compiled of all necessary changes or additions, with specific details, such as "Install 18-inch grab bar across from toilet." In some cases, a social worker or occupational therapist should visit the patient.

Validating Data Received from Patient During Assessment Process

The assessment process is a time of determining the patient's chief complaint or the reason that he or she is seeking care. The nurse may find this information through discussing the patient's history, by physical exam, or both. Data obtained through this process should be as accurate as possible in order to guide the physician in prescribing treatment and to support the nurse's plan of care. Data obtained through assessment should also be validated to identify information that might have been missed on a previous visit, to determine that what the patient is saying matches the symptoms or complaints, and to avoid assumptions on the part of the nurse as to the patient's mental or physical state.

Ensuring Accuracy

When client information does not match assessment or the nurse encounters conflicting information, he or she may use several techniques to **validate the accuracy of the data**. The nurse may repeat his or her assessment and some of the questions asked of the patient, such as repeating a blood pressure reading when results are too low or asking a patient to further describe his or her symptoms. The nurse may also ask another nurse to perform the exam to determine if the results are the same. If the patient's ability to recount information is in question, or the patient's assessment identifies abnormalities that do not change with repeated assessments, the nurse may also check the patient's medical records for possible explanations that will validate the accuracy of the client's assessment.

Obtaining Information About Elderly Patients from Third-Party Sources

Benefits

Families or third-party members who accompany elderly patients on health visits are valuable sources of information. They may provide details when the patient is forgetful or does not understand questions or instructions, and they may provide physical assistance, such as in the case of driving the patient to appointments or helping with mobility. In some cases, family members are responsible for assisting with or providing recommended treatments at home and should be present during the medical visit. Family members who serve as the patient's power of attorney should also be present to understand the patient's condition and to be part of decisions made on behalf of the patient.

Challenges

Families or friends of elderly patients may be valuable sources of information and may be able to provide details when the patient is unsure of or cannot remember circumstances. However, there are times when family or other **third-party sources** may present challenges to caring for or getting history information from an older adult. For example, it may be difficult to direct the discussion so that it is solely focused on the patient, rather than a caregiver or family member's needs. The family member may have other issues such as financial difficulties, a busy schedule, or children present that become distractions during the interview. While third parties are a good source of information, they may be unwilling to allow the older adult to speak for him or herself. Finally, there may be some personal issues, such as urinary incontinence or sexuality, that may be embarrassing for the older patient to discuss in front of a third party.

Obtaining Information from Other Facilities

Patients who change providers may have information **in medical records located at other facilities.** The medical records are the property of the physician at the former facility, but most organizations work together to transfer documents so that healthcare providers may have access to the patient history and data. A nurse can ask the patient about past medical care and then contact past providers to ask about methods of transmitting documents. The information is typically a copy of the original reports, intended only to provide the patient's information. The original information usually remains with the former physician even when the patient is no longer seeking services there. Once the copies of medical records have been obtained, the nurse and physician can use this information to support their own care of the patient and his or her treatments and medications.

Patients Who Normally Reside in Long-Term-Care Facilities

Long-term-care facilities can vary according to their administration and levels of care, just as the residents of these facilities may range from fairly independent to totally reliant on caregivers. The information received from a long-term-care facility should contain the patient's physical history, including information about prior health conditions, prescribed medications, and use of therapy. The patient's social history, such as involved family members, visits from friends, and involvement with activities within the center may also be documented. Finally, a long-term-care facility should provide information about the patient's level of care, that is, whether he or she is in assisted living; requires acute medical care; is completely dependent on staff for activities; or needs to remain in a secured unit, such as those designed for clients with memory loss and dementia.

Signs of Decreased Health Literacy Among Older Adults

Health literacy is defined among patients as the ability to understand health information as presented in order to make informed decisions about one's own health. A person's level of education is not necessarily indicative of health literacy. Nurses must assess for health literacy among older adults to avoid miscommunication, which could potentially cause safety issues, unnecessary treatments, and increased costs. Potential signs of decreased health literacy among older adults include an unwillingness to read or discuss informational materials as presented, forms and paperwork filled out incorrectly, an inability to explain health status or reasons for procedures, deferment to others to make decisions or talk to physicians, distracted or uninterested behavior regarding health care, and perceived noncompliance with medication use or treatment regimens.

Malnutrition

Risk Factors

There are a number of risk factors for malnutrition amongst the elderly population:

- **Hypermetabolism** resulting from various diseases, such as AIDS, and trauma, stress, or infection
- **Weight loss**, especially sudden or loss of 10% of normal weight over a 3-month period
- **Low body weight** of <90% of ideal body weight for age
- **Low body mass index (BMI)** <18.5
- **Immunosuppressive drugs** that interfere with absorption of nutrients
- **Malabsorption** of nutrients caused by diseases, such as chronic failure of kidneys or liver
- **Changes in appetite** that decrease intake of nutrients
- **Food intolerances**, such as lactose intolerance, resulting from lack of enzymes needed to completely digest food so it can be absorbed into the blood stream from the small intestine
- **Dietary restrictions**, such as limiting of protein with kidney failure
- **Functional limitations**, such as inability to feed oneself
- **Lack of teeth or dentures**, limiting intake
- **Alterations of taste or smell** that render food unpalatable

Indications in Older Adults

The assessment of the patient's physical and psychosocial conditions can uncover evidence of **malnutrition** that may be causing complications for the older adult. The nurse can look for warning signs of malnutrition by completing a physical exam and asking the patient some basic questions about his/her diet and eating habits. Warning signs of potential malnutrition include weight loss or low body mass index (BMI); broken or missing teeth, mouth pain, or ill-fitting dentures; immobility and diminished levels of activity, which could result in decreased abilities to access food; polypharmacy; gastrointestinal illness; and increased alcohol consumption.

Poor Hygiene

Poor hygiene in older adults increases the risk of disease and infection and is often attributed to physical impairment (such as poor vision or decreased mobility), depression, or cognitive impairment (Alzheimer's disease or substance abuse). Many older adults may require assistance with hygiene:

- While older adults don't need daily baths, they should bathe 2-3 times weekly. Grab bars, shower or tub seats, tub mats, handheld showers, and proper heating (to avoid chilling the patient) can facilitate more frequent bathing. Mild soap and bath oil may reduce drying of skin. Patients who are fearful of tubs and showers, common with dementia, may receive a sponge bath or Comfort Bath with pre-moistened, warmed towelettes.
- Clothing that is easy to manipulate (such as pull-on pants rather than those with zippers and buttons) and Velcro openings may make it easier for older adults to change clothes.
- Thick-handled toothbrushes or electric toothbrushes may facilitate mouth care.

Companionship

Companionship is a critical need for all ages, but many older adults have little or no companionship even though they may have regular contact with other people. This is especially true for those in nursing homes. Companionship entails talking together, sharing interests, and establishing a relationship based on friendship. Older adults are often quite isolated and may have outlived spouse and friends or are unable to engage in social activities. Caregivers and family may focus on physical needs to the detriment of emotional needs. Some organizations (Friendly Visitors) provide volunteers to visit older adults, and this can provide some degree of companionship, but nurses should discuss this need with the patient and family members, and when time permits, should take even a few minutes to sit and just talk with the patient. Older adults, even those with cognitive impairment, are often eager for interaction and want to share their memories and life stories.

Loneliness and Social Isolation

Social isolation is a pervasive problem and correlates with feelings of **loneliness**. As people age, their sphere of social activity narrows as family (spouse, children, and siblings) and peers die, move to nursing homes, or relocate. Loneliness is especially common among the widowed and, surprisingly, those living with children. Social isolation and loneliness are exacerbated by disease and anxiety. Older adults often have very little interaction with others and may have few visits from family or friends. Loneliness leads to stress-related disorders, such as hypertension, cardiovascular disease, and severe diabetes mellitus. Studies have shown that older women tend to be more isolated than men but that men suffer from more acute loneliness than women. According to the CDC, loneliness and social isolation increase an elderly adult's risk of dementia by 50%, suggesting that loneliness may affect the neurological system negatively. Interventions that are most effective include group activities (social and educational) that allow older adults to interact with others.

Self-Esteem

Low self-esteem is a common problem among older adults who have to deal with so many physical, environmental, and emotional changes. As they lose more and more autonomy, many older adults retreat into depression, passivity, and increasing dependency, feeling that they have nothing to contribute. They may become careless with grooming and exhibit poor hygiene, express negative feelings about themselves ("I'm so dumb"), slump in a posture of defeat, and avoid eye contact. They may fail to complete activities or chores. Strategies to help people **regain self-esteem** include the following:

- Provide companionship and find time to listen to and interact with patients, allowing them time to reminisce. Patients often want to share their life stories, and this helps them to feel their life has had value.
- Provide opportunities for patients to make decisions, and then respect their choices.
- Give positive feedback when earned.
- Ask patients about their feelings and encourage them to express their concerns.

Loss of Independence and Autonomy

The loss of independence and autonomy associated with aging is profoundly disturbing to many older adults:

- Losing independent living increases overall dependency on others, especially if older adults must live with family members or in a long-term care facility.
- Losing the ability to drive can prevent older adults from shopping and engaging in social activities and may increase symptoms of depression. Many people, especially males, do not willingly give up driving and are forced to do so because of safety concerns by family or physicians, and they may become very angry and resentful.
- Role reversal may occur as older adults' children become their care providers and increasingly make decisions for them. This may cause conflicts that are draining to both parties, and some older adults become increasingly dependent and demanding.
- Assistance with IADLs and ADLs is often necessary but may be resisted by the older adult who wants to remain autonomous.

Human Sexuality

Human sexuality is important to adults of all ages. Older adults need and often crave intimacy with others, including sexual intimacy. The intimacy needs of older adults should be addressed by healthcare providers directly during history and physical exams as patients may be embarrassed or reluctant to ask questions. Nurses should not avoid the topic because of personal anxiety and should respect different attitudes and behavior. Assessment should be done in private, ensuring confidentiality. Questioning should progress from general topics ("Do you have a good relationship with your partner?") to more specific questions related to sexual issues ("Is intercourse comfortable for you?"). Older adults may need to know how to deal with physical or environmental limitations. Some older adults engage in risky sexual behavior, putting them at increased risk of HIV or STDs because of decreased immune function, so discussing sexual issues provides an opportunity for education and counseling.

Inappropriate Sexual Behavior

Older adults with dementia or cognitive impairment may exhibit **inappropriate sexual behavior.** They may undress, masturbate, request sexual favors, use obscene language, and behave aggressively. The reason for this regression is not clear and behavior may be out of character for the individual but prompted by a lack of inhibition and decreased reasoning ability. This behavior may be of brief duration during a phase or may persist for prolonged periods (months or years). In some cases, such as disrobing publicly, the person may simply be hot or need to urinate/defecate. People may disrobe and urinate or defecate in inappropriate places, such as a wastebasket, in response to physical need. If people become sexually violent, medication may be prescribed to try to manage behavior, but, in general, medication does little to alleviate inappropriate behavior. Inappropriate behavior is best managed by supervision, distracting the patient, and watching for patterns (such as pulling at clothes) that occur with inappropriate behavior in order to prevent or manage the behavior.

Recreational Drug Use

Illicit/recreational drug use is expected to increase amongst the elderly population as more long-term users (baby boomer generation) are entering older age, and methadone programs and better treatment for HIV/AIDS have prolonged the lives of illicit drug users, many of whom in the past would not have lived to an older age. The stress of dealing with aging and chronic illness causes some older adults to turn to recreational drugs to reduce stress or relieve symptoms. Marijuana (the most frequently abused recreational drug), often taken for "health" reasons, may impair short-term memory, executive functioning, and attention. Treatment for drug use includes behavioral therapy and 12-step programs, although programs specifically designed for older adults are usually more successful.

Prescription Drug Abuse

Abuse of prescription drugs includes taking too few, taking too many, or taking drugs erratically. Older adults, especially women, are particularly vulnerable to abuse of prescription drugs because they have easy access to them (about a third of all prescriptions are for older adults). Because many older adults are isolated and have infrequent contact with healthcare providers, symptoms of prescription drug abuse (such as confusion, falls, or lethargy) may be overlooked or attributed to health conditions, such as Alzheimer's disease. People who abuse alcohol also frequently abuse prescription drugs, so assessment of alcohol abuse should include assessment for drug abuse as well. Over time, patients may seek prescriptions from a number of different doctors. Drugs most commonly abused include narcotic analgesics taken to control chronic pain and CNS depressants to reduce anxiety and improve sleep. Patients often deny abuse of drugs even though evidence is clear. Treatment may include behavioral therapy, medications to relieve withdrawal symptoms, and 12-step or other recovery programs.

Alcohol Abuse

All patients should be assessed for alcohol abuse as part of the initial history and physical exam as well as at subsequent visits, especially if there are health indications (abnormal liver function tests, falls, insomnia) or social indications (family problems, divorce, job loss). There are numerous self-assessment screening tools that ask the patient a number of questions about the frequency and amount of drinking as well as negative consequences. About a third of older adult alcoholics began drinking at an older age, often in response to depression. Social drinking is common in retirement facilities, but alcohol often interacts with drugs and can lead to complications. While studies indicate there may be some health benefits to low consumption of wine, drinking should be guided by the physician after review of medications. The nurse should discuss the assessment and score with the patient and provide information about resources (such as Alcoholics Anonymous and alcohol rehabilitation programs) and health consequences of drinking.

Tobacco Abuse

About 8% of adults over the age of 65 use **tobacco** (primarily cigarettes), and many more are former smokers. Older adult smokers are at particular risk because they often have smoked for more than 40 years and are heavy smokers. Smoking causes 90% of COPD. Smokers are at least two times more likely to die of a stroke or heart attack than non-smokers. Smoking reduces life expectancy by 13-15 years, so patients at any age should be advised to quit completely as quitting can prolong life and improve the quality of life. Simply reducing the use of tobacco has little health benefit, and use usually increases again after a time. Many long-term smokers have numerous health problems related to smoking but are extremely resistant to quitting because of tobacco's addictive qualities. Patients who abuse other substances (alcohol, drugs) are particularly at risk of burns if they fall asleep while smoking.

Addiction in the Elderly Population

Sexual Addiction

Sexual addiction occurs when people become fixated on sex, arousal, and thrill seeking rather than intimacy, often causing them to seek sexual relations with multiple partners (sometimes younger), including prostitutes. Sexual addiction may also take the form of masturbation in response to internet pornography or inappropriate behavior, such as masturbating in public or exposing oneself. Sexual addiction that involves multiple partners increases the danger of both contracting and spreading STDs. Viagra (and other such drugs), while not a cause of sexual addiction, can fuel sexual addiction in males. **Indications of sex addiction** include the following:

- Increasing need for sexual stimulation
- Inability to control urges
- Engaging in more high-risk activities (such as increased contact with prostitutes)
- Utilizing sexual fantasies to cope with stress
- Mood swings
- Neglecting social obligations, family, and friends

Most people are reluctant to disclose sexual addiction, but it should be assessed in those with STDs or those found engaging in inappropriate behavior. Behavioral therapy is indicated.

Gambling Addiction

Older adults often have easy access to gambling (e.g., lotteries, casinos, and online). They may turn to gambling as an outlet for frustration or stress and may not understand the dynamics of addiction before they have squandered their savings. Because of the difficulty finding employment, older adults may not be able to earn money to replace their gambling losses, resulting in increased poverty and stress. Older adults with cognitive impairment may not completely understand the implications of losing money in gambling. Gambling problems may be difficult to identify as older adults may hide gambling because of the stigma attached to it, and they are often reluctant to seek counseling or programs to help them stop gambling. **Signs of gambling** include the following:

- Increased focus on gambling to the exclusion of other activities, including hiding gambling and arguing about gambling with family/friends
- Physical effects such as headaches, increased anxiety, depression, bowel and bladder problems, and constant tiredness
- Financial concerns and lack of basic needs (food, clothing)

Health Promotion: Health Assessment/Data Collection

Data Collection and General Survey

Organs That Maintain Homeostasis in the Body

The organs of homeostatic function include the following:

- **Lungs**: The lungs help maintain acid-base balance by releasing CO_2. They also remove water via expired air.
- **Kidneys**: The kidneys maintain fluid balance in the body by filtering the blood and releasing fluid as needed. Electrolyte levels are maintained in the same way. Wastes and toxins are removed from the blood and body in the urine. The pH of the blood is maintained via the retention of hydrogen ions.
- **Heart**: The heart must pump blood with sufficient force to properly perfuse all organs and to push enough blood through the kidneys for filtering.
- **Adrenal glands**: Aldosterone and cortisol are produced by the adrenals to cause the kidneys to retain sodium and fluids.
- **Pituitary gland**: The pituitary stores and releases antidiuretic hormone (ADH) from the hypothalamus to direct the kidneys to retain fluids to maintain cellular osmotic pressure.
- **Parathyroid glands**: Parathyroid hormone maintains calcium and phosphate levels by causing calcium absorption by the intestines and renal tubules and from the bones as needed.

Daily Gain and Loss of Fluids

The body's fluid gains and losses should be about equal on a daily basis to maintain fluid and electrolyte balance. This can be monitored by measuring **intake** and **output** (I&O), but a number of other factors must be considered as well:

Fluid gains are as follows:

- Food people eat each day contains about 1000 mL of fluid.
- Fluids they drink average 1300 mL per day.
- Metabolic processes produce about 300 mL of fluid per day.

Fluid losses are as follows:

- Fluid is lost via the kidneys by production of 1–2 L of urine daily.
- The skin sweats and this evaporates an average of 600 mL daily, but this can increase up to 1000 mL/hr in hot and dry climates, during fever, during exercise or as a result of burns. Fluid loss can decrease in hot humid conditions.
- Exhaled air accounts for 300–400 mL of fluid loss daily.
- Fluids lost in stools total about 100–200 mL daily.

COMPONENTS OF HEALTH HISTORY

There are several different components that must be included in a nursing **health history**:

- The **biographic element** of the nursing health history includes the patient's name, age, physical address, sex, marital status, occupational status, religious preference, healthcare financing, and regular physician.
- The **chief complaint** is the next aspect of the history and involves the reason the patient is seeking care.
- Following this, the **history of the present illness** details the current health problem, including date of onset, description of symptoms, and any aggravating factors.
- **Past medical history** entails asking about the patient's usual health status, past medical or surgical problems, immunization status, current medications, allergies (including medication allergies), and family history.
- A detailed **family history** is important as it may reveal risk factors for certain medical conditions such as heart disease, diabetes, arthritis, hypertension, or mental disorders.
- The **review of systems** is used to obtain a full, systematic report by the patient on subjective symptoms. For example, in inquiring about the cardiovascular system, the nurse notes positive or negative answers regarding chest pain and other symptoms or problems that are pertinent to heart function and circulation.

SOCIAL DETERMINANTS OF HEALTH

Social determinants of health refer to the non-medical elements of a person's social environment that have a direct impact on his or her physical health and tendencies. The heavy influence of this component of health is reflected in its being listed as one of the five main sections of *Healthy People 2030,* an initiative of the US Department of Health and Human Services (HHS) that aims to allow people to have longer and healthier lives, to reduce health disparities, to create environments that promote health, and to improve the quality of life and health across all age groups. According to HHS, social determinants of health are "the conditions in the environments where people are born, live, learn, work, play, worship, and age that affect a wide range of health, functioning, and quality-of-life outcomes and risks." For these reasons, a health history should inquire into the patient's social determinants of health also:

- The patient's **lifestyle** is an important component of the nursing health history and includes habits, diet, sleep, hobbies, and the patient's ability to perform the activities of daily living.
- A **social history** is the component of the nursing health history that details family relationships, ethnicity, educational level, economic status, and the condition of the patient's home and environment.
- The nursing health history also includes the patient's **psychological status** and the patient's **usual means of obtaining healthcare.**

Obtaining a Health History

The health history assessment and review of systems help to identify nursing care needs:

- First, check the patient's chart for information gathered by other health professionals and note any areas that need clarification prior to the patient interview.
- Use the written or electronic template provided by the facility to record the history, customizing it to the patient.
- Record any changes in this information during the patient's hospital stay.
- Plan the time of the interview with the patient when there are not critical care needs that must be met first.
- Take time to alleviate patient's anxiety and establish rapport and trust.
- Approach the patient with an attitude of respect and sincere caring.
- Listen to the patient and use effective therapeutic communication skills during the interview.
- Review all areas of the health history with the patient and then ask for any other information that may be important. The family may be able to fill in missing information if the patient is unable to do so.

Physical Examination Techniques

The **physical exam** is an important element of nursing assessment. The physical assessment needs to be organized and systematic and should be age- and developmentally-appropriate. The physical exam may be a complete physical exam, a system-specific exam, or an exam of a specific body part. The basic **techniques** of a physical exam are inspection, palpation, auscultation, and percussion. The nurse makes a visual, aural, and olfactory assessment of the patient. This includes paying attention to the patient's skin tone, breathing sounds, and breath odor. Palpation includes techniques for touching the patient's body in order to get physical information such as temperature, skin tone and condition, or swelling in the glands. Auscultation is the examination of sounds within the body, such as heart tones, wheezing or crackling in the lungs, or bowel sounds. Auscultation is usually performed with a stethoscope. Percussion involves making quick taps to parts of the body with the fingers to ascertain the shape and condition of organs, identify areas of tenderness, or assess reflexes.

Palpation

Use of palpation can provide valuable details during physical assessment of the patient:

- Be sure to wash and warm the hands prior to touching the patient.
- Do not use gloves unless you anticipate contact with bodily fluids.
- Explain the process and how it will feel and instruct the patient to relax the muscles if appropriate. Provide warmth and privacy during palpation.
- Use light palpation to feel the cervical lymph nodes and thyroid glands and to feel the superficial blood vessels for thrills.
- Place your hands on the chest to detect heart vibrations and to feel tactile fremitus during speech.
- Palpate the relaxed abdomen to identify structures and their borders and any masses or nodules on otherwise smooth organ surfaces. Of note, the abdomen should be auscultated prior to palpation since palpation may cause bowel sounds that would not otherwise exist and may be misunderstood.
- Utilize both hands to palpate the female reproductive organs by pushing organs into the reach of the other hand.

Palpation to identify organs and structures takes practice. Each patient is different but after you palpate many patients, the similarities in organ borders and consistency can be determined.

Palpating for Tactile Fremitus

The act of speaking causes the chest wall to vibrate. This vibration can be felt by placing your hands lightly on the chest wall over a section of the lungs bilaterally while the patient repeats the letter "e" or the numbers "99." The amount of vibration felt depends on the weight of the patient, the muscle mass of the chest and back, gender, deepness of the voice, and condition of the lungs. **Tactile fremitus** is greater over major airways and normal lung tissue. It is less over lungs full of air or with emphysema or a pneumothorax. Lung consolidation will produce increased fremitus. The nurse should not feel for fremitus over the sternum or scapula. The areas above and below the breasts and above, medial to, and below the scapulae should be tested.

Percussion

Percussion is striking part of the body to set the chest or abdominal wall into motion, producing sound that helps to locate underlying organs and reveal whether they are dense or filled with air or fluid. The sounds produced include:

- **Tympany**: Hollow drum sound produced when the organ contains air (stomach, intestines)
- **Resonance**: Hollow, low-pitched sound of normal lungs
- **Hyperresonance**: Low-pitched sound of lungs with emphysema or pneumothorax (louder than resonance)
- **Dullness**: "thud" heard over dense structures such as the liver
- **Flatness**: sound heard over muscles or bones such as in the thigh

Percussion is performed by placing the middle finger of one hand over the area and striking it with the middle finger of the opposite hand. It can be used to find the margins of an organ or area of pathology by repeatedly striking areas near to each other and listening for changes in sound representing the edge of the organ. The extent of lung consolidation can be determined in this manner.

Auscultation

Auscultation is listening to sounds within the body through either the bell or the diaphragm of the stethoscope. These sounds differ in the following ways:

- **Intensity**: The level of sound in terms of loudness
- **Frequency**: Low or high pitch of the sound
- **Quality**: Helps to distinguish between rumbling and musical-type sounds

The **bell** of the stethoscope is best when listening for the lower frequency sounds of heart murmurs or bruit, with the bell placed lightly on the skin. The **diaphragm** is best for high-pitched sounds, such as heart or lung sounds or bowel sounds, with the diaphragm placed firmly on the skin. The nurse should not touch the tubing or place the end of the stethoscope in contact with cloth or hair, or extra sounds will be heard that may obscure the sounds transmitted.

Vital Signs

Stable Vital Signs

Stable vital signs (those maintained within the normal range for the individual's age) indicate good health (homeostasis). Ill or injured patients have vital signs outside the normal range. The severity of the illness or injury is often indicated by the variability of vital sign measurements. Wide variations mean the patient is unstable. Their vital signs should be checked every five minutes. For stable patients, vital signs can be checked less frequently, depending on the circumstance. The following parameters are considered vital signs:

- Pulse
- Respiration rate
- Blood pressure
- Oxygen saturation
- Temperature

Review Video: Vital Signs and How to Check Them
Visit mometrix.com/academy and enter code: 330799

Pulse

The pulse is a surge of blood through an artery that occurs when the heart contracts (during systole). The key **pulse points** are:

- **Apical**: Over the heart
- **Brachial**: In the elbow bend (most common site for palpation in children under 1 year)
- **Carotid**: In the neck (for pulse checks in unconscious patients; be sure to only palpate one side at a time to maintain perfusion to the brain)
- **Dorsalis pedis**: On top of the foot
- **Facial**: On the jaw under the mouth
- **Femoral**: In the groin (for pulse checks in unconscious patients)
- **Popliteal**: On the back of the knee
- **Posterior tibial**: On the back of the ankle
- **Radial**: On the anterior wrist below the thumb (most common site for palpation in patients older than 1 year)
- **Temporal**: On the temple
- **Ulnar**: On the anterior wrist below the little finger

Pulse **rate** varies by age:

Normal Resting Pulse Rate	Age
60-100 beats per minute	Adult
80-100 beats per minute	Child
100 beats per minute	Toddler
100-140 beats per minute	Infant under one year
up to 150 beats per minute	Newborn (neonate)

Distal Pulse and Pulse Deficit

If a **distal pulse** cannot be felt in the patient's limbs, first utilize a doppler machine to find the pulse. If it still cannot be found, find the apical pulse in the chest. Count to the 5th rib space in the middle of the left side of the chest or midclavicular line. If the apical pulse is regular, count for 30 seconds and record the reading. If the apical pulse is irregular, count for a full minute and record the reading. Report an irregular pulse to the doctor to evaluate for possible pulse deficit. A **pulse deficit** occurs when the radial pulse in the wrist is slower than the apical pulse in the chest. A pulse deficit can indicate that the patient has weak heart contractions, which fail to transmit beats to the peripheral arterial system.

Tachycardia and Bradycardia

Tachycardia is a pulse rate over 100 beats per minute, which may be caused by anxiety, fear, stress, pneumonia, anemia, low blood pressure, dehydration, fever, infection, hyperthyroidism, and heart conditions.

Bradycardia is a resting heart rate less than 60 beats per minute, which may be caused by a heart attack (MI), hypothermia, heat exhaustion, obstructive jaundice, skull fracture, malnutrition, hypothyroidism, and many adverse drug reactions. Olympic athletes may have bradycardia because their hearts are extremely efficient.

Measuring Respirations

Measuring respirations is done to assess the number of times per minute the patient breathes. Typically, when a person is made aware of his breathing, he does not breathe deeply or regularly. Do not tell the patient when measuring the respiration rate, as it may make them aware of their breathing and produce an inaccurate result. The ideal time to measure the patient's respiration rate is after checking the patient's pulse. Count the number of times the patient breathes, counting one rise and fall of the chest wall as one respiration. Count the number of breaths for one minute, noting the depth of the breath and any use of accessory muscles. Record the respiratory rate on the patient's chart.

Indications of Abnormal Respirations

The normal range for respiratory rate for adults is 12-20 breaths per minute. A number of factors may affect the rate of the patient's breathing. The patient may breathe more slowly if resting or if he is positioned on his back. Certain narcotics may also depress the respiratory drive, resulting in fewer breaths per minute. A rapid respiration rate may be caused by increased activity, pain, or stress. An elevated temperature or an infection may cause the patient's respiratory rate to be quicker. Other conditions, such as respiratory distress, fluid overload, or a heart attack, may also cause an elevated respiratory rate.

Blood Pressure

Increased blood pressure contributes to stroke and heart disease. Low blood pressure is associated with shock, trauma, bleeding, or severe infection. Blood pressure is defined by the following parameters:

- Normal adult blood pressure: Systole <120 mmHg, diastole <80 mmHg
- Prehypertension: Systole 120-129, diastole <80
- Hypertension stage 1: Systole 130-139, diastole 80-89
- Hypertension stage 2: Systole ≥140, diastole ≥90
- Hypotension (low blood pressure): 90/50 or less

False BP reading can occur from the following:

- **Incorrect cuff size**: If the patient is obese, use a thigh cuff on the upper arm. Bariatric blood pressure cuffs also exist. If the patient is a child, use a pediatric cuff.
- **Deflating the cuff more rapidly** than 2–3 mmHg per second can inhibit the ability to accurately record both systole and diastole.
- **Venous congestion** makes it difficult to hear the blood pressure sounds. Elevating the patient's arm after positioning the cuff but before inflating it can decrease venous congestion.
- Loud **environmental noises**
- **Operator error**

Aneroid Sphygmomanometer

Blood pressure is measured as systolic and diastolic pressure by means of a stethoscope and an **aneroid sphygmomanometer** (portable blood pressure cuff). For example, if the reading is 120/80 mmHg, 120 is the systole, and 80 is the diastole. The first Korotkoff sound the medical assistant hears is the systole; the last Korotkoff sound is the diastole. Position the blood pressure cuff so it is 1-2 cm from the antecubital fossa and two fingers can slide between the cuff and the arm. The width of the cuff bladder should exceed the diameter of the patient's arm by 20% or more. Place the stethoscope's diaphragm over the patient's brachial artery of the same arm, and insert the earpieces into one's ears. Inflate the cuff quickly, in 7 seconds or less. Deflate the blood pressure cuff slowly, at a rate of 2-3 mmHg per second. Listen for the "lub" and "dub," while mentally noting the mmHg when each sound was made. Remove the cuff and stethoscope. Record the measurement in the patient's chart immediately.

Review Video: Diastolic vs Systolic
Visit mometrix.com/academy and enter code: 898934

Oxygen Saturation

Pulse oximetry non-invasively measures a patient's oxyhemoglobin (oxygen saturation) level using a small clip-like device with a light that measures the oxygen saturation of the site it is attached to. This is a painless method of monitoring an individual's respiratory status and perfusion over a period of time when attached continuously, or in a single moment as part of a physical assessment. Attach the oximeter sensor to one of the patient's first three fingers (index, middle or ring). If the patient's hands are damaged, use a toe or earlobe. Consider using the forehead, nose, or other parts of the foot only as a last resort. Normal range should fall between 95% and 100%, although patients with certain conditions, such as COPD, may have a chronically lower saturation. If a patient's oxygen saturation falls below normal range persistently, the medical assistant must inform the doctor that the patient is hypoxic. Many pulse oximeters also measure the patient's heart rate at the same time. A pulse oximeter is not accurate if the patient is very anemic, has poor circulation (due to being cold or having vascular abnormalities), is edematous, moves a lot, or wears artificial nails or very dark nail polish. Adjust the room temperature, lighting, and move electronic equipment to get a good reading.

Body Temperature

A live patient's body temperature is measured to determine if he or she is storing and releasing heat properly, to detect abnormally high or low body temperatures, and to assess the effectiveness of some types of medications. The coroner measures temperature to determine time of death. Adult normal temperature ranges are as follows:

- Normal range: 97-99 °F (36.1-37.2 °C)
- Hypothermia (too cold): <95 °F (<35 °C)
- Pyrexia (fever): >100.4 °F (>38 °C)
- Hyperpyrexia (lethal fever): >106.7 °F (>41.5 °C)

Temperature is at its lowest around 4:00 a.m. and highest around 6:00 p.m. Temperature spikes often occur after meals. Ovulation in women creates a temperature rise of 0.5-1.0 °F when measured before arising from bed in the morning (basal body temperature). Individual temperature differences in healthy people are due to the rate of metabolism. Patients with hypothyroidism tend to be cold. Body temperature differs at different sites. Normal oral temperature is 98.6 °F, while rectal temperature is 0.5-1.0 °F higher than oral temperature, and axillary temperature is usually 0.5-1.0 °F lower than oral temperature. Do not take the patient's oral temperature for 30 minutes after eating or drinking, as it will be raised with hot food, and lowered with cold drinks.

Head and Neck

Eye Assessment

Assessment of the eyes includes:

- **History**: Ask about blurring, blind spots, floaters, night blindness, halos, pain, photophobia, tearing, allergies, previous ocular problems, use of glasses or contact lenses, and changes in depth perception.
- **Extraocular muscles**: Ask patient to stare straight ahead and shine light from 12 inches. Reflection of light on the corneas should be identical on both eyes. Asymmetry indicates muscle weakness or paralysis.
- **External inspection**: Note symmetry. Use thumbs to pull lower lids down and ask patient to look upward and elevate upper lid at outer aspect and ask patient to look down to examine conjunctiva and sclera. Note redness, pallor, cyanosis, swelling, or excessive tearing. In darkened room, note pupillary response to light and size and symmetry. In lighted room, ask patient to look at a distance and then at an item 8 inches from eyes. Note pupillary constriction and convergence.
- **Ocular fundus (ophthalmoscope)**: Darken room, remove patient's eyeglasses, ask patient to stare at distant object, anchor upper eyelid, hold instrument 10 inches from patient at 15° lateral to patient's line of vision. Note the red reflex and move slowly toward patient, noting abnormalities, such as opaque areas (cataracts), and inspect the optic disc, retinal vessels, and macula.

Vision Assessment

Assessment of vision includes:

- **Visual acuity**: Leave glasses or contact lenses in place and position the patient 20 feet from Snellen chart and shield one eye at a time, asking patient to read the chart down to the smallest line, and record that line as a numeric fraction to indicate errors.
- **Near vision**: Ask patient to read vision screener with text in different sizes. Hold screener approximately 14 inches from the eyes and test one eye at a time with the patient wearing usual glasses or contact lenses.
- **Visual fields**: Stand 2 feet in front of the patient at eye level and ask the patient to look straight ahead and cover one eye. Advance an item (finger, pencil) from the periphery toward the midline from multiple directions and ask the patient to note when the item is first seen. Estimate the angles. Normal findings: upward 50°, temporally 90°, downward 70°, and nasally 60°.

Ear and Hearing Assessment

Assessment of the ears includes:

- **External ear**: Observe for symmetry, size, shape, erythema, crusting, scaling, and discoloration. Move the pinna and tragus to see if they are tender (otitis externa).
- **External ear canal**: Note size, evidence of edema, erythema, or discharge.
- **Internal ear canal and eardrum**: Use an otoscope. Pull the pinna up and back (adults) or down (infants, children under 3) and tilt the patient's head slightly to the opposite side to straighten the ear canal. Insert the otoscope and rotate it to view the entire eardrum. Note any discharge, foreign bodies, edema, or erythema. Note the amount and color of cerumen. Examine the eardrum for color, contour, and perforations.
- **Hearing acuity (estimate)**: Occlude one ear at a time (with a finger), obscure the patient's vision, whisper softly toward the unoccluded ear from 1–2 feet away, using numbers or simple words with equally accented syllables (e.g., "baseball"). Increase intensity of whispers as needed.

Tuning fork tests:

- **Weber test**: Place a vibrating tuning fork on top of the patient's head and ask where sound is heard (should be equal in both ears). An abnormal finding may indicate either conductive or sensorineural hearing loss.
- **Rinne test**: Place a vibrating tuning fork on the mastoid process and measure duration of sound. Then place a tuning fork at the external ear canal. Sound is normally heard twice as long through air as through bone.

Nose and Sense of Smell Assessment

Assessment of the nose and smell includes:

- **History**: Ask about any nasal discharge, frequent URIs, sinusitis, PND, pain, history of trauma, nosebleeds, allergies, and changes in the sense of smell.
- **External inspection**
  - Anterior: Assess nose symmetry or deviation.
  - Lateral: Assess shape.
  - Inferior: Assess the nasal vestibule, applying gentle upward pressure on the tip of the nose to widen the nostrils, noting any difference in size or pain that may indicate local infection.
- **Internal inspection**: Maintaining gentle pressure on the tip, use a penlight to observe for signs of redness, polyps, deviation, or swelling. For further examination, use a nasal speculum or an otoscope, using care to rest the device against the alae nasi (outer aspect) rather than the septum.
- **Obstruction**: Compress one nostril at a time and ask patient to breathe in and note any impaired airflow. Place a flat metal tool beneath the nostrils and ask patient to breathe out and observe for equal misting.
- **Smell (olfactory nerve)**: Ask the patient to close their eyes, and hold one nostril at a time closed. Place an item with a familiar smell (vanilla, alcohol pad, coffee) beneath the nose at approximately 2 cm and ask the patient to identify.

Mouth and Throat Assessment

Assessment of the mouth and throat includes:

- **Preparation**: Ask the patient to remove lipstick and any dentures.
- **Lips**: Note color, texture, moisture, symmetry, scaliness, cracks, and lesions.
- **Mucosa**: Use a tongue blade to improve visualization and note color, nodules, ulcerations, white patches, or other abnormalities.
- **Gums**: Note color and abnormalities such as a black line (lead poisoning), lesions, pallor, gingivitis.
- **Teeth**: Use a gloved thumb and index finger to check for absence of teeth, discoloration, misshapen teeth, or loose teeth.
- **Hard palate**: Note color and architecture. Note presence of *torus palatinus* (midline bony growth), including size and shape.
- **Tongue and floor of mouth**: Ask the patient to stick their tongue out and note symmetry, color, moisture, and texture. Note any ulcerations or nodules. Carefully inspect the sides by grasping the tongue tip with a gauze square and pulling tongue to the side, then palpate for any lesions. Examine the floor of the mouth.
- **Pharynx**: Ask the patient to open their mouth, relax their tongue, and say "ahhh." If visualization is inadequate, use a tongue blade at the midpoint of the tongue. Note that the soft palate rises (10th cranial nerve). Examine the soft palate, uvula, tonsils, and pharynx for signs of swelling, ulceration, pain, and asymmetry. Palpate any suspicious areas, if possible.

Assessment of the Neurological System

Assessment of the neurological system includes:

- Assess the **health history** for any trauma, falls, alcoholism, drug abuse, medications taken, and family history of neurological problems.
- Ask about any presenting **neurological symptoms**, the circumstances in which they occur, whether they fluctuate, and any associated factors, such as seizures, pain, vertigo, weakness, abnormal sensations, visual problems, loss of consciousness, changes in cognition, and motor problems.

Assessment includes determining the level of consciousness and cognition. Posture and movements are assessed for abnormalities. Facial expression and movement are noted. Cranial nerve assessment is done. The patient is assessed for strength, coordination, and balance and the ability to perform ADLs. One should assess for clonus and test all reflexes, including Babinski, gag, blink, swallow, upper and lower abdominal, cremasteric in males, plantar, perianal, biceps, triceps, brachioradialis, patellar and ankle. Peripheral sensation is tested by touching the patient with cotton balls and the sharp and dull ends of a broken tongue blade.

Review Video: What is the Function of the Nervous System
Visit mometrix.com/academy and enter code: 708428

Assessing Functional Status

Functional abilities include the acts needed to meet basic needs and perform *activities of daily living* (ADLs), such as eating and elimination, as well as those *activities that are essential to independent living* (IADLs), such as shopping. A thorough assessment of the patient's functional abilities will identify areas that should be concentrated upon during rehabilitation. One should observe the patient as he/she performs these functions and record the following:

- Degree of independence shown
- Ability to complete activity without rest
- Nerve function
- Muscle function and strength
- Motion
- Coordination
- Cardiac status
- Respiratory status
- Assistance required to complete activity

The facility usually provides one of the tools available to record a functional assessment. The most common tool used is the Functional Independence Measure (FIM). Other tools available include the Barthel Index, the PULSES Profile, and the Patient Evaluation Conference System.

ASA Classification System for the Extent of a Brain Attack Injury

The American Stroke Association developed a **brain attack outcome classification system** to standardize descriptions of stroke injuries:

- **Number of impaired domains** (Potentially affected neurological domains: motor, sensory, vision, language, cognition, and affect): Level 0: no domains impaired; Level 1: one domain impaired; Level 2: two domains impaired; Level 3: greater than 2 domains impaired.
- **Severity of impairment**: A (minimal or no neurological deficit due to stroke); B (mild/moderate deficit); or C (severe deficit). Note: When more than one domain is affected, severity is measured by the domain with the most impairment.

Assessment of function determines the ability to **live independently**:

- **I**: Independent in basic activities of daily living (BADL), such as bathing, eating, toileting, and walking; and instrumental activities of daily living (IADL), such as telephoning, shopping, maintaining a household, socializing, and using transportation
- **II**: Independent in BADL but partially dependent in IADL
- **III**: Partially dependent in BADL (less than 3 areas) and IADL
- **IV**: Partially dependent in BADL (3 or more areas)
- **V**: Completely dependent in BADL (5 or more areas) and IADL

Level III requires much assistance and Levels IV and V cannot live independently.

Administration of the NIHSS

The **National Institutes of Health Stroke Scale (NIHSS)** is administered with careful attention to directions. The examiner should record the answers and avoid coaching or repeating requests, although demonstration may be used with aphasic patients. The scale comprises 11 sections, with scores for each section ranging from 0 (normal) to 2, 3, or 4:

- **Level of consciousness**: Response to noxious stimulation (0–3), request for month and his/her age (0–2), request to open and close eyes, grip and release unaffected hand (0–2)
- **Best gaze**: Horizontal eye movement (0–2)
- **Visual**: Visual fields (0–3)

- **Facial palsy**: Symmetry when patient shows teeth, raises eyebrows, and closes eyes (0–3)
- **Motor, arm**: Drift while arm extended with palms down (0–4)
- **Motor, leg**: Leg drift at 30 degrees while patient supine (0–4)
- **Limb ataxia**: Finger-nose and heel-shin (0–2)
- **Sensory**: Grimace or withdrawal from pinprick (0–2)
- **Best language**: Describes action of pictures (0–3)
- **Dysarthria**: Reads or describes words on list (0–2)
- **Distinction and inattention**: Visual spatial neglect (0–2)

Glasgow Coma Scale

The Glasgow coma scale (GCS) measures the depth and duration of coma or impaired level of consciousness and is used for post-operative assessment. The GCS measures three parameters: best eye response, best verbal response, and best motor response, with a total possible score that ranges from 3 to 15:

Eye opening	4: Spontaneous 3: To verbal stimuli 2: To pain (not of face) 1: No response
Verbal	5: Oriented 4: Conversation confused, but can answer questions 3: Uses inappropriate words 2: Speech incomprehensible 1: No response
Motor	6: Moves on command 5: Moves purposefully respond pain 4: Withdraws in response to pain 3: Decorticate posturing (flexion) in response to pain 2: Decerebrate posturing (extension) in response to pain 1: No response

Injuries/conditions are classified according to the total score: 3–8 Coma; ≤8 Severe head injury likely requiring intubation; 9–12 Moderate head injury; 13–15 Mild head injury.

Review Video: Glasgow Coma Scale
Visit mometrix.com/academy and enter code: 133399

CRANIAL NERVES

	Name	Function	PE Test
I	Olfactory	Smell	Test olfaction
II	Optic	Visual acuity	Snellen eye chart; Accommodation
III	Oculomotor	Eye movement/pupil	Pupillary reflex; Eye/eyelid motion
IV	Trochlear	Eye movement	Eye moves down & out
V	Trigeminal	Facial motor/ sensory	Corneal reflex; Facial sensation; Mastication
VI	Abducens	Eye movement	Lateral eye motion
VII	Facial	Facial expression; Taste	Moves forehead, closes eyes, smile/frown, puffs cheeks; Taste
VIII	Vestibulo-cochlear (Acoustic)	Hearing; Balance	Hearing (Weber/Rinne tests); Nystagmus
IX	Glosso-pharyngeal	Pharynx motor/sensory	Gag reflex; Soft palate elevation
X	Vagus	Visceral sensory, motor	Gag, swallow, cough
XI	Accessory	Sternocleidomastoid and trapezius (motor)	Turns head & shrugs shoulders against resistance
XII	Hypoglossal	Tongue movement	Push out tongue; move tongue from side to side

Thorax, Heart, and Abdomen

Assessment of the Cardiovascular System

Cardiovascular assessment includes questioning the patient for any family history of death at a young age or other cardiovascular diseases. Elderly African-American males are at highest risk for cardiovascular problems. One must question the patient about edema, chest pain, dyspnea, fatigue, vertigo, syncope or other changes in consciousness, weight gain, and leg cramps or pain. If chest pain is a symptom, one must ask about the intensity, timing, location, any radiation, quality, meaning to the patient, factors that aggravate or alleviate the pain, nausea, dyspnea, diaphoresis, or any other accompanying symptoms. Physical assessment includes assessment of vital signs, heart and lung sounds, skin assessment, radial, popliteal, and pedal pulses, circulation and sensation of extremities, and auscultation of the aorta, renal, iliac, and femoral arteries for bruits. Blood should be taken for a lipid profile and electrolytes. The patient must be helped to modify risk factors such as hypertension, smoking, diabetes, obesity, hyperlipidemia, inactivity, and stress.

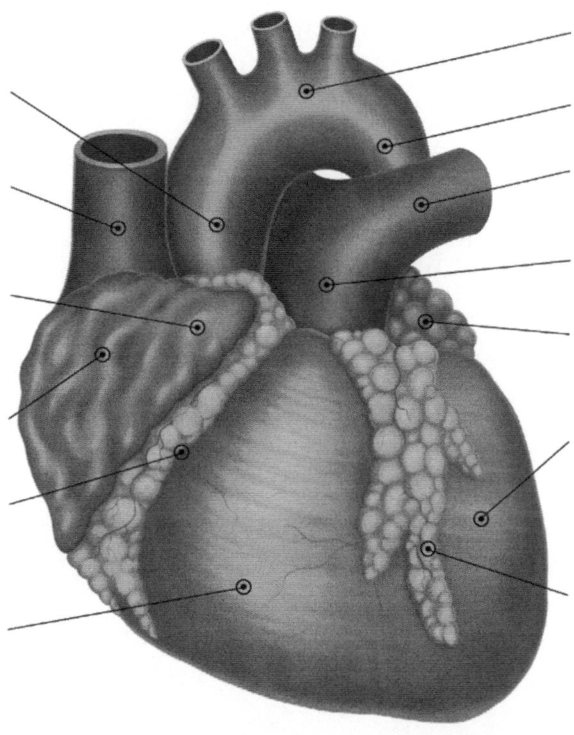

Review Video: Cardiovascular Assessment
Visit mometrix.com/academy and enter code: 323076

Review Video: Functions of the Circulatory System
Visit mometrix.com/academy and enter code: 376581

Review Video: Heart Blood Flow
Visit mometrix.com/academy and enter code: 783139

Review Video: Mnemonics for Heart Anatomy and Physiology
Visit mometrix.com/academy and enter code: 849489

Assessment of Heart Sounds

Auscultation of heart sounds can help to diagnose different cardiac disorders. Areas to auscultate include the aortic area, pulmonary area, Erb's point, tricuspid area, and the apical area. The **normal heart sounds** represent closing of the valves.

The **first heart sound** (S1) "lub" is closure of the mitral and tricuspid valves (heard at apex/left ventricular area of the heart).

The **second heart sound** (S2) "dub" is closure of the aortic and pulmonic valves (heard at the base of the heart). There may be a slight splitting of the S2.

The time between S1 and S2 is systole and the time between S2 and the next S1 is diastole. Systole and diastole should be silent although ventricular disease can cause gallops, snaps, or clicks and stenosis of the valves or failure of the valves to close can cause murmurs. Pericarditis may cause a friction rub.

Additional heart sounds:

- **Gallop rhythms**: S3 commonly occurs after S2 in children and young adults but may indicate heart failure or left ventricular failure in older adults (when heard with patient lying on left side). S4 occurs before S1, during the contracting of the atria when there is ventricular hypertrophy, found in coronary artery disease, hypertension, or aortic valve stenosis.
- **Opening snap**: Unusual high-pitched sound occurring after S2 with stenosis of mitral valve from rheumatic heart disease
- **Ejection click**: Brief high-pitched sound after S1; aortic stenosis
- **Friction rub**: Harsh, grating holosystolic sound; pericarditis
- **Murmur**: Sound caused by turbulent blood flow from stenotic or malfunctioning valves, congenital defects, or increased blood flow. Murmurs are characterized by location, timing in the cardiac cycle, intensity (rated from Grade I to Grade VI), pitch (low to high-pitched), quality (rumbling, whistling, blowing) and radiation (to the carotids, axilla, neck, shoulder, or back).

Review Video: Diastolic vs Systolic
Visit mometrix.com/academy and enter code: 898934

Cardiac Monitoring

Cardiac monitoring includes the evaluation of different intervals and segments on the electrocardiogram:

- **QT interval**: This is the complete time of ventricular depolarization and repolarization, which begins with the QRS segment and ends when the T wave is completed. Typically, duration usually ranges from 0.36–0.44 seconds, but this may vary depending on the heart rate. If the heat rate is rapid, the duration is shorter and vice versa. Certain medications can prolong the QT interval, in such cases monitoring this is critical. A prolonged QT interval puts the patient at risk for R-on-T phenomenon, which can result in dangerous arrhythmias.
- **ST segment**: This is an isoelectric period when the ventricles are in a plateau phase, completely depolarized and beginning recovery and repolarization. Deflection is usually isoelectric. If the ST segment is ≥0.5 mm below the baseline, it is considered depressed and may be an indication of myocardial ischemia. Depression may also indicate digitalis toxicity. If the ST segment is elevated ≥0.3 mm above baseline, this is an indication of myocardial injury.

MAP

The MAP **(mean arterial pressure)** is most commonly used to evaluate perfusion as it shows pressure throughout the cardiac cycle. Systole is one-third and diastole two-thirds of the normal cardiac cycle. The MAP for a blood pressure of 120/60 is calculated as follows:

$$\text{MAP} = \frac{\text{Diastole} \times 2 + \text{Systole}}{3} \frac{60 \times 2 + 120}{3} = \frac{240}{3} = 80$$

Normal range for mean arterial pressure is 70–100 mmHg. A MAP of greater than 60 mmHg is required to perfuse vital organs, including the heart, brain, and kidneys.

Oxygen Saturation as it Relates to Hemodynamic Status

Hemodynamic monitoring includes monitoring **oxygen saturation** levels, which must be maintained for proper cardiac function. The central venous catheter often has an oxygen sensor at the tip to monitor oxygen saturation in the right atrium.

- Increased oxygen saturation may result from left atrial to right atrial shunt, abnormal pulmonary venous return, increased delivery of oxygen or decrease in extraction of oxygen.
- Decreased oxygen saturation may be related to low cardiac output with an increase in oxygen extraction or decrease in arterial oxygen saturation with normal differences in the atrial and ventricular oxygen saturation.

Electrocardiogram

The electrocardiogram records and shows a graphic display of the electrical activity of the heart through a number of different waveforms, complexes, and intervals:

- **P wave**: Start of electrical impulse in the sinus node and spreading through the atria, muscle depolarization
- **QRS complex**: Ventricular muscle depolarization and atrial repolarization
- **T wave**: Ventricular muscle repolarization (resting state) as cells regain negative charge
- **U wave**: Repolarization of the Purkinje fibers

A modified lead II ECG is often used to monitor basic heart rhythms and dysrhythmias. Typical placement of leads for 2-lead ECG is 3–5 cm inferior to the right clavicle and left lower ribcage. Typical placement for a 3-lead ECG is (RA) right arm near shoulder, (LA) V_5 position over 5th intercostal space, and (LL) left upper leg near groin.

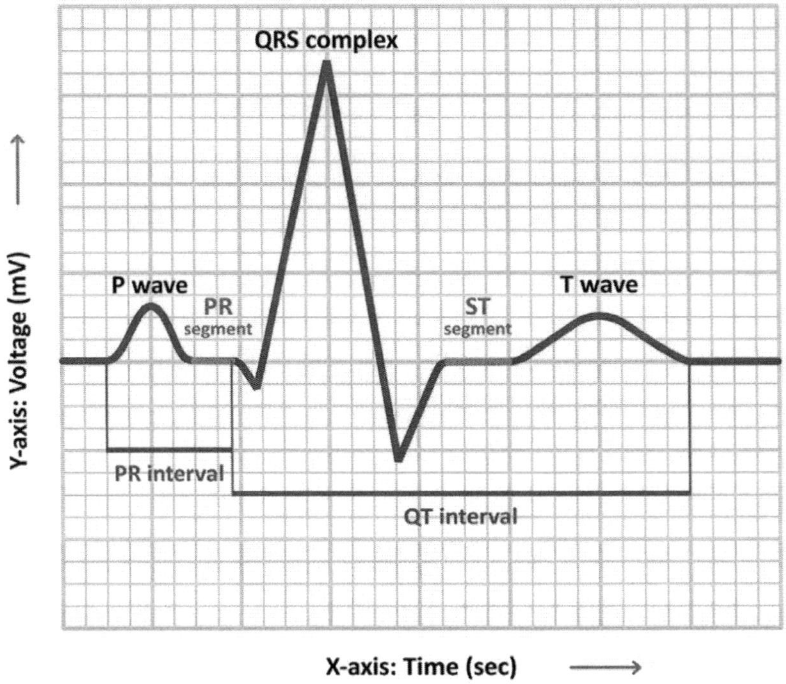

ADMINISTRATION OF 12-LEAD ECG

The electrocardiogram provides a graphic representation of the electrical activity of the heart. It is indicated for chest pain, dyspnea, syncope, acute coronary syndrome, pulmonary embolism, and possible MI. The standard **12 lead ECG** gives a picture of electrical activity from 12 perspectives through placement of 10 body leads:

- 4 limb leads are placed distally on the wrists and ankles (but may be placed more proximally if necessary).
- Precordial leads:
  - V1: Right sternal border at 4th intercostal space
  - V2: Left sternal border at 4th intercostal space
  - V3: Midway between V2 and V4
  - V4: Left midclavicular line at 5th intercostal space
  - V5: Horizontal to V4 at left anterior axillary line
  - V6: Horizontal to V5 at left midaxillary line

In some cases, additional leads may be used:

- Right-sided leads are placed on the right in a mirror image of the left leads, usually to diagnose right ventricular infarction through ST elevation.

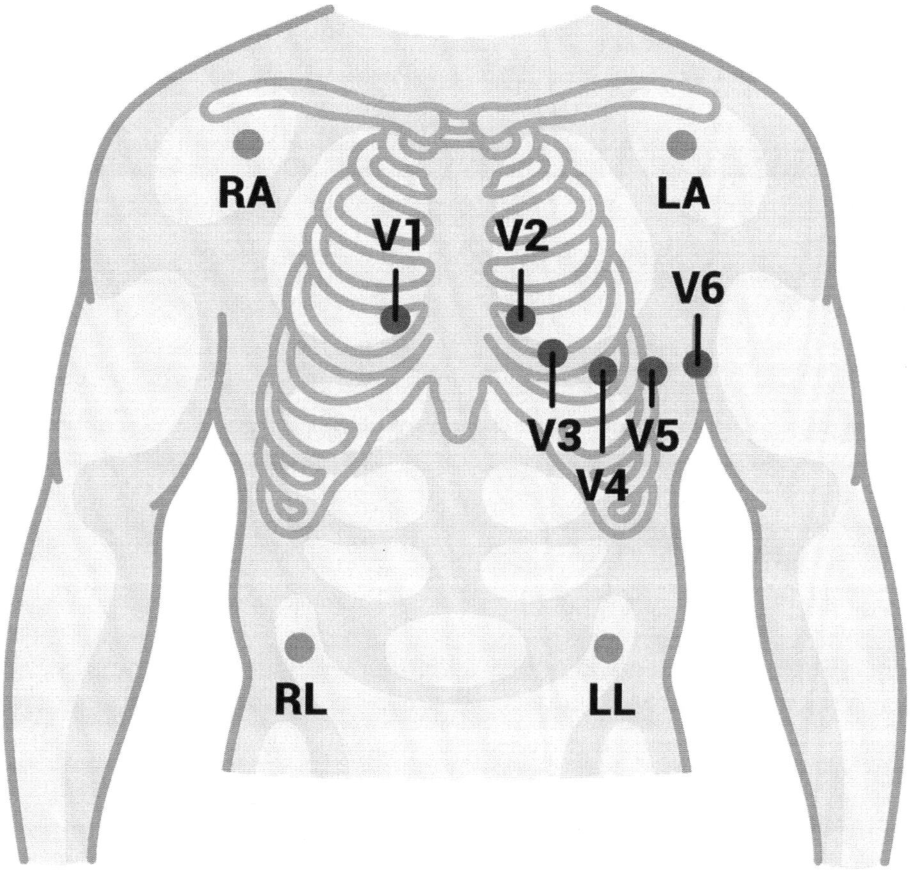

Cardiac Output

Cardiac output (CO) is the amount of blood pumped through the ventricles during a specified period. Normal cardiac output is about 5 liters per minutes at rest for an adult. Under exercise or stress, this volume may multiply 3 or 4 times with concomitant changes in the heart rate (HR) and stroke volume (SV). The basic formulation for calculating cardiac output is the heart rate (HR) per minute multiplied by the stroke volume (SR), which is the amount of blood pumped through the ventricles with each contraction. The stroke volume is controlled by preload, afterload, and contractibility.

$$\mathrm{CO}\left(\frac{\mathrm{mL}}{\mathrm{min}}\right) = \mathrm{HR}\left(\frac{\mathrm{beats}}{\mathrm{min}}\right) \times \mathrm{SV}\ (\mathrm{mL})$$

The heart rate is controlled by the autonomic nervous system. Normally, if the heart rate decreases, stroke volume increases to compensate. The exception to this would be cardiomyopathies, so bradycardia results in a sharp decline in cardiac output.

Cardiac Index

Cardiac index (CI) is the cardiac output (CO) divided by the body surface area (BSA). This is essentially a measure of cardiac output tailored to the individual, based on height and weight, measured in liters/min per square meter of BSA.

- Normal value: 2.2–4.0 L/min/m^2

Stroke Volume

Stroke volume (SV) is the amount of blood pumped through the left ventricle with each contraction, minus any blood remaining inside the ventricle at the end of systole.

- Normal values: 60–100 mL
- Formula:

$$\text{SV (mL)} = \text{CO}\left(\frac{\text{mL}}{\text{min}}\right) \div \text{HR}\left(\frac{\text{beats}}{\text{min}}\right)$$

Pulmonary Vascular Resistance and Ejection Fraction

Pulmonary vascular resistance (PVR) is the resistance in the pulmonary arteries and arterioles against which the right ventricle has to pump during contraction. It is the mean pressure in the pulmonary vascular bed divided by blood flow. If PVR increases, SV decreases.

- Normal value: 1.2–3.0 units or 100–250 dynes/sec/cm^5

Ejection Fraction (EF) is the percentage of the total blood volume of the heart that is pumped out with each beat. Dramatically decreased values indicate heart failure.

- Normal value: 60–70%

Preload and Afterload

Preload refers to the amount of elasticity in the myocardium at the end of diastole when the ventricles are filled to their maximum volume and the stretch on the muscle fibers is the greatest. The preload value is based on the volume in the ventricles. The amount of preload (stretch) affects stroke volume because as stretch increases, the resultant contraction also increases (Frank-Starling Law). Preload may decrease because of dehydration, diuresis, or vasodilation. Preload may increase because of increased venous return, controlling fluid loss, transfusion, or intravenous fluids.

Afterload refers to the amount of systemic vascular resistance to left ventricular ejection of blood and pulmonary vascular resistance to right ventricular ejection of blood. Determinants of afterload include the size and elasticity of the great vessels and the functioning of the pulmonic and aortic valves. Afterload increases with hypertension, stenotic valves, and vasoconstriction.

Assessing Jugular Venous Pressure

Jugular venous pressure (neck-vein) is used to assess the cardiac output and pressure in the right heart as the pulsations relate to changes in pressure in the right atrium. This procedure is usually not accurate if the pulse rate is >100. This is a non-invasive estimation of central venous pressure and waveform. Measurement should be done with the internal jugular if possible; if not, the external jugular may be used.

- **Elevate** the patient's head to 45° (and to 90° if necessary) with patient's head turned to the right.
- Position a **light** at an angle to illuminate veins and shadows.
- Measure the height of the **jugular vein pulsation** above the sternal joint, using a ruler.
    - Normal height is ≤4 cm above sternal angle.

Increased pressure (reflected in a height of >4 cm above the sternal angle) indicates increased pressure in the right atrium, and right heart failure. It may also indicate pericarditis or tricuspid stenosis. Laughing or coughing may trigger the Valsalva response and also cause an increase in pressure.

Additional Cardiac Assessments

The **stress test**, also called an exercise tolerance test, is a commonly used assessment to screen for ischemic heart disease. In this test, the patient is put through exercise with increasing rigor, generally on a treadmill, while attached to an ECG to monitor their heart's rhythm. The patient is assessed for chest pain and dizziness as the rigor level is increased, which is a reflection of the heart's capacity to handle increasing workloads effectively. The stress test is not diagnostic on its own, but provides feedback on the direction of additional testing.

Water-hammer pulse is characterized by the alternation between a bounding heartbeat that is strong and forceful, and then collapse. This could be the result of a heightened stroke volume, decreased peripheral resistance, or these two factors together. To assess for this pulse, the patient is seated and one arm is raised vertically. Upon palpation of the radial pulse in the raised arm, the pulse resembles a tapping in the muscles of the forearm. This is often an indication of aortic regurgitation.

Perfusion Pressure and Pulse Pressure

Coronary perfusion pressure directly affects coronary blood flow, and coronary perfusion occurs during diastole. Coronary artery perfusion pressure is equal to the diastolic blood pressure minus the pulmonary artery occlusion pressure. Normal values are 60–80 mmHg. Goal coronary perfusion when performing CPR to maintain enough perfusion necessary to achieve ROSC (return of spontaneous circulation) is thought to be 15 mmHg. During the cardiac cycle, *aortic pressure* causes the coronaries to be perfused, while *ventricular pressure* compresses the coronaries during systole, decreasing perfusion.

The **pulse pressure** is the difference between systolic and diastolic pressures, and this can be an important indicator. For example, with a decrease in cardiac output, vasoconstriction takes place in the body's attempt to maintain the blood pressure. In this case, the MAP may remain unchanged, but the pulse pressure narrows. Patients should be assessed for changes in pulse pressure that may be precipitated by medications, such as diuretics that alter fluid volume.

Assessment of the Respiratory System

If significant respiratory distress is present, one must stabilize the patient before doing a **respiratory history** or ask family if available:

- Question the patient about risk factors, such as smoking, exposure to smoke or other inhaled toxins, past lung problems, and allergies.
- Ask the patient about symptoms of respiratory problems, such as dyspnea, cough, sputum production, fatigue, ability to do ADLs and IADLs, and chest pain.
- Determine how long symptoms have been present, the length of periods of dyspnea, aggravating and alleviating factors, and the severity of symptoms.

When performing a **physical assessment**, one should assess vital signs, posture, pulse oximetry, check nails for clubbing, do a skin assessment, listen to lung sounds via auscultation and percussion, and look for accessory muscle use, signs of anxiety, and edema. Depending on condition, blood may be drawn for arterial blood gases, electrolytes, and CBC. Sputum cultures may be obtained.

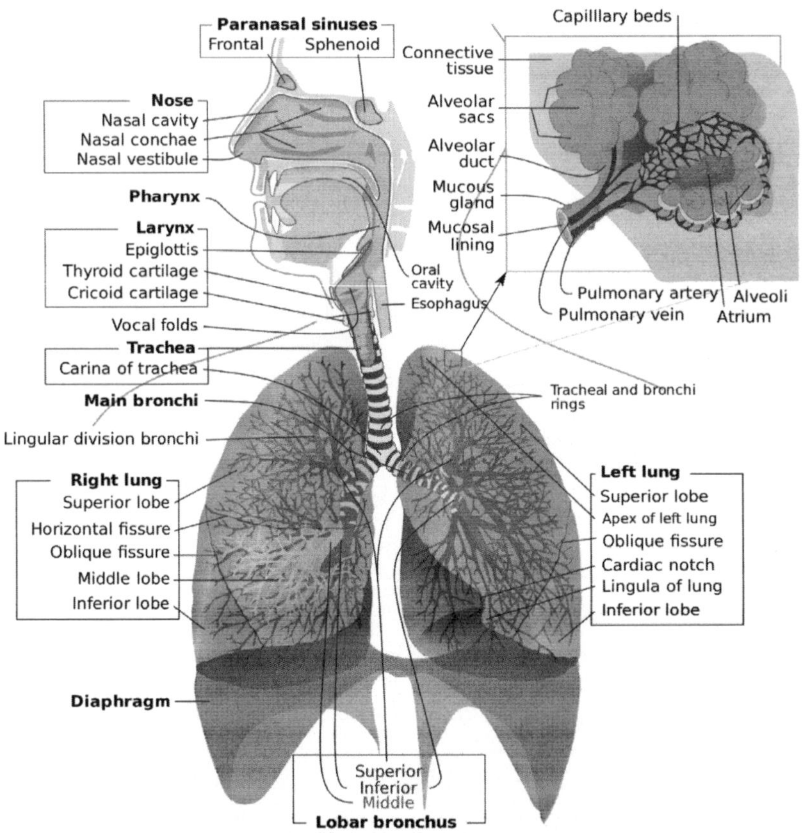

Review Video: Respiratory System
Visit mometrix.com/academy and enter code: 783075

Primary and Secondary Muscles Used for Breathing

Muscles used for breathing are separated into primary and secondary muscle groups.

- The **primary muscle groups** are those that are used in normal, quiet breathing. When patients are in respiratory distress and breathing is more difficult, secondary muscle groups become activated. The muscles considered primary for breathing are the diaphragm and the external intercostal muscles. These muscles act by changing the pressure gradient, allowing the lungs to expand and air to flow in and out.
- The **secondary muscle groups** include the sternocleidomastoid, scaleni, internal intercostals, obliques, and abdominal muscles. These secondary muscle groups work when breathing is difficult, both in inspiration and expiration, in cases such as obstructions or bronchoconstriction. Use of these secondary muscle groups can often be seen on exam and may be described as see-saw or abdominal breathing (when the abdominal muscles are being used during exhalation) or retractions as the muscles activate and can be seen between rigid structures such as bone.

Normal Physiological Airway Clearance

Normal airway clearance is caused by various aspects of the respiratory system. A thin layer of mucus lines the airways as a protective mechanism against debris and helps trap foreign objects before they enter the lower airways. Proper hydration keeps the mucosa adequately moist so it can trap foreign debris. As this debris lands in the mucus, the cilia in the respiratory tract act as an "elevator" to push the debris up to the larynx, where it can either be coughed up or swallowed and digested. An intact cough reflex is necessary for the debris to stimulate the cough, and normal muscle strength and nerve innervation of the diaphragm is required to produce a sufficiently forceful cough.

Ventilation/Perfusion Ratio

In order to maintain homeostasis, the respiratory and cardiac systems need to maintain a careful balance. The **ventilation/perfusion ratio** indicates that ventilation of the lungs and perfusion to the lungs are within a normal balance. A normal ventilation/perfusion ratio is equal to 0.8. A ventilation/perfusion ratio higher than normal is indicative of ventilation that is too high, perfusion that is too low, or some combination of the two. This can occur because of hyperventilation (either physiological or caused by healthcare practitioners due to incorrect ventilator settings), pulmonary embolism, or hypotension. Essentially, a high ventilation/perfusion ratio means that there is more ventilation than perfusion. If the ventilation/perfusion ratio is lower than normal, then ventilation is too low, perfusion is too high, or some combination of the two. This can be caused by atelectasis, pneumonia, or lung disease. Whatever the cause, a low ventilation/perfusion ratio indicates that there is more perfusion than ventilation.

Normal and Abnormal Breath Sound Terms

Normal breath sounds can be divided into three types. Vesicular breath sounds are low, soft sounds that can normally be heard over the peripheral lung space. Bronchovesicular breath sounds are moderate pitch breath sounds that are normally heard in the upper lung fields. Tracheal breath sounds are higher in pitch and heard over the trachea. Abnormal breath sounds are also known as adventitious lung sounds. Wheezes are high-pitched, expiratory sounds caused by air flowing through an obstructed airway. Stridor is also high-pitched, but is usually heard on inspiration in the upper airways. Coarse crackles are caused by an excessive amount of secretions in the airway and can be heard on inspiration and expiration. Fine crackles occur late in the expiratory phase and usually occur when the peripheral airways are being "popped" back open.

Review Video: Lung Sounds
Visit mometrix.com/academy and enter code: 765616

Diagnostics and Tools Used During Pulmonary/Thoracic Trauma Assessment

The diagnostic procedures and tools used during assessment of **pulmonary and thoracic trauma/disease** will vary according to the type and degree of injury/disease, but may include:

- **Thorough physical examination** including cardiac and pulmonary status, assessing for any abnormalities.
- **Electrocardiogram** to assess for cardiac arrhythmias.
- **Chest x-ray** should be done for all those with injuries to check for fractures, pneumothorax, major injuries, and placement of intubation tubes. X-rays can be taken quickly and with portable equipment so they can be completed quickly during the initial assessment.
- **Computerized tomography** may be indicated after initial assessment, especially if there is a possibility of damage to the parenchyma of the lungs.
- **Oximetry and atrial blood gases** as indicated.
- **12-lead electrocardiogram** may be needed if there are arrhythmias for more careful observation.
- **Echocardiogram** should be done if there is apparent cardiac damage.

Capnography with End-Tidal CO_2 Detector

Capnometry utilizes an **end-tidal CO_2 (ETCO) detector** that measures the concentration of CO_2 in expired air, usually through pH sensitive paper that changes color (commonly purple to yellow). Typically, the capnometer is attached to the ETT and a bag-valve-mask (BVM) ventilator. The capnogram provides data in the shape of a waveform that represents the partial pressure of exhaled gas. It is often used to confirm placement of endotracheal tubes as clinical assessment is not always sufficient, and it is a noninvasive mode of monitoring carbon dioxide in the respiratory cycle. Information provided by the capnogram includes:

- $PaCO_2$ level
- Type and degree of bronchial obstruction, such as COPD (waveform changes from rectangular to a fin-like)
- Air leaks in the ventilation system
- Rebreathing precipitated by need for new CO_2 absorber
- Cardiac arrest
- Hypothermia or reduced metabolism

The normal capnogram is a waveform that represents the varying CO_2 level throughout the breath cycle:

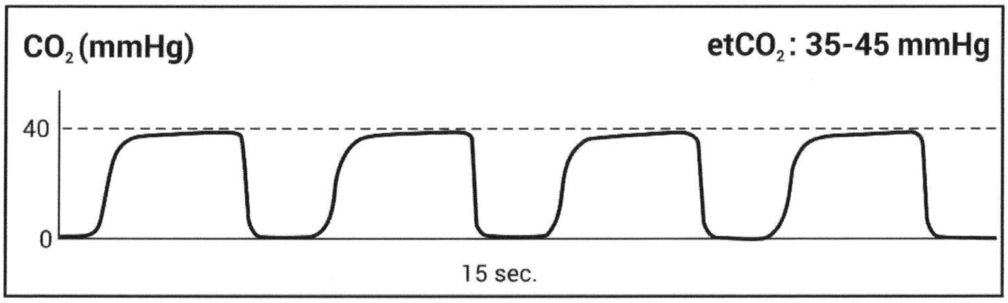

Arterial Blood Gases

Arterial blood gases (ABGs) are monitored to assess effectiveness of oxygenation, ventilation, and acid-base status and to determine oxygen flow rates. Partial pressure of a gas is that exerted by each gas in a mixture of gases, proportional to its concentration, based on total atmospheric pressure of 760 mmHg at sea level. Normal values include:

- Acidity/alkalinity (pH): 7.35–7.45
- Partial pressure of carbon dioxide ($PaCO_2$): 35–45 mmHg
- Partial pressure of oxygen (PaO_2): ≥80 mmHg
- Bicarbonate concentration (HCO_3^-): 22–26 mEq/L
- Oxygen saturation (SaO_2): ≥95%

The relationship between these elements, particularly the $PaCO_2$ and the PaO_2 indicates respiratory status. For example, $PaCO_2$ >55 and the PaO_2 <60 in a patient previously in good health indicates respiratory failure. There are many issues to consider. Ventilator management may require a higher $PaCO_2$ to prevent barotrauma and a lower PaO_2 to reduce oxygen toxicity.

Review Video: Blood Gases
Visit mometrix.com/academy and enter code: 611909

Assessment of the Gastrointestinal System

Assessment of the gastrointestinal system includes:

- Ask about personal and family history of gastrointestinal problems and risk factors, such as alcoholism, smoking, drug and medicine use, and poor dietary habits.
- Ask about symptoms, such as GI discomfort, flatus, nausea, vomiting, diarrhea, and abdominal pain.
- Determine the defecation pattern and ask about weight fluctuations.

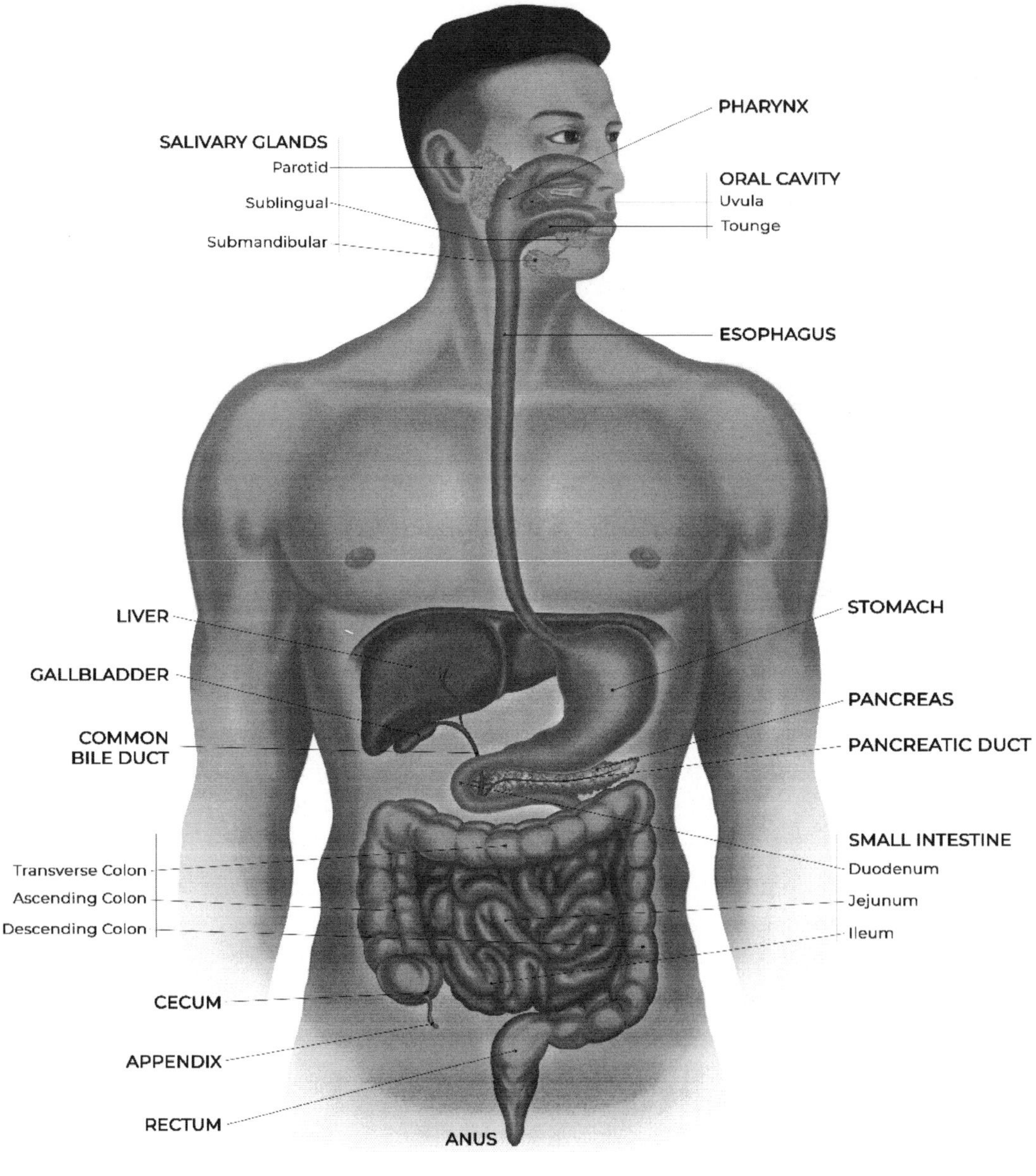

When performing a **physical assessment**, one must assess oral mucosa, tongue, teeth, pharynx, thyroid and parathyroid glands, skin color, moisture, turgor, nodules or lesions, bruises, scars, abdominal shape, and bowel sounds, assessing the abdomen in all 4 quadrants using the stethoscope diaphragm. The number of sounds heard determine if the intestines are functioning:

- **Absent**: no sounds in 3–5 minutes
- **Hypoactive**: only one sound in 2 minutes
- **Normal**: sounds heard every 5–20 seconds
- **Hyperactive**: 5–6 sounds in <30 seconds

One should examine the anal region for fissures, inflammation, tears, and dimples. Blood may be drawn for liver function studies, lipid profile, iron studies, CBC.

Review Video: Gastrointestinal System
Visit mometrix.com/academy and enter code: 378740

Assessment for Gallbladder and Pancreatic Disease

Gallbladder and pancreatic assessments are prompted by the appearance of symptoms. Symptoms of gallbladder disease include epigastric discomfort following fatty food intake, abdominal distension, right upper quadrant pain, which may be colicky, nausea, and vomiting. Pain may occur intermittently.

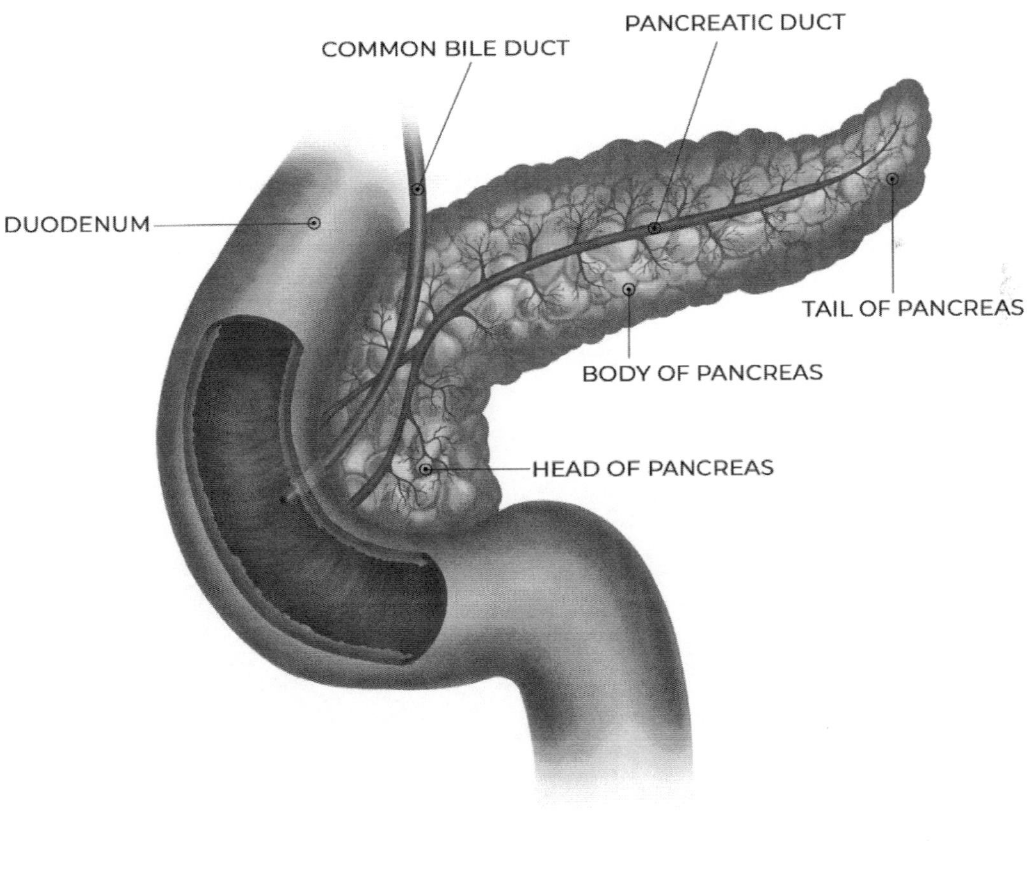

The patient with pancreatitis may have acute onset of severe abdominal pain, back pain, extensive vomiting, and dyspnea. Pancreatitis is most often related to gallstones or alcoholism, so history of alcohol use and examination for gallstones must be done:

- Assess for RUQ tenderness and mass, bowel sounds, and abdominal guarding.
- Assess the vital signs for hypotension, tachycardia, or fever and note any anxiety, agitation, or confusion.
- Note signs of hypoxia.
- Assess the skin for jaundice and bruising on the flanks and near the umbilicus.
- Blood is drawn to assess amylase and lipase, CBC, calcium, glucose, and bilirubin.

Assessment for Liver Disease

The liver must be 70% damaged before lab tests show abnormalities. Assessment of risk factors and early symptoms are important to identify early disease. Risk factors for liver disease include alcoholism and drug abuse, risky sexual practices, exposure to infection or environmental toxins, and travel to countries with poor sanitation. One should question the patient about symptoms of liver disease, such as fatigue, itching, abdominal pain, anorexia, weight gain, fever, blood in stools or black stools, sleep problems, lack of menstruation, and lack of libido. Physical assessment includes checking vital signs and skin for scratches, pallor, jaundice, dryness, bruising, petechiae, abdominal veins and spider angiomas, and red palms:

- Assess for gynecomastia, abdominal distension, fluid waves, bowel sounds, liver margins, tenderness, consistency, and hardness and sharpness of the edge.
- Examine extremities for wasting, edema, and weakness.
- Assess neurological system for cognitive status, tremors, balance problems, slurred speech.
- Identify testicular atrophy.
- Blood should be drawn for serum enzymes and proteins, bilirubin, ammonia, clotting factors, and lipid profile.

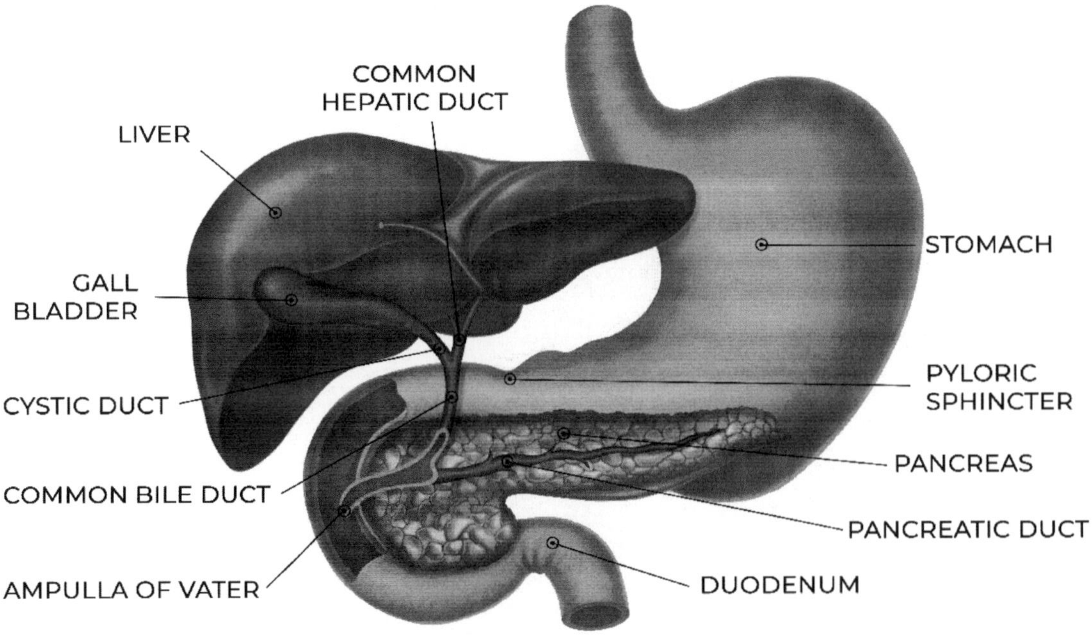

Assessment of Nutritional Status

Assessment of nutritional status begins with an assessment of the patient's intake. The patient is asked to report intake for the previous 24 hours. This may indicate the need for a **food diary** over a period of time:

- Compare the patient's nutritional intake with the requirements of the USDA's MyPlate.
- Measure height and weight and check against a BMI table to help determine nutritional status.
- Measure waist circumference.
- Assess the patient for physical signs of poor nutrition such as muscle wasting, obesity, hair breakage and loss, poor skin turgor, ulcers, bruising, and loss of subcutaneous tissue.
- Assess mucous membranes and condition of teeth, abdomen, extremities, and thyroid gland.

Nutritional status is connected to endocrine disease, infections, other acute and chronic diseases, digestion, absorption, excretion, and storage of nutrients, so these areas must also be assessed. Blood testing should include proteins, transferrin, electrolytes, vitamins A and C, carotene, and CBC. Test urine for creatinine, thiamine, riboflavin, niacin, albumin, and iodine.

Assessing Nutritional Status of Hospitalized Patients

Assessing the nutritional status of the hospital inpatient is an important part of forming a care plan. The two screening tools that are most commonly used are the **subjective global assessment (SGA)** and the **prognostic nutritional index (PNI)**. The SGA provides a nutritional assessment based on both the patient history and current symptoms. The patient is asked about any changes in weight and is also asked questions about his or her diet. The presence of symptoms that may lead to weight loss and poor nutritional status, such as diarrhea, nausea, and vomiting, as well as water retention (edema) and muscle wasting (cachexia), is also included in the SGA. The PNI is also used as an indicator of malnutrition and is especially helpful in predicting survival in cancer patients and determining how well a patient will recover from surgery. The PNI results from a calculation involving the measurement of serum albumin and absolute lymphocyte count.

Assessment of Kidneys and Urinary Tract

Assessment of kidneys and urinary tract includes:

- Assess the health history for family urinary system disease and risk factors, such as previous urinary disease, increased age, immobility, hypertension, diabetes, chemical exposure, chronic disease, radiation to the pelvis, STIs, alcohol or drug use, and complications of pregnancy and delivery.
- Determine daily fluid intake.
- Question symptoms such as flank or abdominal pain, hesitancy, urgency, difficulty or straining with voiding, difficulty emptying the bladder, urinary incontinence, fatigue, SOB, exercise intolerance from anemia, fever, chills, blood in the urine, and GI symptoms.

Physical assessment includes vital signs, kidney and bladder palpation, and percussion over the bladder after urination:

- Palpate for ascites and edema.
- Measure the DTRs and check gait and ability to walk heel-to-toe.
- Examine the genitalia and check the urethra and vagina for herniation, irritation, or tears.

Urine specimen is obtained via clean catch midstream technique for analysis and culture if indicated. Blood is taken for a CBC, and in males, prostate-specific antigen (PSA) levels will also be measured via blood specimen.

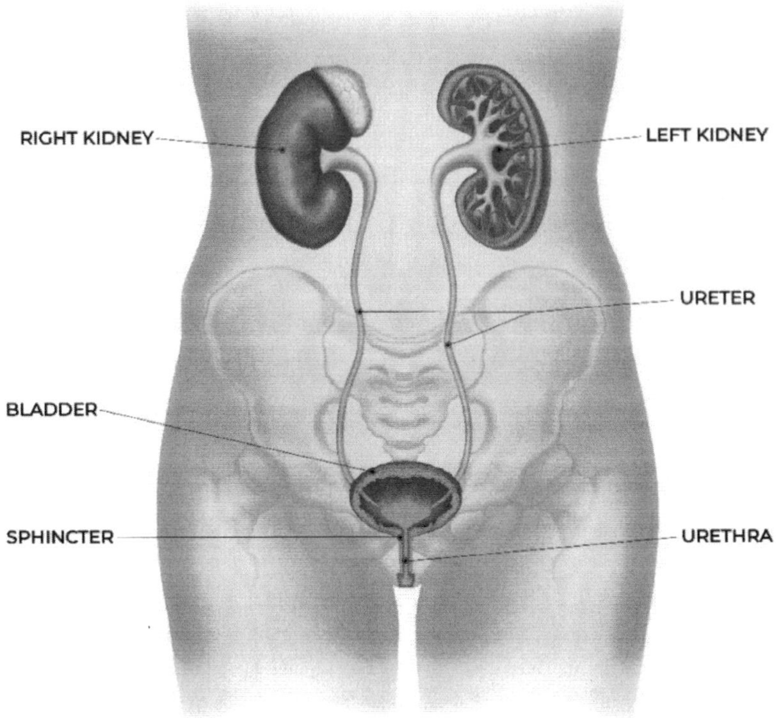

Review Video: Urinary System
Visit mometrix.com/academy and enter code: 601053

Kidney Regulatory Functions Regarding Fluid Balance

Kidney regulatory functions include maintaining **fluid balance**. Fluid excretion balances intake with output, so increased intake results in a large output and vice versa:

- **Osmolality** (the number of electrolytes and other molecules per kg/urine) measures the concentration or dilution. With dehydration, osmolality increases; with fluid retention, osmolality decreases. With kidney disease, urine is dilute and the osmolality is fixed.
- **Specific gravity** compares the weight of urine (weight of particles) to distilled water (1.000). Normal urine is 1.010–1.025 with normal intake. High intake lowers the specific gravity, and low intake raises it. In kidney disease, it often does not vary.
- **Antidiuretic hormone** (ADH/vasopressin) regulates the excretion of water and urine concentration in the renal tubule by varying water reabsorption. When fluid intake decreases, blood osmolality rises, and this stimulates the release of ADH, which increases reabsorption of fluid to return osmolality to normal levels. ADH is suppressed with increased fluid intake, so less fluid is reabsorbed.

Assessing Sexual Health and Preferences

Bringing up the topic of sex gives a patient permission to ask questions and openly discuss **sexual concerns**:

- Ask for permission to ask questions about sexual health and preferences during the gynecological/urological portion of the health history.
- If the patient refuses, go on with the rest of the health history, otherwise continue.
- Ask first if the person has sex with men, women, or both.
- Be nonjudgmental and do not assume that those who are elderly or disabled do not have sex. Use layman terms according to the patient's age and education level.
- Ask if the person is having any problems with relationships or sexual intercourse.
- Ask if the person has ever been forced to have sex or if is afraid of anyone close to them.
- End by asking if there are any questions about expression of sexual feelings, contraception, safe sex practices, or risky behavior.
- Refer those with problems to their doctor, or a gynecologist, urologist, or sex therapist.

Integumentary and Peripheral Vascular Systems

General Skin Assessment

Skin color varies according to ethnicity. Color changes should be assessed to determine if they are local or extend over the entire body, and if they are permanent or transient. Pallor may indicate stress, impaired oxygenation, and vasoconstriction. Erythema may indicate vasodilation, local inflammation, and blushing. Cyanosis indicates impaired oxygenation, and jaundice indicates increased bilirubin.

Temperature is typically assessed by touching the skin with the back of the hand. Skin should be warm and equal bilaterally. Hypothermia may indicate impaired circulation, intravenous infusion, and immobilized limb (such as in a cast). Hyperthermia may indicate fever, infection, and excessive exercise.

Review Video: Skin Assessment
Visit mometrix.com/academy and enter code: 794925

Effects of Age on Skin

Age is an important consideration when evaluating the skin because the characteristics of the skin change as people age.

- An **infant's** skin is thinner than an adult's because, while the epidermis is developed, the dermis layer is only about 60% of that of an adult and continues to develop after birth. The skin of premature infants is especially friable, allowing for transepidermal water loss and evaporative heat loss.
- During **adolescence**, the hair follicles activate, the thickness of the dermis decreases about 20%, and epidermal turnover time increases, so healing slows.
- As people **continue to age**, Langerhans' cells decrease in number, making the skin more prone to cancer, and the inflammatory reactions decrease. The sweat glands, vascularity, and subcutaneous fat all decrease, interfering with thermoregulation and contributing to dryness and irritation of the skin. The epidermal-dermal junction flattens, resulting in skin that is prone to tearing. The elastin in the skin degrades with age and solar exposure. The thinning of the hypodermis can lead to pressure injuries.

Review Video: Integumentary System
Visit mometrix.com/academy and enter code: 655980

Braden Scale

The Braden scale is a risk assessment tool that has been validated clinically as predictive of the risk of patient's developing pressure injuries. It was developed in 1988 by Barbara Braden and Nancy Bergstrom and is in wide use. The scale scores six different areas with five areas scored 1–4 points, and one area 1–3 points. The lower the score, the greater the risk.

Area	Score of 1	Score of 2	Score of 3	Score of 4
Sensory perception	Completely limited	Very limited	Slightly limited	No impairment
Moisture	Constantly moist	Very moist	Occasionally moist	Rarely moist
Activity	Bed	Chair	Occasional walk	Frequent walk
Mobility	Immobile	Limited	Slightly limited	No limitations
Nutritional pattern	Very poor	Inadequate	Adequate	Excellent
Friction and shear	Problem	Potential problem	No apparent problem	

Assessment of Lower Extremities

Assessment of lower extremities includes a number of different elements:

- **Appearance** includes comparing limbs for obvious differences or changes in skin or nails as well as evaluating for edema, color changes in skin, such as pallor or rubor. Legs that are thin, pale, shiny, and hairless indicate peripheral arterial disease.
- **Perfusion** should be assessed by checking venous filling time and capillary refill, skin temperature (noting changes in one limb or between limbs), bruits (indicating arterial narrowing), pulses (comparing both sides in a proximal to distal progression), ankle-brachial index and toe-brachial index.
- **Sensory function** includes the ability to feel pain, temperature, and touch.
- **Range of motion** of the ankle must be assessed to determine if the joint flexes past 90° because this is necessary for unimpaired walking and aids venous return in the calf.
- **Pain** is an important diagnostic feature of peripheral arterial disease, so the location, intensity, duration, and characteristics of pain are important.

Assessment of Pulse and Bruit

Evaluation of the pulses of the **lower extremities** is an important part of assessment for peripheral arterial disease/trauma. Pulses should be first evaluated with the patient in supine position and then again with the legs dependent, checking bilaterally and proximal to distal to determine if intensity of pulse decreases distally. Pedal pulses should be examined at both the posterior tibialis and the dorsalis pedis. The pulse should be evaluated as to the rate, rhythm, and intensity, which is usually graded on a 0 to 4 scale:

0+= pulse absent
1+= weak, difficult to palpate
2+= normal as expected
3+= full
4+= strong and bounding

Pulses may be **palpable** or **absent** with peripheral arterial disease. Absence of pulse on both palpation and Doppler probe does indicate peripheral arterial disease.

Bruits may be noted by auscultating over major arteries, such as femoral, popliteal, peroneal, and dorsalis pedis, indicating peripheral arterial disease.

Assessing Perfusion of Lower Extremities

Assessment of perfusion can indicate venous or arterial abnormalities:

- **Venous refill time**: Begin with the patient lying supine for a few moments and then have the patient sit with the feet dependent. Observe the veins on the dorsum of the foot and count the seconds before normal filling. Venous occlusion is indicated with times greater than 20 seconds.
- **Capillary refill**: Grasp the toenail bed between the thumb and index finger and apply pressure for several seconds to cause blanching. Release the nail and count the seconds until the nail regains normal color. Arterial occlusion is indicated with times of more than 2–3 seconds. Check both feet and more than one nail bed.
- **Skin temperature**: Using the palm of the hand and fingers, gently palpate the skin, moving distally to proximally and comparing both legs. Arterial disease is indicated by decreased temperature (coolness) or a marked change from proximal to distal. Venous disease is indicated by increased temperature about the ankle.

ABI

Procedure

The ankle-brachial index **(ABI) examination** is done to evaluate peripheral arterial disease of the lower extremities.

1. Apply BP cuff to one arm, palpate brachial pulse, and place conductivity gel over the artery.
2. Place the tip of a Doppler device at a 45-degree angle into the gel at the brachial artery and listen for the pulse sound.
3. Inflate the cuff until the pulse sound ceases and then inflate 20 mmHg above that point.
4. Release air and listen for the return of the pulse sound. This reading is the brachial systolic pressure.
5. Repeat the procedure on the other arm and use the higher reading for calculations.
6. Repeat the same procedure on each ankle with the cuff applied above the malleoli and the gel over the posterior tibial pulse to obtain the ankle systolic pressure.
7. Divide the ankle systolic pressure by the brachial systolic pressure to obtain the ABI.

Sometimes, readings are taken both before and after 5 minutes of walking on a treadmill.

Interpreting Results

Once the ABI examination is completed, the ankle systolic pressure must be divided by the brachial systolic pressure. Ideally, the BP at the ankle should be equal to that of the arm or slightly higher. With peripheral arterial disease the ankle pressure falls, affecting the ABI. Additionally, some conditions that cause calcification of arteries, such as diabetes, can cause a false elevation.

Calculation is simple:

$$\text{ABI} = \frac{\text{Ankle systolic}}{\text{Brachial systolic}}$$

The degree of disease relates to the **score**:

- >1.4: Abnormally high, may indicate calcification of vessel wall
- 1.0–1.4: Normal reading, asymptomatic
- 0.9–1.0: Low reading, but acceptable unless there are other indications of PAD
- 0.8–0.9: Likely some arterial disease is present
- 0.5–0.8: Moderate arterial disease
- < 0.5: Severe arterial disease

Musculoskeletal and Neurosensory Systems

Assessing Risk of Falling

Many factors must be examined and combined to determine the **fall risk** status of a patient. They include age, sensory deficits, mobility problems, neurological disorders, past history of falling, cognitive impairment, and depression. Some medications, such as those associated with postural hypotension and psychotropic medications, may increase the danger of falls. The presence of dizziness, acute or chronic illness, poor physical status, elimination requirements, medications, and environmental concerns contribute to the risk for falls.

Multiple factors increase risk, so careful history and physical exam are necessary as part of assessment. When the presence of risk factors shows a risk for falls, this information should be communicated to other caregivers by wristband, colored markers on doors, care plans, or other effective means. The factors are then modified as much as possible. The patient should be re-evaluated as their condition changes or after a fall to determine the cause.

Assessing Patients with Disabilities

A patient with **disabilities** may find it very difficult to obtain screening for health problems due to inaccessibility:

- Work with the patient to resolve barriers to obtain weight, mammography, bone density tests, and pap/pelvic exams on a regular basis.
- Ask how to best assist the patient during the assessment.
- Observe the patient carefully for nonverbal communication, such as grimacing.
- If sensation is affected, warn the patient before touching any part of the body.
- Always address all areas of the patient's history, including sexual history.
- Use an interpreter that is not a family member if needed.
- Give the patient extra time to respond to questions when there is aphasia or other communication problems.
- Address the impact of the disability on the ability to perform ADLs, health status in general, access to healthcare, financial status, emotional status, work, community roles, and family wellbeing.

Pathophysiology of Pain

Nociceptors

Nociceptors are the primary neurons, or **sensory receptors**, responding to stimuli in the skin, muscle, and joints, as well as the stomach, bladder, and uterus. These neurons have specialized responses for mechanical, thermal, or chemical stimuli. The **neuron stimulation** is a direct result of tissue injury and follows four stages: **transduction** where a change occurs, **transmission** where the impulse is transferred along the neural path, **modulation** or translation of the signal, and **perception** by the patient. When injury occurs, the nociceptors initiate the process that begins **depolarization of the peripheral nerve**. Nociceptors may consist of either A-fiber axons or C-fiber axons. The message travels along the neural pathway and creates a perception of pain. A-fiber axons carry these pain messages at a much faster rate than C-fiber axons.

Nociceptive Pain

Nociceptive pain is an umbrella term for pain caused by **stimulation of the neuroreceptor**. This stimulation is a direct result of tissue injury. The severity of pain is proportionate to the extent of the injury. Nociceptive pain can be subdivided into two classifications: somatic and visceral pain.

Somatic pain is located in the cutaneous tissues, bone joints, and muscle tissues. **Visceral pain** is specific to internal organs protected by a layer of viscera, such as the cardiovascular, respiratory, gastrointestinal, or genitourinary systems. Both types are treatable with opioids.

Visceral Pain

Visceral pain is associated with the internal organs. It can be very different depending on the affected organ. Not all internal organs are sensitive to pain (some lack **nociceptors**, such as the spleen, kidney, and pancreas), and may withstand a great deal of damage without causing pain. Other internal organs, such as the stomach, bladder, and ureters, can create significant pain from even the slightest damage. Visceral pain generally has a **poorly defined area**. It is also capable of referring pain to other remote locations away from the area of injury. It is described as a squeezing or cramping: a deep ache within the internal organs. The patient may complain of a generalized sick feeling or have nausea and vomiting. Visceral pain generally responds well to treatment with **opioids**.

Review Video: Visceral Pain
Visit mometrix.com/academy and enter code: 430402

Somatic Pain

Somatic pain refers to messages from pain receptors located in the **cutaneous or musculoskeletal tissues**. When the pain occurs within the musculoskeletal tissue, it is referred to as **deep somatic pain**. Metastasizing cancers commonly cause deep somatic pain. **Surface pain** refers to pain concentrated in the **dermis and cutaneous layers** such as that caused by a surgical incision. Deep somatic pain is generally described as a dull, throbbing ache that is well focused on the area of trauma. It responds well to **opioids**. Surface somatic pain is also directly focused on the injury. It is frequently described as sharper than deep somatic pain. It may also present as a burning or pricking sensation.

Review Video: Somatic Pain
Visit mometrix.com/academy and enter code: 982772

Review Video: Somatic Nervous System
Visit mometrix.com/academy and enter code: 100382

Neuropathic Pain

Neuropathic pain results from injury to the **nervous system**. This can result from cancer cells compressing the nerves or spinal cord, from actual cancerous invasion into the nerves or spinal cord, or from chemical damage to the nerves caused by chemotherapy and radiation. Other causes include diabetes- and alcohol-related damage, trauma, neuralgias, or other illnesses affecting the neural path either centrally or peripherally. When the nerves become damaged, they are unable to carry accurate information. This results in more severe, distinct **pain messages**. The nerves may also relay pain messages long after the original cause of the pain is resolved. It can be described as sharp, burning, shooting, shocking, tingling, or electrical in nature. It may travel the length of the nerve path from the spine to a distal body part such as a hand, or down the buttocks to a foot. NSAIDs and opioids are generally ineffective against neuropathic pain, though adjuvants may enhance the therapeutic effect of opioids. Nerve blocks may also be used.

Review Video: Neuropathic Pain
Visit mometrix.com/academy and enter code: 780523

Adverse Systemic Effects of Pain

Acute pain causes adverse systemic effects that can negatively affect many body systems.

- **Cardiovascular**: Tachycardia and increased blood pressure is a common response to pain, causing increased cardiac output and systemic vascular resistance. In those with pre-existing cardiovascular disease, such as compromised ventricular function, cardiac output may decrease. The increased myocardial need for oxygen may cause or worsen myocardial ischemia.
- **Respiratory**: Increased need for oxygen causes an increase in minute ventilation and splinting due to pain, which may compromise pulmonary function. If the chest wall movement is constrained, tidal volume falls, impairing the ability to cough and clear secretions. Bed rest further compromises ventilation.
- **Gastrointestinal**: Sphincter tone increases and motility decreases, sometimes resulting in ileus. There may be an increased secretion of gastric acids, which irritates the gastric lining and can cause ulcerations. Nausea, vomiting, and constipation may occur. Reflux may result in aspiration pneumonia. Abdominal distension may occur.
- **Urinary**: Increased sphincter tone and decreased motility result in urinary retention.
- **Endocrine**: Hormone levels are affected by pain. Catabolic hormones such as catecholamine, cortisol, and glucagon increase, and anabolic hormones such as insulin and testosterone decrease. Lipolysis increases along with carbohydrate intolerance. Sodium retention can occur because of increased ADH, aldosterone, angiotensin, and cortisol. This in turn causes fluid retention and a shift to extracellular space.
- **Hematologic**: There may be reduced fibrinolysis, increased adhesiveness of platelets, and increased coagulation.
- **Immune**: Leukocytosis and lymphopenia may occur, increasing risk of infection.
- **Emotional**: Patients may experience depression, anxiety, anger, decreased appetite, and sleep deprivation. This type of response is most common in those with chronic pain, who usually have different systemic responses from those with acute pain.

Core Principles of Pain Assessment and Management

According to the Joint Commission, assessing pain should be a priority in patient care, and organizations must establish **policies** for assessment and treatment of pain and must educate staff members about these policies. The Joint Commission considers a **plan of care** regarding pain control an essential patient right. Hospitals should be consistent in the use of the same assessment tools throughout the organization, specific to different patient populations (for example, pediatrics and geriatrics). The latest standards (2018) of evidence-based practice include the following:

- Organizations must establish a clinical leadership team to oversee pain management and safe prescription of opioids.
- Patients must be involved in planning and setting goals and should receive education regarding safe use of opioid and non-opioid medications.
- Patients should be screened for pain in all assessments, including visits to the emergency department.
- Patients at high risk for opioid misuse or adverse effects must be identified and monitored.
- Healthcare providers should have access to prescription drug monitoring safety databases, such as the prescription databases provided by most states.
- Organizations must provide performance improvement educational programs regarding pain assessment and management and must collect and analyze data on its pain assessment and management.

Areas Addressed When Assessing Pain

Information concerning a patient's pain can be gathered from a variety of sources, including observations, interviews with the patient and family, medical records, and observations of other health care providers. However, it is important to remember that each patient's pain is **subjective** and **personal**. Pain is defined as whatever the patient says it is. Having the patient give parameters of quality, location, duration, speed of onset, and intensity can all be beneficial in forming a treatment plan based on the patient's needs. Pain is also influenced by psychological, social, and spiritual factors. Behavioral, psychological, and subjective assessment information such as physical demeanor and vital signs can be helpful in further defining a patient's pain parameters.

Physical Signs of Pain

The best assessment of the patient's pain is **the patient's own report**. All other information is assessed as supporting this report. However, when this method is restricted or unavailable, **physical signs and symptoms** can help the nurse's assessment capabilities. It is important to be familiar with the patient's **baseline** or resting information to give a clear picture of the changes the body may go through when experiencing significant pain. Systolic blood pressure, heart rate, and respirations may all increase above the patient's normal parameters. Tightness or tension may be felt in major muscle groups. Posturing can also occur: the patient may guard areas of the body, curl themselves up into a fetal position, or hold only certain body portions rigid. Calling out, increased volume in speech, and moaning can also be indicators. Facial expressions, such as flat affect or grimacing, and distraction from their surroundings also indicate a significant increase in stressful stimuli.

Importance of Pain Assessments in Advanced Disease

As many as 90% of all **advanced disease patients** will experience some level of pain. The hospice and palliative care philosophy focuses on the relief of pain and provision for comfort measures for all patients who desire it to improve quality of life. Each patient has the right to accept or refuse treatment for their pain. This becomes difficult when the patient is unable to **communicate** their desires and pain level. It can be assumed that if a patient was experiencing pain when able to communicate, they will continue to experience pain when the ability to communicate has been compromised—pain will be present even in an unconscious state. Changes from previous behavioral, psychological, and subjective and objective assessment data provide the supporting information for continued pain assessments in a nonverbal patient.

Pain Assessment Tools

ABCDE Mnemonic Approach to Pain Assessment

The Agency for Healthcare Policy and Research recommends use of the **ABCDE method** for assessing and managing pain:

- **Asking** the patient about the extent of pain and assessing systematically.
- **Believing** that the degree of pain the patient reports is accurate.
- **Choosing** the appropriate method of pain control for the patient and circumstances.
- **Delivering** pain interventions appropriately and in a timely, logical manner.
- **Empowering** patients and family by helping them to have control of the course of treatment.

The **5 key elements of pain assessment** include:

- **Quality**: Words are used to describe pain, such as *burning*, *stabbing*, *deep*, *shooting*, and *sharp*. Some may complain of pressure, squeezing, and discomfort rather than pain.
- **Intensity**: Use of a 0–10 scale or other appropriate scale to quantify the degree of pain.
- **Location**: Where does the patient indicate pain?
- **Duration**: Is it constant; does it come and go; is there breakthrough pain?
- **Aggravating/alleviating factors**: What increases the intensity of pain and what relieves the pain?

Review Video: Assessment Tools for Pain
Visit mometrix.com/academy and enter code: 634001

Review Video: How to Accurately Assess Pain
Visit mometrix.com/academy and enter code: 693250

Unidimensional Tools for Pain Assessment

Unidimensional tools for pain assessment focus on one aspect only: the patient's level of pain. Tools include:

- **Visual analog/numeric rating scale**: A 1–10 rating scale presented visually or verbally from which the patient chooses a number to describe the degree of pain the patient is experiencing. Zero represents no pain, 1 very mild pain, and 10 the most severe pain the patient can imagine.
- **Descriptive**: Pain is described in simple terms that a patient can choose from: mild, moderate, or severe. This may be especially helpful for patients from other countries or cultures where the 1–10 scale is not generally used.
- **FACES**: A chart shows a facial expression scale of simple drawings showing faces with different emotions, such as happiness, fear, and pain. Used primarily for children over age 3 and for nonverbal adults, although both a child's and an adult's version are available. A revised version applies numeric values to expressions so that pain can be assessed according to a numeric rating scale as well.

Multidimensional Tools for Pain Assessment

Multidimensional tools used for pain assessment assess various aspects of pain in addition to its impact on mental health, sleep, and functional status. Tools include:

- **Multidimensional pain inventory**: The patient begins by identifying a significant other and then answering 20 questions (rating scale 0–6) about the current rate of pain, the degree of interference in daily life, the ability to work, satisfaction from social/recreational activities, support level of the significant other, mood, pain during the previous week, changes brought about by pain, concerns of the significant other, ability to deal with pain, irritability, and anxiety.
- **Brief pain inventory**: Patients are assessed on the severity of pain (on a 1–10 scale), location of pain, impact of pain on daily function, pain medication, and amount of pain relief in the past 24 hours or the past week. They are asked if the pain interferes with general activity, walking, normal work, mood, interpersonal relations, sleep, or enjoyment of life.

- **McGill pain questionnaire**: The patient marks areas of internal and external pain on body diagrams and selects appropriate adjectives for 20 different sections regarding sensory, affective, and evaluative perceptions. For example, the questionnaire allows the patient to indicate if the pain is "flickering, quivering, pulsing, throbbing, beating, or pounding." The patient also rates present pain intensity (PPI) from 0 (none) to 5 (excruciating).

Assessment Tools for Cognitively Impaired or Nonverbal Patients

The following are types of assessment tools available for use with cognitively impaired or nonverbal patients:

- **Discomfort Scale for Dementia of the Alzheimer Type (DS-DAT)**: For use with elderly persons experiencing dementia, decreased cognition, and decreased verbalization
- **Assessment of Discomfort in Dementia Protocol (ADD)**: Particularly designed for use with patients exhibiting difficult behaviors
- **Checklist of Nonverbal Pain Indicators (CNPI)**: Pain measurement with cognitive impairment
- **Noncommunicative Patient's Pain Assessment Instrument (NOPPAIN)**: Specifically for use by nursing assistants
- **Pain Assessment for the Dementing Elderly (PADE)**: Assessing physical pain behaviors
- **Pain Assessment Tool in Confused Older Adults (PATCOA)**: Focuses on the observation of nonverbal cues
- **Pain Assessment in Advanced Dementia (PAINAD)**: Adapted from the DS-DAT
- **Pain Assessment Checklist for Seniors with Limited Ability to Communicate (PACSLAC)**: To assess common and subtle symptoms
- **Abbey Pain Scale**: For late-stage dementia in nursing home environments

Pain Assessment of Neonates/Infants

Pain assessment of neonates and infants depends on careful observation of a number of characteristics. The Neonate/Infant Pain Scale (NIPS) assesses 6 areas with a score >3 indicating pain. Five areas are scored 0-1, depending upon the degree of stress. Crying, which is often the most indicative of pain, is scored 0-2:

Characteristic	0	1	2
Expression on face	Rested, normal	Negative, tightened muscles, grimace	
Crying	None	Intermittent, moaning, whimper	Loud, shrill continuous crying
Respiratory patterns	Relaxed, normal	Changes include irregular breathing, tachypnea, holding breath, gagging	
Upper extremities	Relaxed, random movement	Tense, rigid, or rapid extending and flexing.	
Lower extremities	Relaxed, random movement	Tense, rigid, or rapid extending and flexing.	
Arousal state	Quiet, awake or asleep with random leg movements	Restless, fussing, thrashing about.	

Assessing Pain in Pediatric Patients

When assessing the pediatric patient, the nurse must take into consideration the **chronological and developmental age** of the child. These factors help determine which measure the child might use to express pain, as well as treatments that might prove most successful. Assessment parameters must also include the presence of and parameters surrounding chronic illness, as well as neurological impairment. The nurse must identify the underlying cause of the pain, what nonpharmacological measures have been tried for pain control, and what methods can be used to deliver pharmacological interventions. The weight of the child in kilograms determines the appropriate dosages of medications. If the child is able to speak, do the child and the parents speak the same language as the health care provider, and are there any other obvious barriers to communication or pain relief measures?

Review Video: How to Properly Assess Pediatric Pain
Visit mometrix.com/academy and enter code: 264352

Preteen/Adolescent Pain Scale

Pain is subjective and may be influenced by the individual's pain sensation threshold (the smallest stimulus that produces the sensation of pain) and tolerance threshold (the maximum degree of pain that a person can tolerate). The most common current pain assessment tool for preteens and adolescents is the 1-10 pain scale:

- 0 = no pain
- 1-2 = mild pain
- 3-5 = moderate pain
- 6-7 = severe pain
- 8-9 = very severe pain
- 10 = excruciating pain

However, assessment also includes information about onset, duration, and intensity. Identifying pain triggers and what relieves the pain is essential when developing a pain management plan. Children may show very different behaviors when they are in pain. Some may cry and moan with minor pain, and others may seem indifferent even when they are truly suffering. Thus, judging pain by behavior alone can lead to the wrong conclusions.

Non-Communicating Children's Pain Checklist

The **Non-Communicating Children's Pain Checklist** (NCCPC) is designed for children ages 3-8 who are cognitively impaired, but a modified version may be used for children recovering from anesthesia. The checklist contains 7 categories with sub-listings that are each scored: 0 (not occurring), 1 (occurring occasionally), 2 (occurring fairly often), 3 (occurring frequently), and NA (not applicable).

- **Vocal**: Moaning, whining, crying, screaming, yelling, or using a specific word for pain
- **Social**: Uncooperative, unhappy, withdrawn, seeking closeness, or can't be distracted
- **Facial**: Furrowed brow, eye changes, not smiling, lips tight or quivering, or clenching or grinding teeth.
- **Activity**: Not moving and quiet or agitated and fidgety.
- **Body and limbs**: Floppy, tense, rigid, spastic, pointing to a part of body that hurts, guarding part of the body, flinching, or positioning body to show pain.
- **Physiological**: Shivering, pallor, increased perspiration, tears, gasping, or holding breath
- **Eating and sleeping**: Eating less or sleeping significantly more or less than usual

The child is usually observed for 2 hours and then scored. All scores are then added together. A score of ≥7 indicates pain.

QUESTT Pediatric Pain Assessment Tool

QUESTT is designed to focus on assessment, action, and consequent reassessment for results.

- **Question** both the child and parent about the pain experience.
- **Use** assessment tools and rating scales that are appropriate to the developmental stage and situation and understanding of the child.
- **Evaluate** the patient for both behavioral and physiological changes.
- **Secure** the parent's participation in all stages of the pain evaluation and treatment process.
- **Take the cause of the pain into consideration** during the evaluation and choice of treatment methods.
- **Take action** to treat the pain appropriately, and then evaluate the results on a regular basis.

Barriers to Optimal Pain Assessments

Barriers to optimal pain assessments include:

- **Professional**: Health care providers may lack knowledge about pain assessment and management of different patient populations or may carry out assessments based on personal perceptions rather than validated pain assessment instruments. Some may be concerned about managing adverse effects or the patient's development of tolerance or addiction. In other cases, healthcare providers may lack empathy for patients' suffering. Lack of cultural awareness may affect interpretation of pain. For example, patients in cultures that encourage expression of pain may be assessed as having more pain than patients from cultures that value stoicism.
- **System**: The organization may lack clear policies regarding pain assessment and management, and may not have established clear guidelines for consistent use of pain assessment instruments. Additionally, supervision and accountability may be inadequate, and the organization may be concerned about costs and reimbursement for treatment.
- **Patient**: For personal or cultural reasons, patients may minimize or overstate the degree of pain, interfering with assessment. Some patients may be concerned about addiction or the effects of drugs on cognition (confusion, disorientation, lethargy) or other side effects (constipation, nausea, itching). Some may want to protect family from knowing the extent of pain.
- **Family**: Cultural biases may influence how the family responds to a patient's pain, and this can influence the patient's response as well. Families may lack understanding of the role of pain assessment and management. Some lack understanding about the difference between addiction and pain control at the end of life.
- **Society**: Concerns about drug abuse and addiction often permeate society and influence societal attitudes toward pain control and appropriate drugs to use. Laws and regulations may make access to certain drugs, such as those derived from marijuana, difficult or impossible to obtain.

Influential Factors in Pain Perception

Factors that can influence the perception of pain include:

- **Emotional state/attitude**: Patients who are extremely upset or anxious may be so overwhelmed they don't feel the pain, or they may experience pain as more severe than those who are relaxed and calm. If patients expect to suffer from pain, they are also more likely to report severe pain than patients who expect that their pain will be controlled.
- **Cultural expectations**: Perception may vary according to cultural beliefs about pain. For example, if a patient believes that pain is punishment, the patient may agonize over past sins. If a patient believes that pain is fate and reflects karma, then the patient may feel that bearing pain is necessary.
- **Pain threshold**: Different patients simply perceive and experience pain to different degrees. What may be a minor pain to one individual may be severe to another.

Effects of Gender on Pain Experience

Gender can affect pain sensitivity, tolerance, distress, and exaggeration of pain, and the patient's willingness to report pain, as well as displayed nonverbal cues concerning the pain experience. Studies indicate that women generally have **lower pain thresholds** and **less tolerance** for noxious stimuli or pain factors that hinder them from doing things they enjoy. Women seek help for pain-related problems sooner than men and respond better to therapy. Women also experience more **visceral pain** than men. Men are more prone to experience **somatic pain** and show more stoicism regarding pain experiences than women. **Neuropathic pain** seems to be experienced equally between men and women. Nurses need to be careful that biases concerning gender experiences with pain do not skew their assessments of pain. However, they need to be aware that pain experiences are always individual and may differ between the sexes.

Psychological Factors in Experience of Pain

Psychological factors that may influence a patient's experience of pain include:

- **Fear**: The fear of pain and the anticipation of having pain are factors in how much pain a person feels, because the fear stimulates areas of the brain that focus attention on the body so that the patient experiences an increased sensation of pain. Fear also causes muscles to tense, blood pressure to increase, and the heart rate to increase, and all of these can exacerbate the perception of pain. While pain medications may be necessary, practicing relaxation and mindfulness exercises may help to reduce anxiety and have a positive effect.
- **Depression**: The same neurotransmitters that transmit sensations of pain are also those that transmit moods, so many people with depression present first with complaints of pain or discomfort, and this can result in chronic pain if the depression is not resolved. In some cases, pain may lead to depression, but then the depression worsens the pain so it becomes a cycle of worsening discomfort. Patients may benefit from cognitive behavioral therapy or medication such as SSRIs.

Pain Documentation in Medical Records

Recommendations for **pain documentation** in the medical record include:

- Describe the time of onset, the location of pain, the character of the pain, and the degree of pain, using a validated pain assessment instrument (either a self-reporting instrument, such as the visual analog scale, or one based on observation, such as PAINAD).

- Document all interventions, both pharmacological (opioids, adjuvants) and nonpharmacological (positioning, massage, relaxation exercises), including the time, the dosage, and the method of administration.
- Assess and document the initial response to the medication based on the expected response time. For example, an IV medication should take effect almost immediately, but oral medications may take up to 20 minutes to take effect.
- Assess and document the duration of response based on the expected duration of the medication. For example, if a medication response is expected to last for 6 hours, the patient's pain level should be assessed at least every 2 hours and more frequently if the rate of pain increases.
- Describe any adverse effects, such as itching or nausea.

Review Video: Documentation of Pain Management
Visit mometrix.com/academy and enter code: 760328

Psychosocial Integrity

Psychosocial Assessment

Elements of the Psychosocial Assessment

A psychosocial assessment should provide additional information to the physical assessment to guide the patient's plan of care and should include:

- Previous hospitalizations and experience with healthcare
- Psychiatric history: Suicidal ideation, psychiatric disorders, family psychiatric history, history of violence and/or self-mutilation
- Chief complaint: Patient's perception
- Complementary therapies: Acupuncture, visualization, and meditation
- Occupational and educational background: Employment, retirement, and special skills
- Social patterns: Family and friends, living situation, typical activities, support system
- Sexual patterns: Orientation, problems, and sex practices
- Interests/abilities: Hobbies and sports
- Current or past substance abuse: Type, frequency, drinking pattern, use of recreational drugs, and overuse of prescription drugs
- Ability to cope: Stress reduction techniques
- Physical, sexual, emotional, and financial abuse: Older adults are especially vulnerable to abuse and may be reluctant to disclose out of shame or fear
- Spiritual/cultural assessment: Religious/spiritual importance, practices, restrictions (such as blood products or foods), and impact on health/health decisions

Cognitive Assessment

Individuals with evidence of dementia, delirium, or short-term memory loss should have cognition assessed. The **mini-mental state exam (MMSE)** or the **mini-cog test** are both commonly used. These tests require the individual to carry out specified tasks and are used as a baseline to determine change in mental status.

MMSE:

- Remembering and later repeating the names of 3 common objects
- Counting backward from 100 by 7s or spelling "world" backward
- Naming items as the examiner points to them
- Providing the location of the examiner's office, including city, state, and street address
- Repeating common phrases
- Copying a picture of interlocking shapes
- Following simple 3-part instructions, such as picking up a piece of paper, folding it in half, and placing it on the floor

A score of ≥24/30 is considered a normal functioning level.

Mini-cog:

- Remembering and later repeating the names of 3 common objects
- Drawing the face of a clock, including all 12 numbers and the hands, and indicating the time specified by the examiner

A score of 3–5 (out of 5) indicates a lower chance of dementia but does not rule it out.

Confusion Assessment Method

The Confusion Assessment Method is an assessment tool intended to be used by those without psychiatric training in order to assess the progression of delirium in patients. The tool covers 9 factors, some factors have a range of possibilities, and others are rated only as to whether the characteristic is present, not present, uncertain, or not applicable. The tool also provides room to describe abnormal behavior. Factors indicative of delirium include:

- **Onset**: Acute change in mental status
- **Attention**: Inattentive, stable, or fluctuating
- **Thinking**: Disorganized, rambling conversation, switching topics, illogical
- **Level of consciousness**: Altered, ranging from alert to coma
- **Orientation**: Disoriented (person, place, and time)
- **Memory**: Impaired
- **Perceptual disturbances**: Hallucinations, illusions
- **Psychomotor abnormalities**: Agitation (tapping, picking, moving) or retardation (staring, not moving)
- **Sleep-wake cycle**: Awake at night and sleepy in the daytime

**The Confusion Assessment Method indicates delirium if there is an acute onset, fluctuating inattention, and disorganized thinking OR altered level of consciousness.*

Hamilton Anxiety Scale

The Hamilton Anxiety Scale (HAS or HAMA) is utilized to evaluate the anxiety related symptomatology that may be present in adults as well as children. It provides an evaluation of overall **anxiety** and its degree of severity. This includes **somatic anxiety** (physical complaints) and **psychic anxiety** (mental agitation and distress). This scale consists of 14 items based on anxiety produced symptoms. Each item is ranked 0–4 with 0 indicating no symptoms present and 4 indicating severe symptoms present. This scale is frequently utilized in psychotropic drug evaluations. If performed before a particular medication has been started and then again at later visits, the HAS can be helpful in adjusting medication dosages based in part on the individual's score. It is often utilized as an outcome measure in clinical trials.

Beck Depression Inventory

The Beck Depression Inventory (BDI) is a widely utilized, self-reported, multiple-choice questionnaire consisting of 21 items, which measures the **degree of depression**. This tool is designed for use in adults ages 17–80. It evaluates physical symptoms such as weight loss, loss of sleep, loss of interest in sex, fatigue, and attitudinal symptoms such as irritability, guilt, and hopelessness. The items rank in four possible answer choices based on an increasing severity of symptoms. The test is scored with the answers ranging in value from 0–3. The total score is utilized to determine the degree of depression. The usual ranges include: 0–9 no signs of depression, 10–18 mild depression, 19–29 moderate depression, and 30–63 severe depression.

Evaluation for Suicidal or Homicidal Thoughts

During a risk assessment two of the most important areas to evaluate are the patient's **risk for self-harm or harm to others**. The staff member performing the assessment should very closely evaluate for any descriptions or thoughts the patient may have concerning these risks. Direct questioning on these subjects should be performed and documented. Close evaluation of any delusional thoughts the patient may be having should be carefully evaluated. Does the patient believe he or she is being instructed by others to perform either of these acts? Safety of the patient and others needs to be a top priority and carefully documented. If the patient indicates that they are having these thoughts or ideas, they must be placed in either suicidal or assault precautions with close monitoring per facility protocol.

Suicide Risk Assessment

A suicide risk assessment should be completed and documented upon admission, with each shift change, at discharge, or any time suicidal ideations are suggested by the patient. This risk assessment should evaluate some of the following criteria:

- Would the patient sign a contract for safety?
- Is there a suicide plan? How lethal is the plan?
- What is the elopement risk?
- How often are the suicidal thoughts, and have they attempted suicide before?

Any associated symptoms of hopelessness, guilt, anger, helplessness, impulsive behaviors, nightmares, obsessions with death, or altered judgment should also be assessed and documented. The higher the score the higher the risk for suicide.

Alcohol Use Assessment

The **Clinical Instrument for Withdrawal for Alcohol (CIWA)** is a tool used to assess the severity of alcohol withdraw. Each category is scored 0–7 points based on the severity of symptoms, except #10, which is scored 0–4. A score <5 indicates mild withdrawal without need for medications; for scores ranging 5–15, benzodiazepines are indicated to manage symptoms. A score >15 indicates severe withdrawal and the need for admission to the unit.

- Nausea/Vomiting
- Tremor
- Paroxysmal Sweats
- Anxiety
- Agitation
- Tactile Disturbances
- Auditory Disturbances
- Visual Disturbances
- Headache
- Disorientation or Clouding of Sensorium

The **CAGE** tool is used as a quick assessment to identify problem drinkers. Moderate drinking, (1–2 drinks daily or one drink a day for older adults) is usually not harmful to people in the absence of other medical conditions. However, drinking more can lead to serious psychosocial and physical problems. One drink is defined as 12 ounces of beer/wine cooler, 5 ounces of wine, or 1.5 ounces of liquor.

- **C** – *Cutting Down*: "Do you think about trying to cut down on drinking?"
- **A** – *Annoyed at Criticism*: "Are people starting to criticize your drinking?"
- **G** – *Guilty feeling*: "Do you feel guilty or try to hide your drinking?"
- **E** – *Eye opener*: "Do you increasingly need a drink earlier in the day?"

"Yes" on one question suggests the possibility of a drinking problem. "Yes" on ≥2 indicates a drinking problem

Screening for Risk-Taking Behavior

The ability to assess outcomes and respond appropriately to risks are part of the decision-making process. Decision making can be impaired in patients with mental health disorders such as depression, anxiety, bipolar disorder, and personality disorders, as well as in patients who have experienced a brain injury or have a dependence on drugs or alcohol. Health care providers should screen patients for the presence of high-risk behaviors. This may be accomplished through a self-administered questionnaire or through a patient interview with a trained clinician. Examples of **high-risk behaviors** include substance use/abuse, high risk sexual behaviors, high risk driving behaviors such as drinking and driving, speeding or riding with a drunk driver, and violence related behaviors. Patients with an increased response to risk taking may exhibit signs of impulsivity and sensation seeking. Conversely, other patients may exhibit abnormally cautious behavior.

Indicators of Abuse That May Be Identified in the Patient History

The healthcare provider should always be aware of the presence of any **indicators** that may present a potential for or an actual situation that involves **abuse**. These indicators may present in the **patient's history**. Some examples of indicators concerning their primary complaint may include the following: vague description about the cause of the problem, inconsistencies between physical findings and explanations, minimizing injuries, long period of time between injury and treatment, and over-reactions or under-reactions of family members to injuries. Other important information may be revealed in the family genome, such as family history of violence, time spent in jail or prison, and family history of violent deaths or substance abuse. The patient's health history may include previous injuries, spontaneous abortions, or history of pervious inpatient psychiatric treatment or substance abuse.

During the collection of the patient history, the financial history, the patient's family values, and the patient's relationships with family members can also reveal actual or potential **abuse indicators**.

- The **financial history** may indicate that the patient has little or no money or that they are not given access to money by a controlling family member. They may also be unemployed or utilizing an elderly family member's income for their own personal expenses.
- **Family values** may indicate strong beliefs in physical punishment, dictatorship within the home, inability to allow different opinions within the home, or lack of trust for anyone outside the family.
- **Relationships** within the family may be dysfunctional. Problems such as lack of affection between family members, co-dependency, frequent arguments, extramarital affairs, or extremely rigid beliefs about roles within the family may be present.

During the collection of the patient history, the sexual, social, and psychological history of the patient should be evaluated for any signs of actual or potential abuse.

- The **sexual history** may reveal problems such as previous sexual abuse, forced sexual acts, sexually transmitted infections (STIs), sexual knowledge beyond normal age-appropriate knowledge, or promiscuity.
- The **social history** may reveal unplanned pregnancies, social isolation as evidenced by lack of friends available to help the patient, unreasonable jealousy of significant other, verbal aggression, belief in physical punishment, or problems in school.
- During the **psychological assessment** the patient may express feelings of helplessness and being trapped. The patient may be unable to describe their future, become tearful, perform self-mutilation, have low self-esteem, and have had previous suicide attempts.

Observations That May Indicate Abuse

During the initial assessment, observations may also be made by the provider that can provide vital information about actual or potential abuse. **General observations** may include finding that the patient history is far different from what is objectively viewed by the provider or that there is a lack of proper clothing or lack of physical care provided. The home environment may include lack of heat, water, or food. It may also reveal inappropriate sleeping arrangements or lack of an environmentally safe housing situation. Observations concerning **family communications** may reveal that the abuser answers all the questions for the whole family or that others look to the controlling member for approval or seem fearful of others. Family members may frequently argue, interrupt each other, or act out negative nonverbal behaviors while others are speaking. They may avoid talking about certain subjects that they feel are secretive.

Indicators of Abuse That May Be Evident During the Physical Assessment

During the **physical assessment** the provider should always be aware of any **indicators of abuse**. These indicators may include increased anxiety about being examined or in the presence of the abuser; poor hygiene; looks to abuser to answer questions for them; flinching; over or underweight; presence of bruises, welts, scars or cigarette burns; bald patches on scalp for pulling out of hair; intracranial bleeding; subconjunctival hemorrhages; black eye(s); hearing loss from untreated infection or injury; poor dental hygiene; abdominal injuries; fractures; developmental delays; hyperactive reflexes; genital lacerations or ecchymosis; and presence of STIs, rectal bruising, bleeding, edema, or poor sphincter tone.

Domestic Violence

Men, women, elderly, children, and the disabled may all be victims of **domestic violence**. The violent person harms physically or sexually and uses threats and fear to maintain control of the victim. The violence does not improve unless the abuser gets intensive counseling. The abuser may promise not to do it again, but the violence usually gets more frequent and worsens over time. The provider should ask all patients in private about abuse, neglect, and fear of a caretaker. If abuse is suspected or there are signs present, the state may require **reporting**:

- Give victims information about community hotlines, shelters, and resources.
- Urge them to set up a plan for escape for themselves and any children, complete with supplies in a location away from the home.

- Assure victims that they are not at fault and do not deserve the abuse.
- Try to empower them by helping them to realize that they do not have to take abuse and can find support to change the situation.

Review Video: Domestic Violence
Visit mometrix.com/academy and enter code: 530581

Assessment of Domestic Violence

According to the guidelines of the Family Violence Prevention Fund, **assessment** for domestic violence should be done for all adolescent and adult patients, regardless of background or signs of abuse. While females are the most common victims, there are increasing reports of male victims of domestic violence, both in heterosexual and homosexual relationships. The person doing the assessment should be informed about domestic violence and be aware of risk factors and danger signs. The interview should be conducted in private (special accommodations may need to be made for children <3 years old). The manager's office, bathrooms, and examining rooms should have information about domestic violence posted prominently. Brochures and information should be available to give to patients. Patients may present with a variety of physical complaints, such as headache, pain, palpitations, numbness, or pelvic pain. They are often depressed and may appear suicidal and may be isolated from friends and family. Victims of domestic violence often exhibit fear of spouse/partner, and may report injury inconsistent with symptoms.

Steps to Identifying Victims of Domestic Violence

Identifying and assisting victims of domestic violence involves the following steps:

1. **Inquiry**: Non-judgmental questioning should begin with asking if the person has ever been abused—physically, sexually, or psychologically.
2. **Interview**: The person may exhibit signs of anxiety or fear and may blame himself or report that others believe he is abused. The person should be questioned if she is afraid for her life or for her children.
3. **Question**: If the person reports abuse, it's critical to ask if the person is in immediate danger or if the abuser is on the premises. The interviewer should ask if the person has been threatened. The history and pattern of abuse should be questioned, and if children are involved, whether the children are abused. Note: State laws vary, and in some states, it is mandatory to report if a child was present during an act of domestic violence as this is considered child abuse. The provider must be aware of state laws regarding domestic and child abuse, and all healthcare providers are mandatory reporters.
4. **Validate**: The interviewer should offer support and reassurance in a non-judgmental manner, telling the patient the abuse is not his or her fault.
5. **Give information**: While discussing facts about domestic violence and the tendency to escalate, the interviewer should provide brochures and information about safety planning. If the patient wants to file a complaint with the police, the interviewer should assist the person to place the call.
6. **Make referrals**: Information about state, local, and national organizations should be provided along with telephone numbers and contact numbers for domestic violence shelters.
7. **Document**: Record keeping should be legal, legible, and lengthy with a complete report and description of any traumatic injuries resulting from domestic violence. A body map may be used to indicate sites of injury, especially if there are multiple bruises or injuries.

Injuries Consistent with Domestic Violence

There are a number of characteristic **injuries** that may indicate domestic violence, including ruptured eardrum; rectal/genital injury (burns, bites, or trauma); scrapes and bruises about the neck, face, head, trunk, arms; and cuts, bruises, and fractures of the face. The pattern of injuries associated with domestic violence is also often distinctive. The bathing-suit pattern involves injuries on parts of body that are usually covered with clothing as the perpetrator inflicts damage but hides evidence of abuse. Head and neck injuries (50%) are also common. Abusive injuries (rarely attributable to accidents) are common and include bites, bruises, rope and cigarette burns, and welts in the outline of weapons (belt marks). Bilateral injuries of arms/legs are often seen with domestic abuse. Defensive injuries are indicative of abuse.

Defensive injuries to the back of the body are often incurred as the victim crouches on the floor face down while being attacked. The soles of the feet may be injured from kicking at perpetrator. The ulnar aspect of hand or palm may be injured from blocking blows.

Identifying and Reporting Neglect of the Basic Needs of Adults

Neglect of the basic needs of adults is a common problem, especially among the elderly, adults with psychiatric or mental health problems, or those who live alone or with reluctant or incapable caregivers. In some cases, **passive neglect** may occur because an elderly or impaired spouse or partner is trying to take care of a patient and is unable to provide the care needed, but in other cases, **active neglect** reflects a lack of caring which may be considered negligence or abuse. Cases of neglect should be reported to the appropriate governmental agency, such as adult protective services. Indications of neglect include the following:

- Lack of assistive devices, such as a cane or walker, needed for mobility
- Misplaced or missing glasses or hearing aids
- Poor dental hygiene and dental care or missing dentures
- Patient left unattended for extended periods of time, sometimes confined to a bed or chair
- Patient left in soiled or urine- and feces-stained clothing
- Inadequate food, fluid, or nutrition, resulting in weight loss
- Inappropriate and unkempt clothing, such as no sweater or coat during the winter and dirty or torn clothing
- A dirty, messy environment

Therapeutic Communication

Therapeutic Communication

Facilitating Communication

Therapeutic communication begins with respect for the patient/family and the assumption that all communication, verbal and nonverbal, has meaning. Listening must be done empathetically. The following are some techniques that facilitate communication.

Introduction:

- Make a personal introduction and use the patient's name: "Mrs. Brown, I am Susan Williams, your nurse."

Encouragement:

- Use an open-ended opening statement: "Is there anything you'd like to discuss?"
- Acknowledge comments: "Yes," and "I understand."
- Allow silence and observe nonverbal behavior rather than trying to force conversation. Ask for clarification if statements are unclear.
- Reflect statements back (use sparingly): Patient: "I hate this hospital." Nurse: "You hate this hospital?"

Empathy:

- Make observations: "You are shaking," and "You seem worried."
- Recognize feelings:
  - Patient: "I want to go home."
  - Nurse: "It must be hard to be away from your home and family."
- Provide information as honestly and completely as possible about condition, treatment, and procedures and respond to the patient's questions and concerns.

Exploration:

- Verbally express implied messages:
  - Patient: "This treatment is too much trouble."
  - Nurse: "You think the treatment isn't helping you?"
- Explore a topic but allow the patient to terminate the discussion without further probing: "I'd like to hear how you feel about that."

Orientation:

- Indicate reality:
  - Patient: "Someone is screaming."
  - Nurse: "That sound was an ambulance siren."
- Comment on distortions without directly agreeing or disagreeing:
  - Patient: "That nurse promised I didn't have to walk again."
  - Nurse: "Really? That's surprising because the doctor ordered physical therapy twice a day."

Collaboration:

- Work together to achieve better results: "Maybe if we talk about this, we can figure out a way to make the treatment easier for you."

Validation:

- Seek validation: "Do you feel better now?" or "Did the medication help you breathe better?"

Avoiding Non-therapeutic Communication

While using therapeutic communication is important, it is equally important to avoid interjecting **non-therapeutic communication**, which can block effective communication. *Avoid the following:*

- Meaningless clichés: "Don't worry. Everything will be fine." "Isn't it a nice day?"
- Providing advice: "You should..." or "The best thing to do is...." It's better when patients ask for advice to provide facts and encourage the patient to reach a decision.
- Inappropriate approval that prevents the patient from expressing true feeling or concerns:
    - Patient: "I shouldn't cry about this."
    - Nurse: "That's right! You're an adult!"
- Asking for an explanation of behavior that is not directly related to patient care and requires analysis and explanation of feelings: "Why are you so upset?"
- Agreeing with rather than accepting and responding to patient's statements can make it difficult for the patient to change his or her statement or opinion later: "I agree with you," or "You are right."
- Making negative judgments: "You should stop arguing with the nurses."
- Devaluing the patient's feelings: "Everyone gets upset at times."
- Disagreeing directly: "That can't be true," or "I think you are wrong."
- Defending against criticism: "The doctor is not being rude; he's just very busy today."
- Changing the subject to avoid dealing with uncomfortable topics;
    - Patient: "I'm never going to get well."
    - Nurse: "Your family will be here in just a few minutes."
- Making inappropriate literal responses, even as a joke, especially if the patient is at all confused or having difficulty expressing ideas:
    - Patient: "There are bugs crawling under my skin."
    - Nurse: "I'll get some bug spray,"
- Challenging the patient to establish reality often just increases confusion and frustration:
    - "If you were dying, you wouldn't be able to yell and kick!"

Communicating with Patients with Disabilities

Guidelines for communicating with individuals with disabilities:

- Do not assume that the person with disabilities also has impaired cognition.
- Always treat the person with respect and dignity.
- Use first names with the patient if asked to do so, but start out formally as with any patient.
- Offer to shake hands even when a prosthesis is present.
- Be patient if communication is impaired.
- Offer assistance, but allow the patient to tell you what is helpful; otherwise don't assist.
- When a wheelchair is used, sit down so the patient does not have to strain their neck to speak with you.
- If providing directions, consider the obstacles that may be in the way and assist the person to find an appropriate way around them.

Communication with Patients with Cognitive Disabilities

The person with cognitive disabilities may be easily distracted, so verbal communication should be attempted in a quiet area:

- Address people with dignity and respect.
- Do not try to discuss abstract ideas but stick with concrete topics.
- Keep words and sentences very simple and try rephrasing when necessary. People may have difficulty in distinguishing your spoken words and deriving the meaning from them.
- Be very patient with people's attempts to speak to you since they may have difficulty in processing thoughts and changing them into spoken words.
- Use objects around you and gestures to illustrate your words since the patient may also use pointing and gesturing when unable to find the words to communicate with you. The person may prefer written communication, although some may be unable to read.
- Use touch to convey your regard during communication, as this is recognized by the patient as reassurance of your care and concern for them.
- Give a few instructions at a time as to not overwhelm them.

Communicating with Deaf or Hearing-Impaired Patients

Communicating with a person with deafness or hearing impairment:

- Try to communicate in a quiet environment if possible.
- Wave or touch the person to let him or her know you are trying to communicate.
- Determine the method the person uses to communicate: sign language, lip reading, hearing devices, or writing.
- Fingerspell or use some signs if able to do so.
- Address the person directly when you speak even though the person may be looking at an interpreter or your lips.
- Look at the person as the interpreter tells you what was said.
- Speak slowly so the interpreter can keep up with you.
- If the person reads lips, face the person and speak clearly and normally, using normal volume.
- If writing a communication, do not speak while writing.
- Do not be afraid to check that the person understands you, and ask questions if you do not understand the person.

Communication with People with Low Vision or Blindness

Communicating with a person with low vision or blindness:

- Greet the person with low vision or blindness, identifying yourself and others present.
- Always say goodbye when you are leaving.
- Alert the person to written communications, such as warning signs or printed notices.
- Face the person and touch briefly on the arm to let the person know you are speaking to him or her if you are in a group.
- Speak at normal loudness.
- Make any directions given specific in terms of the length of walk and obstacles, such as stairs.
- Use the position of hands on a clock face to give directions (potatoes at 3 o'clock) as well as using *right* or *left*.
- Mention sounds that the person may hear in transit or on arrival at a destination.

Communicating with a Patient on a Ventilator

When a patient on a ventilator is conscious, he or she may still be able to communicate by blinking, nodding, shaking the head, or pointing to a picture or word board:

- If the person is able to write, try to reposition the IV line to leave the dominant hand free to communicate.
- Discuss the need for communication with the physician and ask if a valve or an electric larynx can be used to permit speech.
- Help the patient practice lip reading of single words.
- Remember the patient's glasses or hearing aids when attempting to communicate.
- Enlist the aid of a speech therapist if there is frustration on the part of the patient and family due to communication difficulty.

Communicating with Persons with Speech Problems Due to a Stroke

Methods to communicate with stroke patients with speech problems:

- **Dysarthria**: Patients have problems forming the words to speak them aloud. Give them time to communicate, offer them a picture board or other means of communicating, and give encouragement to family members who are frustrated with the difficulty of trying to communicate.
- **Expressive aphasia**: The patients' efforts at speech come out garbled when they try to say sentences, but single words may be clear. Encourage the patients to try to write and to practice the sounds of the alphabet. Resist the urge to finish sentences for the patients.
- **Receptive aphasia**: The patients have a problem comprehending the speech they hear. Communicate in simple terms and speak slowly. Test comprehension of the written word as an alternative method of communication.
- **Global aphasia**: The patient has both receptive and expressive aphasia. Use simple, clear, slow speech augmented by pictures and gestures.

Communication Problems of Patients with Parkinson's Disease

Parkinson's disease causes problems with speaking in the majority (75–90%) of patients. The reason for this is not clear but may relate to increasing rigidity and changes in movement. Speech is often very low-pitched or hoarse, given in a monotone and with a soft voice. Speech production may decrease because of the effort required to speak. **Speech therapy** can develop exercises for the patient that can assist them in remembering to speak slowly and carefully, as patients are not always aware that their **communication** is impaired:

- Allow time for the patient to communicate, asking for repetition if you do not understand the message.
- Help family by teaching ways to facilitate communication with the patient and encouraging them to assist the patient to do the exercises provided by the therapist.
- If speech volume is very low, suggest amplification devices that can be obtained through speech therapy.

Communication with Patients with Psychiatric Problems

Persons with psychiatric disorders appreciate being addressed with respect, dignity, and honesty:

- Speak simply and clearly, repeating as necessary.
- Encourage patients to discuss their concerns regarding treatment and medications to improve compliance.
- Use good eye contact and be attentive to your body language messages.
- Be alert, but unless the person is known to be violent, try to relax and listen to them.
- Don't try to avoid words or phrases pertaining to psychiatric problems, but if you do say something inappropriate, apologize honestly to the patient.
- Offer patients outlets for their thoughts and feelings.
- Learn more about their disorder and ways to use therapeutic communication to help them with their problem, such as re-orienting them as needed.

Cultural Competence

Different cultures view health and illness from very different perspectives, and patients often come from a mix of many cultures, so the nurse must be not only accepting of cultural differences but must be sensitive and aware. There are a number of characteristics that are important for a nurse to have **cultural competence**:

- **Appreciating diversity**: This must be grounded in information about other cultures and understanding of their value systems.
- **Assessing own cultural perspectives**: Self-awareness is essential to understanding potential biases.
- **Understanding intercultural dynamics**: This must include understanding ways in which cultures cooperate, differ, communicate, and reach understanding.
- **Recognizing institutional culture**: Each institutional unit (hospital, clinic, office) has an inherent set of values that may be unwritten but is accepted by the staff.
- **Adapting patient service to diversity**: This is the culmination of cultural competence as it is the point of contact between cultures.

Coping

Functional Coping Strategies of Families

Some families utilize a number of functional coping strategies to deal with stress. These families exhibit resilience in difficult situations. Strategies include:

- The family gathers information, increases organization, discusses issues, and tries to jointly solve problems.
- Family members draw together as a strengthened family unit to deal with stressful situations.
- The family attempts to carry on as normal a routine as possible while making accommodations as needed for a child who is ill. This provides the child with a sense of security.
- The family accepts those things that cannot be changed rather than wasting energy trying to deny or alter reality.
- The family communicates openly and directly, avoiding family secrets and including the child in discussions as appropriate to the child's age.
- The family uses humor to deflect stress.
- The family uses resources outside of the immediate family for support, such as extended family, spiritual advisors, and community agencies.

Dysfunctional Coping Strategies of Families

Some families are not resilient when dealing with stressful situations and exhibit dysfunctional coping strategies, which include:

- Family members may resort to substance abuse, such as alcohol and/or drugs, rather than facing problems. This adds to the family dysfunction and negatively affects all members.
- The family may take out frustrations through domestic violence, aimed at the child or other family members. This can include physical, sexual, or mental abuse and can create an environment of fear within the family.
- The family denies problems and refuses to acknowledge that family dynamics have changed, attempting to carry on as usual.
- The family uses threats, aggression, and/or withholding of affection to retain control and maintain the family unit.
- The family may blame vulnerable members, such as the child, for the stressful situation, often scapegoating the member that they "blame" rather than dealing with the real problems.

Self-Concept and Sexuality

Sexuality

Sexuality is an integral part of each individual's personality and refers to all aspects of being a sexual human. It is more than just the act of physical intercourse. A person's sexuality is often apparent in what they do, in their appearance, and in how they interact with others. There are four main aspects of sexuality:

- **Genetic identity** or one's chromosomal gender
- **Gender identification** or how one perceives oneself with regard to male or female
- **Gender role** or the attributes of one's cultural role
- **Sexual orientation** or the gender to which one is attracted

Assessing and attempting to conceptualize a person's sexuality will lead to a broader understanding of the client's beliefs and allow for a more holistic approach to providing care.

Gender Identity

Gender identity is the gender to which the individual identifies, which may or may not be the gender of birth (natal gender). Most children begin to express identification and behaviors associated with gender between ages 2 and 4. The degree to which this identification is influenced by genetics and environment is an ongoing debate because, for example, female children are often socialized toward female roles (dresses, dolls, pink items). Societal pressure to conform to gender stereotypes is strong, so gender dysphoria, which is less common in early childhood than later, may be suppressed. At the onset of puberty, sexual attraction may further complicate gender identity although those with gender dysphoria most often have sexual attraction to those of the same natal gender, so a natal boy who identifies as a girl is more likely to be sexually attracted to boys than to girls. Later in adolescence, individuals generally experiment with sexual behavior and solidify their gender identity.

Influence of Sexual Orientation on Behaviors

The degree to which sexual orientation influences behavior may vary widely depending on the individual. For example, some gay males may be indistinguishable in appearance and general behavior from heterosexual males while others may behave in a stereotypically flamboyant manner. The same holds true for lesbians, with some typically feminine in appearance and behavior and others preferring a more masculine appearance. The typical heterosexual model (two people in a stable relationship) is increasingly practiced by homosexual couples while others prefer less traditional practices. Depending on the degree of acceptance that LGBTQ individuals encounter, they may hide their sexual orientation or maintain a heterosexual relationship in order to appear straight. LGBTQ individuals are at higher risk of depression and suicide, especially if they experience rejection because of their sexual orientation or have been taught that it is sinful. LGBTQ individuals with multiple sexual partners (especially males) are at increased risk for STIs, including HIV/AIDS.

Coming Out Process

The coming out process is the act of revealing LGBTQ sexual orientation to family and friends. This generally occurs during adolescence or early adulthood although some may delay coming out for decades or never do so. Individuals may come out to select groups of people. For example, friends may be aware of an individual's orientation but not family or co-workers. Coming out can be frightening for many people, especially if they have reason to fear rejection or fear for their safety. Stages in coming out typically progress in the following order:

Stage	Actions and feelings involved
Confusion	The individual may be unsure of feelings or be in denial.
Exploration	The individual begins to question orientation and wonder about LGBTQ people.
Breakthrough	The individual accepts the likelihood of being LGBTQ and seeks others of the same orientation.
Acceptance	The individual accepts orientation and begins to explore and read about the LGBTQ culture.
Pride	The individual begins to exhibit pride in orientation and may reject straight culture or exhibit stereotypically LGBTQ behaviors.
Synthesis	The individual comes to terms with the reality of the LGBTQ orientation, is at peace with their identity, and is generally out to family, friends, and co-workers.

Practice Issues When Working with LGBTQ Clients

Possible practice issues with LGBTQ clients include, but are not limited to, the following:

- Stigmatization and violence
- Internalized homophobia
- Coming out
- AIDS
- Limited civil rights
- Orientation vs. preference (biology vs. choice)

Problematic treatment models for treating gay and lesbian people include the following:

- The moral model for treatment is religiously oriented and views homosexuality as sinful.
- Reparative or conversion psychotherapy focuses on changing a person's sexual orientation to heterosexual. Traditional mental health disciplines view this type of treatment as unethical and as having no empirical base.

Cultural and Spiritual Nursing Care

Influencing Factors on Outlook in Long-Term Care

Culture

Culture is defined as the behavior and belief systems of a particular group of people. A person's cultural outlook is shaped by ethnicity, gender, and age. It affects their outlook on all things, including health care. It can affect the types of foods patients might eat while sick, their behaviors during illness, and their attitude about death and dying. The patient's cultural beliefs should be taken into account when planning care. If the patient's cultural beliefs are not taken into account, it may increase the patient's stress level, hindering the healing process.

Religion

Religion is the set of beliefs that a person has regarding the nature of the universe. The patient's religion may dictate the level of participation in their care, including what treatments they may and may not accept. Religion can also aid in the patient's ability to cope during the recovery period following serious illness or injury. The patient's religious outlook should be taken into account when planning the patient's care. Failure to do so may result in the patient's refusal to participate in the care or withdrawal from the hospital setting altogether.

Appropriate Action If a Patient Asks for a Priest

During times of illness or injury, it is not uncommon for a patient to request to see a priest or a person of authority within their church. If a patient makes such a request, the charge nurse or appropriate staff should be contacted immediately to assist with the request. The first step is to find out if there is a specific person the patient wishes to see. Most hospitals and extended-care facilities have an on-call clergyperson who can be notified if the patient does not have a specific person to call.

Caring for Muslim Patients

It is important to ask the **Muslim patient** if they have any specific dietary restrictions. Many strict practicing Muslims will eat only specially slaughtered fish, chicken, and beef. Most Muslims will not eat pork products. Try to avoid handing a Muslim patient anything with the left hand, as that is the hand that is reserved for performing perineal care on oneself. Muslims place a strong emphasis on cleanliness. Many Muslims wish to wash with soap and water after using the bedpan and toilet paper. They should also be provided with fresh water to wash with prior to their prayers. If possible, female patients should be cared for by female staff.

Caring for Christian Patients

It is important to ask if the **Christian patient** has any dietary restrictions. Though most Christians do not have dietary restrictions as a result of their faith, some may have self-imposed dietary restrictions. Some Catholic patients may wish to fast during Lent. During their stay, some Catholic or Orthodox Christian patients may choose to receive communion or give confession during their hospitalization. Some patients may request to receive Last Rites if they are critically ill or dying. It is important to notify the charge nurse or appropriate staff immediately if the patient requests to see a priest while at the hospital. In many cases, the patient or family will know a priest they would want to call.

Caring for Hindu Patients

It is important to inquire about any specific dietary needs of the **Hindu patient**. Most Hindus are vegetarian or vegan; even those that do eat meat may refuse to eat beef or pork. After using the bedpan, many Hindu patients want to wash their perineal area using clean water after using toilet paper. This should be made available if requested. Some Hindus may prefer to wash in the shower rather than sitting in the bath. Members of the Hindu faith particularly value privacy; if possible, the patient should be cared for by staff of the same gender. Some Hindu patients may prefer to die while lying on the ground to maintain closeness between the individual and Mother Earth. If necessary, a Hindu priest may be called in to perform holy rites for the patient.

Caring for Jewish Patients

Orthodox Jews eat only kosher meat and typically avoid dishes in which milk and meat have been prepared together. Other types of foods that are forbidden include pork products, meat from birds of prey, and shellfish. Most **Jewish patients** prefer to wash their hands and say a brief prayer prior to eating; they should be provided them with an opportunity to do so. Jewish men may prefer to remain bearded or may choose to shave using an electric razor rather than a razor blade. Jewish patients observe specific practices regarding death. The family will notify their Synagogue of the patient's impending death; if there is no family present, the health care staff should do so. After the death, three members of the family typically wash the body. Burial should take place within 24 hours after dying.

Caring for Mormon Patients

Many Mormons follow a set of dietary restrictions put forward in the *Word of Wisdom*. It teaches against the use of stimulants, such as coffee, tea, and other caffeinated beverages. Though most Mormons are not strict vegetarians, they do tend to eat meat sparingly. Some Mormons may wear a special undergarment that should be treated with the utmost privacy. It can be removed for laundering and washing but is otherwise worn at all times. Though Mormons do not have specific rites or rituals regarding a dying patient, the family should be allowed to spend as much time as possible with the patient in their final hours. If the patient wears the sacred undergarment, it should be put back on the body after postmortem care has been performed.

Caring for Buddhist Patients

It is important to inquire about a **Buddhist patient's** dietary needs on admission as many Buddhist patients are vegetarians or vegans. Many Buddhists fast on specific days, including the days of the New Moon and Full Moon. On fasting days, a Buddhist will only eat at specific times. The medical staff should collaborate with the patient on these days to ensure they get their meal tray at appropriate times. The type of rituals surrounding death and dying varies depending on the patient's traditions. The patient may request a Buddhist monk or nun to perform chants in order to assist in the patient's passing. If possible, the body should not be touched until 3–8 hours after death.

Spiritual Assessments

HOPE Mnemonic

HOPE is a simple mnemonic used as a guideline for the spiritual assessment:

H	Hope	What sources of hope (who or what) do you have to turn to?
O	Organized	Are you a part of an organized religion or faith group? What do you gain from membership in this group?
P	Personal	What spiritual practices (prayer, meditation) are most helpful?
E	Effects	What effects do your beliefs play on any medical care or end-of-life issues and decisions? Do you have any beliefs that may affect the type of care the health care team can provide you with?

FICA Mnemonic

FICA is another abbreviated spiritual assessment tool:

F	Faith	Do you have a faith or belief system that gives your life meaning?
I	Importance	What importance does your faith have in your daily life?
C	Community	Do you participate and gain support from a faith community?
A	Address	What faith issues would you like me to address in your care?

Spirit Mnemonic

SPIRIT (Maugens) is a mnemonic used for a spiritual assessment tool:

S	Spiritual	Do you have a formal religious affiliation?
P	Personal	Which practices and beliefs do you personally accept and practice? Does spirituality play a part in your daily life?
I	Integration	Do you participate in a spiritual community and receive support from that community?
R	Ritual	Are there specific practices and restrictions in your religious convictions that would affect your healthcare choices?
I	Implication	Are there aspects of your spirituality you would like me to keep in mind during your care?
T	Terminal events	As you prepare for the end of life, how does your faith affect the decisions you make or how you feel about death?

Spiritual Care at the End of Life

The patient's basic beliefs should be assessed in order to provide holistic care as the end of life approaches. **Spiritual care** must be provided according to the patient's religion and/or philosophy of choice, and must remain unbiased from the caregiver's own beliefs. If the patient does not wish to have spiritual counseling, it should not be pressed upon them. Advice and comfort can be provided by anyone known to the patient. Spiritual care is intended to relieve spiritual suffering and to explore answers to significant questions that the patient and family may have. Even those who do not have a formal religion affiliation or philosophical practice may experience questions and may search for meaning and comfort at the end of life.

The caregiver must assess prior and present religious affiliations, along with individual beliefs about God and the afterlife. The information must include devotional practices, rituals, and routines, and identify the degree of involvement and support available from the patient's chosen religious community. This spiritual assessment opens the door for effective spiritual caregiving, and it allows patients and their families to access spiritual coping strategies and support mechanisms. The holistic assessment addresses the patient's ability to resolve meaningful spiritual questions, identifying deeper understandings and retaining hope, strength, and peace. Questions can include the patient's interpretation of the meaning and purpose of their life, the role of family, and personal strengths and connections to various spiritual communities and to nature. Provisions should be made to explore spiritual relationships and to provide support for loss and crisis, as desired by the patient and family.

Addressing Emotional and Spiritual Health

Strategies to address emotional and spiritual health include:

- Remain observant and note both verbal and nonverbal communication.
- Address the patient by the surname unless asked to do otherwise, avoiding terms such as "honey" and "dear."
- Take the time to converse with the patient before broaching serious subjects.
- Use a pleasant and soft tone of voice when talking with the patient.
- Note indications of spiritual beliefs, such as Bibles, Korans, offering bowls, prayer beads, rosaries, and religious symbols as well as prayers, meditation, chants, signs of the cross, and fasts.
- Ask the meaning of unfamiliar symbols or items.
- Respect personal space, including noting how close the patient and family members stand to others.
- Avoid judgmental statements or attitudes toward traditions and practices that are different from those common to Western culture.
- Assist with religious or spiritual rituals and practices if requested.
- Ask the patient and family members if their needs are being met and about what issues are important to them.

Grief, Loss, and Palliative Care

Grief

Grief is an emotional response to a **loss** that begins at the time a loss is anticipated and continues on an individual timetable. While there are identifiable stages or tasks, it is not an orderly and predictable process. It involves overcoming anger, disbelief, guilt, and a myriad of related emotions. The grieving individual may move back and forth between stages or experience several emotions at any given time. Each person's grief response is unique to their own coping patterns, stress levels, age, gender, belief system, and previous experiences with loss.

Kubler-Ross's Five Stages of Grief

Kubler-Ross taught the medical community that the dying patient and family welcomes open, honest discussion of the dying process and felt that there were certain **stages** that patients and family go through. The stages may not occur in order, but may vary or some may be skipped. Stages include:

- **Denial**: The person denies the diagnosis and tries to pretend it isn't true. During this time, the person may seek a second opinion or alternative therapies. They may use denial until they are better able to emotionally cope with the reality of the disease or changes that need to be made. Patients may also wish to save family and friends from pain and worry. Both patients and family may use denial as a coping mechanism when they feel overwhelmed by the reality of the disease and threatened losses.
- **Anger**: The person is angry about the situation and may focus that rage on anyone.
- **Bargaining**: The person attempts to make deals with a higher power to secure a better outcome to their situation.
- **Depression**: The person anticipates the loss and the changes it will bring with a sense of sadness and grief.
- **Acceptance**: The person accepts the impending death and is ready to face it as it approaches. The patient may begin to withdraw from interests and family.

Review Video: The Five Stages of Grief
Visit mometrix.com/academy and enter code: 648794

Anticipatory Grief

Anticipatory grief is the mental, social, and somatic reactions of an individual as they prepare themselves for a **perceived future loss**. The individual experiences a process of intellectual, emotional, and behavioral responses in order to modify their self-concept, based on their perception of what the potential loss will mean in their life. This process often takes place ahead of the actual loss, from the time the loss is first perceived until it is resolved as a reality for the individual. This process can also blend with past loss experiences. It is associated with the individual's perception of how life will be affected by the particular diagnosis as well as the impending death. Acknowledging this anticipatory grief allows family members to begin looking toward a changed future. Suppressing this anticipatory process may inhibit relationships with the ill individual and contribute to a more difficult grieving process at a later time. However, appropriate anticipatory grieving does not take the place of grief during the actual time of death.

Disenfranchised Grief

Disenfranchised grief occurs when the loss being experienced cannot be openly acknowledged, publicly mourned, or socially supported. Society and culture are partly responsible for an individual's response to a loss. There is a **social context** to grief; if a person incurring the loss will be putting himself or herself at risk if grief is expressed, disenfranchised grief occurs. The risk for disenfranchised grief is greatest among those whose relationship with the individual they lost was not known or regarded as significant. This is also the situation found among bereaved persons who are not recognized by society as capable of grief, such as young children, or needing to mourn, such as an ex-spouse or secret lover.

Grief vs. Depression

Normal grief is preoccupied with self-limiting to the loss itself. Emotional responses will vary and may include open expressions of anger. The individual may experience difficulty sleeping or vivid dreams, a lack of energy, and weight loss. Crying is evident and provides some relief of extreme emotions. The individual remains socially responsive and seeks reassurance from others.

Depression is marked by extensive periods of sadness and preoccupation often extending beyond 2 months. It is not limited to the single event. There is an absence of pleasure or anger and isolation from previous social support systems. The individual can experience extreme lethargy, weight loss, insomnia, or hypersomnia, and has no recollection of dreaming. Crying is absent or persistent and provides no relief of emotions. Professional intervention is required to relieve depression.

Loss

Loss is the blanket term used to denote the absence of a valued object, position, ability, attribute, or individual. The aspect of **loss** as it is associated with the death of an animal or person is a relatively new definition. Loss is an individualized and subjective experience depending on the **perceived attachment** between the individual and the missing aspect. This can range from little or no value of attachment to significant value. Loss also can be represented by the **withdrawal of a valued relationship** one had or would have had in the future. Depending on the unique and individual responses to the perception of loss and its significance, reactions to the loss will vary. Robinson and McKenna summarize the aspects of loss in three main attributes:

- Something has been removed.
- The item removed had value to that person.
- The response is individualized.

Mourning

Mourning is a public grief response for the death of a loved one. The various aspects of the mourning process are partially determined by **personal and cultural belief systems**. Kagawa-Singer defines mourning as "the social customs and cultural practices that follow a death." Durkheim expands this to include the following: "mourning is not a natural movement of private feelings wounded by a cruel loss; it is a duty imposed by the group." Mourning involves participation in religious and culturally appropriate customs and rituals designed to publicly acknowledge the loss. These rituals signify they are adjusting to the change in their relationships created by the loss, as well as mark the beginning of the reorganization and forward movement of their lives.

Bereavement

Bereavement is the emotional and mental state associated with having suffered a **personal loss**. It is the reactions of grief and sadness initiated by the loss of a loved one. Bereavement is a normal process of feeling deprived of something of value. The word bereave comes from the root "reave" meaning to plunder, spoil, or rob. It is recognized that the lost individual had value and a defining role in the surviving individual's life. Bereavement encompasses all the acts and emotions surrounding the feeling of loss for the individual. During this grieving period, there is an increased mortality risk. A **positive bereavement experience** means being able to recognize the significance of the loss while still recognizing the resilience and value of life.

Risk Factors Complicating Bereavement

The caregiver should assess for multiple **life crises** that take energy away from the grieving process. An important factor is the grieving individual's history with past grieving experiences. Assess for other recent, unresolved, or difficult losses that may need to be addressed before the individual can move toward resolution of the current loss. Age, mental health, substance abuse, extreme anger, anxiety, or dependence on the individual facing the end of life can add additional stressors and handicap natural coping mechanisms. Income strains, community support, outside and personal responsibilities, the absence of cultural and religious beliefs, the difficulty of the disease process, and age of the loved one lost can also present additional risk factors.

Interventions for Patients and Family Experiencing Loss and Grief

Loss is painful and frightening. Loss can occur through death or loss of health, self-esteem, or relationships. Loss can also occur from threats, such as fire, flood, theft, or severe weather. The severity of the loss, preparation for it, and the maturity, stability, and coping mechanisms of the person all affect the grieving process. Multiple losses and substance abuse can complicate grief and recovery. Previous life experience and cultural and religious beliefs can help in resolution of grief. Many emotions are triggered, and if the loss is not acknowledged, the person may become depressed or develop health problems. **Interventions** for those experiencing grief and loss include:

- Teach patients to recognize symptoms, such as SOB, empty feelings in the chest or abdomen, deep sighing, lethargy, and weakness as signs of grief.
- Assist the patient and family to heal themselves by accepting the loss, recognizing the pain from it, making changes to adapt to and assimilate the loss, and moving toward new relationships and activity.
- Refer to groups or counseling for more intense support if needed.

Supporting Families and Patients as They Receive Bad News

It is often best if the patient can **receive bad news** while being **supported** by family, friends, physicians, nurses, support staff, social workers, and clergy if they so desire. However, the patient may not want family members or others to be present, and this too should be respected.

- Provide privacy and ensure that there will be no interruptions.
- Provide seating for all participants.
- Do not provide too much information at once, as the opening statement may be all that the patient can comprehend at one time.
- Allow time for reactions before providing more information.
- Wait for the patient to signal the need for more information and then provide an honest answer in layman's terms. Information may not be absorbed and may need to be repeated as the patient and family are ready for it later after the initial conference.
- Use techniques of therapeutic communication. People may need others to sit and listen and provide comforting empathy many times before having a conversation about problem solving.

Spirituality

Spirituality provides a connection of the self to a higher power and a way of finding meaning in life experiences. It provides guidance for behavior and can help to clarify one's purpose in life. It can offer hope to those who are ill or facing loss and grief and can give comfort, support, and guidance. **Spirituality** is not always connected to a religion and is highly individualized. A person may lose faith and confidence in his/her spiritual beliefs during trying times:

- Ask patients about their spiritual beliefs.
- Listen attentively and do not offer opinions about their beliefs or share your own unless invited.
- Show respect for their views and offer to obtain spiritual support by calling a spiritual leader or setting up a spiritual ritual that has meaning for them.

This support can help them to regain their beliefs and endure illness by helping them to rise above their suffering and find meaning in this experience.

Palliative and Hospice Care

Palliative care attempts to make the rest of the patient's life as comfortable as possible by treating distressing symptoms to keep them controlled. It does not attempt to cure but only to control discomfort caused by the disease. Palliative care does not require terminal illness/prognosis and can be implemented for any patient with chronic disease and suffering.

Hospice care uses palliative care as it supports the patient and family through the dying process. Hospice teams support the daily needs of the patient and family and provide needed equipment, medical expertise, and medications to control symptoms. They offer spiritual, psychological, and social support to the patient and family as needed and desired. Assistance with end-of-life planning is given to help the patient and family accomplish goals important to them. Bereavement support is also given. The team consists of the attending physician, hospice physician advisor, nurses, social worker, clergy, hospice aides, and volunteers. Hospice care is given in the home when the patient has family who are willing to assume care with the assistance of the hospice team. Hospice care also occurs in hospice facilities, hospitals, and extended care facilities. To qualify for Hospice care, the patient must be deemed terminal and given a 6-month or less life expectancy by two separate physicians. Should the patient survive 6 months in hospice, they can be extended for two 90-day periods, and then an unlimited number of 60-day periods per physician order.

PALLIATIVE SURGERY

Palliative surgery is sometimes carried out to reduce pain and symptoms although in most cases it does not appreciably prolong life. Palliative surgery may be **cancer-directed**, such as palliative nephrectomy with renal cell carcinoma, partial or total gastrectomy for gastric cancer, or endoscopic paranasal debulking for facial metastasis, and aimed at removing cancerous tissue. Decompression of the vertebra (in the case of bony metastases) and arthroplasty of the femur may be carried out to reduce pain and the risk of pathological fractures. Palliative surgery may also be **non-cancer-directed**, which includes procedures that do not remove cancerous tissue, such as palliative colonic splinting and nerve block procedures. Patients may undergo pleurodesis, thoracentesis, thoracotomy, paracentesis, and pericardiocentesis to relieve discomfort. The risks and pain associated with surgical procedures must be balanced against improvement in the quality of life with consideration of the expected length of survival.

PALLIATIVE STENTS

A stent is a small tube, usually metal or plastic, that is inserted into a duct, vessel, or canal to maintain patency and relieve symptoms associated with cancer that is causing obstruction. These stents are usually placed with microsurgical techniques. **Common stents** include:

- **Pancreatic stents**: These open the bile duct to allow drainage in order to reduce jaundice and associated discomforts, to reduce pain, and to improve digestion.
- **Duodenal stents**: These are placed to maintain patency of the duodenum, which is often obstructed with pancreatic cancer, as an alternative to stomach bypass surgery and/or to relieve nausea and vomiting. Patients may be restricted to soft foods and fluids after the procedure.
- **Liver stents**: These are placed in the bile duct system to allow bile to drain into the small intestine in order to relieve jaundice and symptoms of liver failure.
- **Colonic stents**: These stents are placed to relieve colorectal blockage and relieve symptoms of bowel obstruction.
- **Ureteral stents**: These stents can be used to prevent urinary retention when ureters are obstructed.

Complications of stents may include infection, perforation, hemorrhage, and migration of the stent. Over time, obstruction may recur, especially with malignancies.

PALLIATIVE RADIATION

Palliative radiation is used to reduce pain and symptoms. Most palliative radiation is done with external beam radiation therapy. **Radiotherapy** uses include:

- **Bone pain**: Radiotherapy may be utilized to reduce tumor mass, such as with multiple myeloma and bony metastasis, and to reduce pain and risk of fractures, with relief often occurring within days of treatment.
- **Pericardial effusions**: Radiotherapy is most effective in reducing effusions with radiosensitive tumors (leukemias, lymphomas).
- **Hemoptysis associated with lung cancer**: Radiotherapy can control hemoptysis in up to 80% of patients with inoperative lung cancer.

- **Spinal cord compression**: Radiotherapy is the primary treatment to relieve compression and reduce symptoms.
- **Brain tumor**: Radiotherapy may reduce the size of the tumor and associated symptoms, such as headaches and nausea.

Radiation does pose some risks of adverse effects that must be considered in relation to quality of life. Depending on the site of radiation, adverse effects may include fatigue, local skin irritation and burns, hair loss, GI upset (nausea, vomiting, dysphagia, diarrhea), dysuria, depressed immune system, and anemia.

Palliative Chemotherapy

Palliative chemotherapy is used primarily to reduce symptoms and pain by decreasing tumor size, which reduces compression of surrounding tissues, and to prolong life when cancer is advanced. Many chemotherapeutic agents are available, and adverse effects associated with use vary widely but can include nausea and vomiting, anorexia, hair loss, weakness, fatigue, and impaired immune system. **Palliative chemotherapy** is often given in conjunction with palliative radiation. Patients should be well-informed before deciding on a course of palliative chemotherapy and should understand how many cycles will be needed (usually 2 full cycles are given before deciding whether the treatment is effective), how long the cycles will be, what type of adverse effects to expect, what reduction in symptoms is anticipated, and how long studies show that the treatment prolongs life. If the prolongation of life and symptom relief is minimal, the trade-off for decreased quality of life must be considered.

Palliative Sedation

Palliative sedation differs from physician-assisted suicide in that it is primarily intended to provide comfort and alleviate suffering, and the hastening of death that may occur is a secondary effect while the primary purpose of physician-assisted suicide is to bring about a patient's death (even though it is also intended to provide comfort and alleviate suffering). These are legal distinctions. In most states, physician-assisted suicide is illegal, but the US Supreme Court has upheld the rights of individuals to have **palliative sedation** to alleviate symptoms. Midazolam (Versed) 0.5-6.0 mg/hr intravenously is often used for palliative sedation for patients who are highly agitated and in severe uncontrolled pain. Midazolam is a very short-acting benzodiazepine with action beginning within 5 minutes and peaking at 20-60 minutes. Propofol, another IV agent, is also used, with starting doses of 0.25 mg/kg/hr. Palliative sedation is indicated for patients when other medications and therapies have been unable to control their refractory symptoms, such as intractable pain, severe nausea and vomiting, feeling of suffocation, and seizures.